Pharmacy and Pharmaceutical Science

Pharmacy and Pharmaceutical Science

Edited by Jesse Hanson

hayle
medical

New York

Hayle Medical,
750 Third Avenue, 9th Floor,
New York, NY 10017, USA

Visit us on the World Wide Web at:
www.haylemedical.com

ISBN: 978-1-63241-787-9

Cataloging-in-Publication Data

Pharmacy and pharmaceutical science / edited by Jesse Hanson.
p. cm.
Includes bibliographical references and index.
ISBN 978-1-63241-787-9
1. Pharmacy. 2. Pharmacology. 3. Drugs. 4. Pharmaceutical industry. I. Hanson, Jesse.
RS153 .P43 2019
615--dc23

Table of Contents

Chapter 20   **Sustained-release study on Exenatide loaded into mesoporous silica nanoparticles: in vitro characterization and in vivo evaluation** 170
Cuiwei Chen, Hongyue Zheng, Junjun Xu, Xiaowei Shi,
Fanzhu Li and Xuanshen Wang

Chapter 21   **Linagliptin versus sitagliptin in patients with type 2 diabetes mellitus** 178
Khosro Keshavarz, Farhad Lotfi, Ehsan Sanati, Mahmood Salesi,
Amir Hashemi-Meshkini, Mojtaba Jafari, Mohammad M. Mojahedian,
Behzad Najafi and Shekoufeh Nikfar

Chapter 22   **^{99m}Tc-radiolabeled GE11-modified peptide for ovarian tumor targeting** 189
Najmeh Rahmanian, Seyed Jalal Hosseinimehr, Ali Khalaj, Zohreh Noaparast,
Seyed Mohammad Abedi and Omid Sabzevari

Chapter 23   **Fabrication and biological evaluation of chitosan coated hyaluronic acid-docetaxel conjugate nanoparticles in CD44$^+$ cancer cells** 198
Nazanin Shabani Ravari, Navid Goodarzi, Farhad Alvandifar, Mohsen Amini,
Effat Souri, Mohammad Reza Khoshayand, Zahra Hadavand Mirzaie,
Fatemeh Atyabi and Rassoul Dinarvand

    Permissions

    List of Contributors

    Index

Preface

This book has been an outcome of determined endeavour from a group of educationists in the field. The primary objective was to involve a broad spectrum of professionals from diverse cultural background involved in the field for developing new researches. The book not only targets students but also scholars pursuing higher research for further enhancement of the theoretical and practical applications of the subject.

The practice of preparing, compounding and dispensing pharmaceutical drugs is called pharmacy. The three main sub-fields of pharmacy are pharmaceutics, medicinal chemistry and pharmacognosy, and pharmacy practice. Other branches of pharmacy include pharmacology and pharmacoinformatics. All the interdisciplinary areas of study associated with the action, design, disposition, or delivery of pharmaceutical drugs fall under the broad category of pharmaceutical sciences. There is an application of knowledge from diverse fields, like biology, epidemiology, chemistry, chemometrics, physics, mathematics and chemical engineering in the field of pharmaceutical sciences. Pharmacogenomics is an important area of study, which falls under the scope of pharmaceutical sciences. It involves the study of the role of genome in drug response. This book includes some of the vital pieces of work being conducted across the world, on various topics related to pharmacy and pharmaceutical science. It explores all the important aspects of these fields in the present day scenario. The extensive content of this book provides the readers with a thorough understanding of the subject.

It was an honour to edit such a profound book and also a challenging task to compile and examine all the relevant data for accuracy and originality. I wish to acknowledge the efforts of the contributors for submitting such brilliant and diverse chapters in the field and for endlessly working for the completion of the book. Last, but not the least; I thank my family for being a constant source of support in all my research endeavours.

Editor

Comparison of clinical results of two pharmaceutical products of riboflavin in corneal collagen cross-linking for keratoconus

Hassan Hashemi[1*], Mohammad Amin Seyedian[1], Mohammad Miraftab[1], Hooman Bahrmandy[1], Araz Sabzevari[2] and Soheila Asgari[1]

Abstract

Background: To compare the 6-month results of two formulations of Riboflavin provided by Sina Darou, Iran, and Uznach, Switzerland, in corneal collagen cross-linking (CXL) for keratoconus patients.

Findings: Considering the results of the previous study about the similarity of the formulations and the active ingredients of the two types of Riboflavin, they were used in the CXL procedure of 60 keratoconic eyes (30 eyes in each group). After 6 months, the mean improvement of UCVA (0.239), BCVA (0.707), and MRSE (0.513) did not differ significantly between the two groups. The mean decrease in max- K (0.731), mean- K (0.264), central corneal thickness (0.759), and Q-value (0.669) did not show any significant difference between the two groups. The two groups had no significant difference in endothelial cell count decrease (0.229). The Sina Darou formulation decreased corneal hysteresis more than the Swiss formulation (P = 0.057) but there were no significant differences in the mean decrease of corneal resistance factor between the two groups (P = 0.117).

Conclusions: Based on the early results, the results of visual acuity, refraction, and corneal topography using Sina Darou and Uznach formulations of Riboflavin showed that both were effective in CXL. However, considering the relatively significant difference in corneal hysteresis changes between the two groups, this study will continue to report the long-term results.

Keywords: Riboflavin, Pharmaceutical product, Sina Darou, Cross linking, Keratoconus, Clinical trial

Background

Collagen cross linking (CXL) with Riboflavin has shown desirable effects on the arrest of keratoconus [1-3]. In this procedure, riboflavin produces free radicals under the effect of UV. These radicals create new covalent bonds in the stroma which strengthen the corneal tissue [1]. Riboflavin enhances UVA absorbance as a photosensitizer [4] and reduces cellular damage [5]. Therefore, the use of riboflavin in CXL is of extreme importance. In a primary study, we showed that the formulation and the amount of the active ingredient of riboflavin produced in Sina Darou, Iran, were similar to riboflavin produced in Uznach, Switzerland. Fluorometry and high

performance liquid chromatography were used to compare the amount of the active ingredient of the two products. After calculating the area under curve of the absorption rate of the active ingredient of the two products, statistical analysis showed no significant difference between them. In the present study, the efficacy of the two pharmaceutical products was compared in order to recommend the use of the Iranian product, which is more available and has lower costs, instead of the Swiss product.

Finding
Methods
In this parallel clinical trial, 60 eyes of 60 keratoconus patients that received CXL were compared in two groups. The flowchart of the passage of participants is shown in Figure 1. Iranian riboflavin 0.1% (Sina Darou, Iran) was used during CXL in group A and Swiss

* Correspondence: hhashemi@norc.ac.ir
[1]Noor Ophthalmology Research Center, Noor Eye Hospital, No. 96 Esfandiar Blvd., Vali'asr Ave., Tehran, Iran
Full list of author information is available at the end of the article

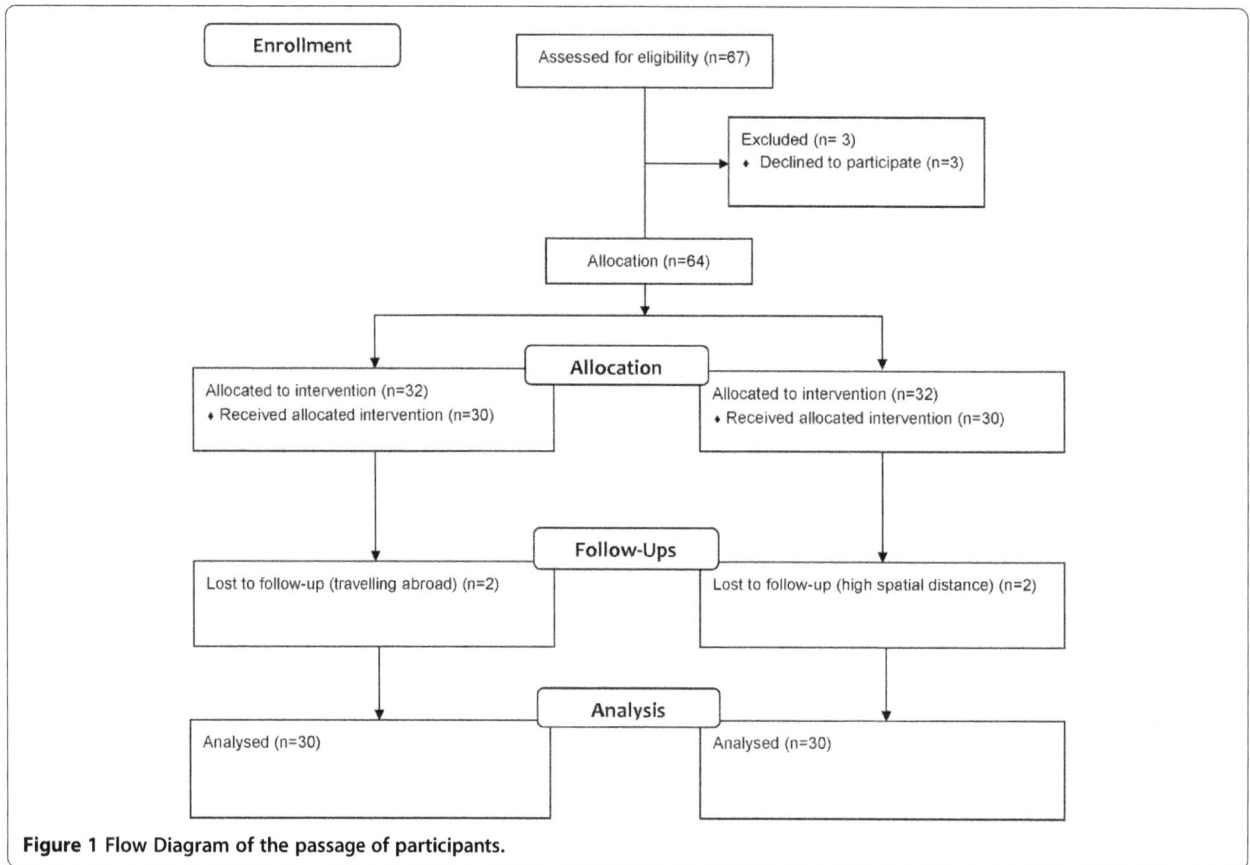

Figure 1 Flow Diagram of the passage of participants.

riboflavin 0.1% (Streuli Pharmaceuticals, Uznach, Switzerland) was used in group B. The patients were allocated to the groups consecutively. The inclusion criteria were the clinical and paraclinical diagnosis of progressive keratoconus, age 15–35 years, keratometry less than 55 D, and a central corneal thickness (CCT) more than 400 micron. Patients with other ocular diseases or a history of ocular surgery were excluded from the study. Participants discontinued the use of the hard and soft contact lens 3 weeks and 3 days prior to the surgery, respectively.

At first, a written informed consent was obtained from each participant. Noor review board approved the study. Iranian Registry of Clinical Trials also approved the study (registration number: IRCT201212034333N2).

The method of the surgery has been already reported [3]. After local anesthesia, the epithelium of the central 7 mm of the cornea was removed in 3–4 vertical strips that measured about 2 mm in width sparing a strip measuring approximately 1 mm. An epithelial strip was also horizontally removed from the lower one third of the cornea. Then, Iranian or Swiss riboflavin 0.1% drops in dextran 20% were instilled on the cornea every 3 minutes for 30 minutes in the intervention and control group, respectively. After the saturation of riboflavin in the anterior chamber, irradiation (wavelength 370 nm,

power 3 mW/cm^2) was started at 5 cm using UVX system (IROC, Zürich, Switzerland). During 30 minutes of irradiation, riboflavin instillation was repeated every three minutes. Then, the corneal surface was irrigated with sterile balanced saline solution, a soft bandage contact lens (Night & Day, Ciba Vision, Duluth, GA) was placed on it, and chloramphenicol 0.5% (Sina Darou, Iran) was administered. Post surgical regimen included chloramphenicol 0.5% four times daily, betamethasone 0.1% (Sina Darou, Iran), and preservative free artificial tears (Hypromelose, preservative free) as required. The patients were examined on days 1 and 3 after surgery, and the lens was removed if healing was observed. After removing the lens, chloramphenicol was discontinued while betamethasone twice daily was continued for another week. If epithelial healing was not observed, daily visits continued until the epithelium healed completely. No complications were noticed during or after surgery. Corneal haze related to the surgery was completely removed before the third month.

The patients received ophthalmic examination and paraclinical evaluation before the procedure and 1, 3, and 6 months after it. Paraclinical tests included uncorrected visual acuity (UCVA) and best spectacle corrected visual acuity (BSCVA) using a Snellen chart, and manifest refraction spherical equivalent (MRSE) using an

Auto refractometer (Topcon KR-8800, Japan). We used Pentacam (Oculus Optikgerate GmbH, Germany) to evaluate corneal topographic indices, an ocular response analyzer (ORA; Reichert Ophthalmic Instruments, Buffalo, USA) to assess corneal biomechanical properties, and a non-contact specular microscope (Konan Medical, Hyogo, Japan) to investigate endothelial cell count (ECC). The corneal biomechanical properties and ECC were evaluated twice, once before the surgery and once six months after the procedure.

We used repeated measure analysis of variance to evaluate the trend of the changes in each group and between the two groups. The results are shown as mean ± SD. The level of significance was set at 0.05.

Results

Sixty eyes of 60 patients (60% male) with a mean age of 24.32 ± 4.59 were evaluated. The patients received Iranian (group A) and Swiss (group B) riboflavin in 2 groups. The differences of all of the baseline indices were not statistically significant between the two groups.

The mean UCVA showed an improving trend in group A until the end of the 6th month (P = 0.168) while in group B, it resumed its improving trend after a decrease in the third month (P = 0.577). The trend of the 6-month results did now a significant difference between the two groups (P = 0.239). The mean BCVA showed a decrease in both groups one month after the procedure but improved afterwards, although it was not significant. The trend of the BCVA changes was not significant between the two groups (P = 0.707).

After 6 months, MRSE decreased in group A but remained stable in group B. In general, the mean 6-month changes of MRSE was not significant between the two groups (P = 0.513). The trend of the changes of the above-mentioned indices is shown in Table 1.

Despite an increase in max-K in the first follow up, it had a decreasing trend thereafter. The flattening was significant in neither group. In general, the decreasing trend of max-K was similar in both groups until the end of the sixth month (P = 0.731). Mean-K also showed the same decreasing trend with no significant difference between the two groups (P = 0.264). CCT showed a small insignificant decrease in both groups with no significant difference in 6 months (P = 0.759). The Q-value insignificantly shifted toward a prolate shape (more positive) in both groups but the 6-month trend of the changes showed no significant difference between the two groups (P = 0.669) (Figure 2).

Mean ± SD of corneal hysteresis (CH) was 7.70 ± 1.63 before the procedure in Group A which decreased to 6.76 ± 1.54 mmHg six months after the surgery (P = 0.008). In group B, CH decreased from 7.38 ± 2.10 to 7.23 ± 1.56 mmHg (P = 0.630). The decrease in CH between the two groups was borderline significant (P = 0.057).

Mean ± SD of corneal resistance factor (CRF) decreased from 7.02 ± 1.90 to 6.32 ± 1.30 mmHg in group A (P = 1.000) and from 6.80 ± 2.03 to 6.80 ± 1.84 mmHg in group B (P = 1.000); the difference between the two groups was not significant (P = 0.117).

The mean ± SD of ECC in group A was 2815.4 ± 243.1 and 2415.8 ± 317.8 cell/mm^2 before and after the surgery, respectively (P < 0.001). In group B, ECC decreased from 2751.0 ± 261.2 to 2467.0 ± 255.9 cell/mm^2 (P < 0.001). The decrease in ECC showed no significant difference between the two groups (P = 0.229).

Discussion

CXL decreases or arrests the progression of keratoconus. After CXL, the corneal rigidity increases by up to 4.5 times [6] and the effects of the strengthening remain for a long time [2,3]. Although there are still concerns regarding

Table 1 Comparison of the results between two groups of keratoconus patients receiving Iranian and Swiss riboflavin

	Riboflavin	No of eyes	Pre operation	After surgery 1 months	3 months	6 months	P-value*
UCVA (logMAR)	Sina Darou, Iran	30	0.82 ± 0.66	0.60 ± 0.52	0.52 ± 0.39	0.45 ± 0.36	0.239
	Uznach, Switzerland	30	0.82 ± 0.55	0.67 ± 0.54	0.79 ± 0.54	0.73 ± 0.51	
BCVA (logMAR)	Sina Darou, Iran	30	0.23 ± 0.28	0.25 ± 0.21	0.24 ± 0.19	0.19 ± 0.13	0.707
	Uznach, Switzerland	30	0.22 ± 0.18	0.27 ± 0.22	0.24 ± 0.19	0.20 ± 0.21	
Sphere (diopter)	Sina Darou, Iran	30	−1.53 ± 2.56	−1.70 ± 2.43	−1.80 ± 2.45	−1.42 ± 2.36	0.937
	Uznach, Switzerland	30	−1.59 ± 1.82	−1.64 ± 2.45	−1.57 ± 2.33	−1.63 ± 2.33	
Cylinder (diopter)	Sina Darou, Iran	30	−2.48 ± 1.77	−2.93 ± 2.07	−2.17 ± 2.17	−2.36 ± 1.79	0.242
	Uznach, Switzerland	30	−2.65 ± 1.94	−2.83 ± 1.88	−3.20 ± 2.04	−2.77 ± 1.93	
Spherical equivalent (diopter)	Sina Darou, Iran	30	−2.77 ± 2.51	−3.16 ± 3.02	−2.88 ± 3.13	−2.60 ± 2.85	0.513
	Uznach, Switzerland	30	−2.96 ± 2.28	−3.10 ± 2.78	−3.16 ± 2.75	−3.01 ± 2.70	

*Related to the comparison of the trend of the changes between the two groups using repeated measure ANOVA.

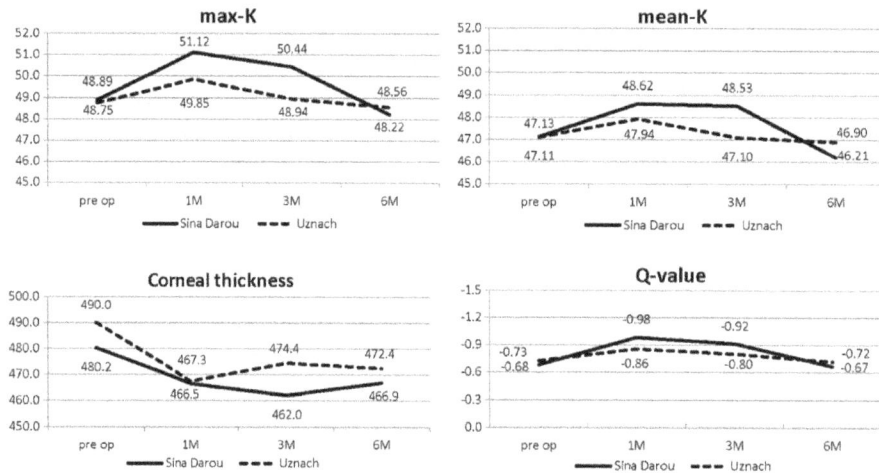

Figure 2 The temporal changes of max-K, mean-K, corneal thickness and Q-value between two groups of keratoconus patients receiving Iranian and Swiss riboflavin.

regression due to the unknown collagen turnover time in the cornea [7,8], the 5-year results of treatment [3] can reduce the concern to a great extent. In this procedure, riboflavin produces free radicals under the effect of UV. These radicals create new covalent bonds in the stroma which strengthen the corneal tissue [1].

The role of riboflavin in this procedure is to increase UV absorbance and protection against its destructive effects on the cornea and lower layers. In vivo, riboflavin decreases the cytotoxic effects of UVA by up to 10 times [5]. On the other hand, it increases UV absorbance by up to 95% [4]. Without riboflavin, only 25-35% of UV is absorbed in the cornea [9] and reaches 50% in the lens which is undesirable [10]. This absorbance rate is influenced by riboflavin concentration. UV absorbance increases linearly in concentrations up to 0.04% while higher concentrations have no effect on absorbance [11].

CXL is considered a desirable treatment option and besides efficacy, it minimizes the cytotoxic effects on the epithelium with no cellular damage in the corneal endothelium and lens. During the procedure, epithelial cellular death occurs to a depth of approximately 300 micron; however, due to their high repopulation property, they regenerate after 6 months [12-14] with no dramatic effects on the treatment outcome [15,16]. On the other hand, the regeneration speed is very low in the endothelial cells and their damage is irreversible [11]. Clinical studies have shown that the cellular damage of CXL in the epithelium is within acceptable ranges and have reported no pathological damage from the endothelium to the retina after CXL [11,16,17]. Therefore, riboflavin is a mainstay of treatment.

Imported riboflavin is now used in Iran. Easier accessibility and lower costs persuaded us to use the Iranian riboflavin (Sina Darou). A preliminary study showed that

both drugs were similar in formulation and active ingredient.

The clinical use of the drug in our study showed its efficacy, and the trend of the changes of vision, refraction, and topography was similar in both groups. In other words, although refraction, vision, and keratometry of the patients were deteriorating in the past year, development of the collagen bands arrested the process 6 months after the surgery with even improvement in some patients. The rate of the changes was similar in both groups, and also similar to a previous study we conducted using Swiss riboflavin [3]. Some studies reported that vision and refraction remained stable without significant changes [18] while some other studies reported a significant improvement in vision and refraction [19,20]. Of course, differences in the follow-up period, participants' age, and study population may be the reasons for the different results.

In shorter follow-up, it should be kept in mind that the results of paraclinical tests may be affected by the corneal haze of CXL.

In our study, corneal keratometry changed similarly in both groups, showing that the process of protrusion and steepening stopped similarly in both treatment groups. Therefore, the inter- and intra-fibril bands were well developed in the group that received Iranian riboflavin. Wollensak et al. [1] reported that max-K decreased by 2.01 D in a follow-up period of 3 months to 4 years. In our study, the decrease was 0.6 and 0.3D in the Iranian and Swiss riboflavin groups, respectively. The reason for the difference could be different surgical methods; wollensak et al. removed the 7 mm central cornea while we removed a number of epithelial strips. Comparative studies should be designed and performed to evaluate this hypothesis.

CH, CRF, and ECC significantly decreased in the group that received Iranian riboflavin. Since the cytotoxic effects of the procedure on the epithelial cells continues for up to 6 months [12-14], the results of the procedure after one year or more should be used to evaluate CH, CRF, and ECC changes.

Of course, it should be noticed that despite laboratory reports of increased corneal rigidity following CXL, numerous clinical studies have found no change in the corneal biomechanical properties after CXL and different follow-ups have shown that the corneal biomechanical changes are stable without improvement [21-26].

Conclusion

In general, it could be stated that vision, refraction, and corneal topography following CXL using Iranian (Sina Darou) and Swiss riboflavin are similar based on the 6-month results. However, considering the different decreases in CH, we require long-term studies to replace Swiss riboflavin with the Iranian one. Therefore, this study will continue to report the long-term results.

Abbreviations
CXL: Collagen cross linking; MRSE: Manifest refraction spherical equivalent; BCVA: Best corrected visual acuity; UCVA: Uncorrected visual acuity; max K: Maximum keratometry; CCT: Central corneal thickness; ECC: Endothelial cell count; CH: Corneal hysteresis; CRF: Corneal resistance factor.

Competing interests
The authors declare that they have no competing interests.

Authors' contributions
HH, MA, MM and HB have designed and supervised the project and advised on writing the paper. AS has performed primary study (laboratory study). SA analyzed the data and wrote the manuscript. HH, MA, MM and HB finalized the manuscript. All authors read and approved the final manuscript.

Acknowledgements
This research was supported by a grant from the Noor Ophthalmology Research Center.

Author details
[1]Noor Ophthalmology Research Center, Noor Eye Hospital, No. 96 Esfandiar Blvd., Vali'asr Ave., Tehran, Iran. [2]Faculty of Pharmacy, Tehran University of Medical Sciences, Tehran, Iran.

References
1. Wollensak G, Spoerl E, Seiler T: Riboflavin/ultraviolet-a-induced collagen crosslinking for the treatment of keratoconus. Am J Ophthalmol 2003, 135:620–627.
2. Raiskup-Wolf F, Hoyer A, Spoerl E, Pillunat LE: Collagen crosslinking with riboflavin and ultraviolet-A light in keratoconus: long-term results. J Cataract Refract Surg 2008, 34:796–801.
3. Hashemi H, Seyedian MA, Miraftab M, Fotouhi A, Asgari S: Corneal collagen cross-linking with riboflavin and ultraviolet A irradiation for keratoconus: long-term results. Ophthalmology 2013, 120:1515–1520.
4. Sporl E, Schreiber J, Hellmund K, Seiler T, Knuschke P: Studies on the stabilization of the cornea in rabbits. Ophthalmologe 2000, 97:203–206.
5. Wollensak G, Spoerl E, Reber F, Seiler T: Keratocyte cytotoxicity of riboflavin/UVA-treatment in vitro. Eye (Lond) 2004, 18:718–722.
6. Wollensak G, Spoerl E, Seiler T: Stress–strain measurements of human and porcine corneas after riboflavin-ultraviolet-A-induced cross-linking. J Cataract Refract Surg 2003, 29:1780–1785.
7. Jankov Ii MR, Jovanovic V, Delevic S, Coskunseven E: Corneal collagen cross-linking outcomes: review. Open Ophthalmol J 2011, 5:19–20.
8. Jankov Ii MR, Jovanovic V, Nikolic L, Lake JC, Kymionis G, Coskunseven E: Corneal collagen cross-linking. Middle East Afr J Ophthalmol 2010, 17:21–27.
9. Tsubai T, Matsuo M: Ultraviolet light-induced changes in the glucose-6-phosphate dehydrogenase activity of porcine corneas. Cornea 2002, 21:495–500.
10. Michael R: Development and repair of cataract induced by ultraviolet radiation. Ophthalmic Res 2000, 32(Suppl 1):1–44.
11. Spoerl E, Mrochen M, Sliney D, Trokel S, Seiler T: Safety of UVA-riboflavin cross-linking of the cornea. Cornea 2007, 26:385–389.
12. Caporossi A, Baiocchi S, Mazzotta C, Traversi C, Caporossi T: Parasurgical therapy for keratoconus by riboflavin-ultraviolet type A rays induced cross-linking of corneal collagen: preliminary refractive results in an Italian study. J Cataract Refract Surg 2006, 32:837–845.
13. Mazzotta C, Traversi C, Baiocchi S, Sergio P, Caporossi T, Caporossi A: Conservative treatment of keratoconus by riboflavin-uva-induced cross-linking of corneal collagen: qualitative investigation. Eur J Ophthalmol 2006, 16:530–535.
14. Mencucci R, Marini M, Paladini I, Sarchielli E, Sgambati E, Menchini U, Vannelli GB: Effects of riboflavin/UVA corneal cross-linking on keratocytes and collagen fibres in human cornea. Clin Experiment Ophthalmol 2010, 38:49–56.
15. Spoerl E, Wollensak G, Seiler T: Increased resistance of crosslinked cornea against enzymatic digestion. Curr Eye Res 2004, 29:35–40.
16. Wollensak G, Spoerl E, Wilsch M, Seiler T: Endothelial cell damage after riboflavin-ultraviolet-A treatment in the rabbit. J Cataract Refract Surg 2003, 29:1786–1790.
17. Wollensak G, Sporl E, Reber F, Pillunat L, Funk R: Corneal endothelial cytotoxicity of riboflavin/UVA treatment in vitro. Ophthalmic Res 2003, 35:324–328.
18. Goldich Y, Marcovich AL, Barkana Y, Mandel Y, Hirsh A, Morad Y, Avni I, Zadok D: Clinical and corneal biomechanical changes after collagen cross-linking with riboflavin and UV irradiation in patients with progressive keratoconus: results after 2 years of follow-up. Cornea 2012, 31:609–614.
19. El-Raggal TM: Riboflavin-ultraviolet A corneal cross-linking for keratoconus. Middle East Afr J Ophthalmol 2009, 16:256–259.
20. Kanellopoulos AJ: Collagen cross-linking in early keratoconus with riboflavin in a femtosecond laser-created pocket: initial clinical results. J Refract Surg 2009, 25:1034–1037.
21. Asri D, Touboul D, Fournie P, Malet F, Garra C, Gallois A, Malecaze F, Colin J: Corneal collagen crosslinking in progressive keratoconus: multicenter results from the French national reference center for keratoconus. J Cataract Refract Surg 2011, 37:2137–2143.
22. Gkika M, Labiris G, Giarmoukakis A, Koutsogianni A, Kozobolis V: Evaluation of corneal hysteresis and corneal resistance factor after corneal cross-linking for keratoconus. Graefes Arch Clin Exp Ophthalmol 2012, 250:565–573.
23. Greenstein SA, Fry KL, Hersh PS: In vivo biomechanical changes after corneal collagen cross-linking for keratoconus and corneal ectasia: 1-year analysis of a randomized, controlled, clinical trial. Cornea 2012, 31:21–25.
24. Sedaghat M, Naderi M, Zarei-Ghanavati M: Biomechanical parameters of the cornea after collagen crosslinking measured by waveform analysis. J Cataract Refract Surg 2010, 36:1728–1731.
25. Spoerl E, Terai N, Scholz F, Raiskup F, Pillunat LE: Detection of biomechanical changes after corneal cross-linking using ocular response analyzer software. J Refract Surg 2011, 27:452–457.
26. Vinciguerra P, Albe E, Mahmoud AM, Trazza S, Hafezi F, Roberts CJ: Intra- and postoperative variation in ocular response analyzer parameters in keratoconic eyes after corneal cross-linking. J Refract Surg 2010, 26:669–676.

2

Crocin suppresses multidrug resistance in MRP overexpressing ovarian cancer cell line

Shadi Mahdizadeh[1], Gholamreza Karimi[2], Javad Behravan[3,4], Sepideh Arabzadeh[3], Hermann Lage[5] and Fatemeh Kalalinia[3,6*]

Abstract

Background: Crocin, one of the main constituents of saffron extract, has numerous biological effects such as anti-cancer effects. Multidrug resistance-associated proteins 1 and 2 (MRP1 and MRP2) are important elements in the failure of cancer chemotherapy. In this study we aimed to evaluate the effects of crocin on MRP1 and MRP2 expression and function in human ovarian cancer cell line A2780 and its cisplatin-resistant derivative A2780/RCIS cells.

Methods: The cytotoxicity of crocin was assessed by the MTT assay. The effects of crocin on the MRP1 and MRP2 mRNA expression and function were assessed by real-time RT-PCR and MTT assays, respectively.

Results: Our study indicated that crocin reduced cell proliferation in a dose-dependent manner in which the reduction in proliferation rate was more noticeable in the A2780 cell line compared to A2780/RCIS. Crocin reduced MRP1 and MRP2 gene expression at the mRNA level in A2780/RCIS cells. It increased doxorubicin cytotoxicity on the resistant A2780/RCIS cells in comparison with the drug-sensitive A2780 cells.

Conclusion: Totally, these results indicated that crocin could suppress drug resistance via down regulation of MRP transporters in the human ovarian cancer resistant cell line.

Keywords: Crocin, Multidrug resistance, MRP1, MRP2, A2780, A2780/RCIS

Background

Cancer is a leading cause of death in the world that broadly affects more and less economically developed countries [1]. Using different chemotherapy regimens is a common method in cancer treatment, but there is some limitation on the effectiveness of chemotherapy that leads to poor therapeutic results [2]. One of the most important reasons of treatment failure during chemotherapy is the multidrug resistance (MDR) phenomenon. The MDR tumors are resistant to chemotherapeutic agents which are structurally and functionally different from the initial anticancer drug. Typical MDR occurs through overexpression of the membrane efflux proteins that pump anticancer drugs out of the cells [3]. These pharmaceutical transporter proteins belong to the ATP-binding cassette transporters family (ABC family) [4, 5]. One important class of the ABC family is the human multidrug resistance-associated protein (MRP) family which contains seven members. Several members of the MRP family especially MRP1 and MRP2 are involved in the detoxification and protection of the host against xenobiotic materials. They are also assumed to cause drug resistance through their ability in transporting a wide range of anticancer drugs out of the cells and their presence in many different types of tumors [6].

In the last decades, different research explored new botanical candidates with potential anti-cancer effects that has opened a window to developing safer and more effective anti-cancer therapies [7, 8]. *Crocus sativus* is a plant of the Iridaceae family. Stigmas of *Crocus sativus* flowers (saffron) contain various chemical substances [9]. Crocin is a major glycosylated carotenoid found in saffron [10] that has various pharmacological effects like protecting the myocardial cell against hypoxia damage [11], antioxidant [12, 13], anti-atherosclerosis

---

* Correspondence: kalaliniaf@mums.ac.ir

[3]Biotechnology Research Center, School of Pharmacy, Mashhad University of Medical Sciences, P. O. Box 91775-1365, Mashhad, Iran

[6]Medical Genetic Research Center, Mashhad University of Medical Sciences, Mashhad, Iran

Full list of author information is available at the end of the article

[14, 15], antidepressant [16] and anti-inflammatory effects [17, 18]. In addition, different studies have shown anticancer activities of crocin against human leukemia, breast, colorectal, and bladder cancer cell lines [19–23]. Based on these facts, it is expected that crocin could potentially be used clinically for the prevention and treatment of cancer in the near future.

It has shown that crocin inhibits Lipopolysaccharides (LPS)-induced nitric oxide (NO) release from brain microglial cells and reduces the LPS-stimulated productions of tumor necrosis factor-alpha, interleukin-1 beta, and intracellular reactive oxygen species, which effectively cause decreased NF-kappa B activation [17, 24]. On the other hand, it has been previously showed that sulindac, the nonsteroidal anti-inflammatory drug, generates oxidative stress via induction of reactive oxygen species (ROS) production, which finally leads to the higher expression of MRP1 and MRP3 in human colorectal cancer cell lines [25]. These evidences suggest that crocin might affect the protein expression of MDR proteins. In the present study, we aimed to evaluate the effects of crocin on the expression and function of MRP1 and MRP2 in the human ovarian carcinoma cell lines A2780 and its cisplatin-resistant derivative A2780/ RCIS cells (MRP2-overexpressing cell line).

Methods
Materials
Fetal bovine serum (FBS) and RPMI 1640 with L-glutamine were purchased from Gibco (USA) and Biosera (UK), respectively. MTT, DMSO, trypan blue, doxorubicin and penicillin G/streptomycin were obtained from Sigma-Aldrich (Germany). Crocin was generously provided by Dr. Seyed Ahmad Mohajeri (Pharmaceutical Research Center, Mashhad University of Medical Sciences, Iran). RNA tripure isolation kit was obtained from Roche Applied Science, Germany and Real-time EXPRESS One-Step SYBR GreenER™ Kit was purchased from Invitrogen, USA. The MRP-overexpressing, cisplatin-resistant ovarian cancer cell line, A2780/RCIS and its parental cisplatin sensitive cell line A2780 were generously provided by Professor Herman Lage (Molecular Pathology Department, Charite Campus Mitte, Berlin, Germany).

Preparation of the crocin solution
Total crocin was extracted and crystallized from saffron stigmas and its purity was tested with HPLC and was more than 96 % [26]. Crocin was dissolved in DMSO (dimethyl sulfoxide) and PBS to a final concentration of 1024 mM and stored at –20 °C. The drug was freshly diluted to its final concentration (10, 20, 40, 60, 80 and 100 μM) in culture medium prior to the start of each experiment.

Cell culture and treatment
Cells were cultured in RPMI-1640 contained FBS 10 % (v/v), penicillin (100 U/mL), and streptomycin (100 μg/mL) at 37 °C in humidified air containing CO_2 5 %. For MTT and real-time PCR studies, ovarian cancer cells were incubated for 4–72 h with crocin (0–100 μM). For MRP activity analysis, all cell lines were co-treated with different concentrations of crocin (0–100 μM) and doxorubicin (0–500 nM) for 4–72 h. This study was obtained the approval of the Research Ethics Committee of Mashhad University of Medical Sciences (code No: IR.MUMS.REC.1390.301).

MTT cytotoxicity assay
Drug sensitivity of the A2780 cell line and drug-resistant cell line A2780/RCIS were confirmed by MTT assay. Cells were seeded at an initial density of 10^4 cells/well in 96-well plates. The plates were incubated at 37 °C in a 5 % CO_2-supplemented atmosphere for 24 h. Subconfluent cells were treated with different concentrations of crocin and doxorubicin in a final volume of 100 μl of standard growth medium in each well. The control wells had DMSO in the growth medium at equal volumes to those used for the test compounds. Cell viability was measured after 4–72 h, using 3-(4, 5-dimethylthiazol-2-yl)-2, 5-diphenyl tetrazolium bromide (MTT). The reduced MTT dye was solubilized with DMSO (100 μl/well) and absorbance was determined on an ELISA plate reader (BioTek, Bad Friedrichshall, Germany) with a test wavelength of 550 nm and a reference wavelength of 630 nm. Each experiment was performed in triplicate and was repeated at least three times. The percentage of cell proliferation was calculated using the ratio of $OD_{test}/OD_{control}$.

Real-Time RT-PCR
Total cellular RNA was extracted using tripure isolation reagent. The total amount of RNA was measured using a NanoDrop 1000 spectrophotometer (Thermo Fisher Scientific, Wilmington, DE) and the acceptable purity was in the range of 1.8-2.2 for the A260/A230 and A260/A280 ratios. Real-time RT-PCR was performed to measure the expression levels of MRP1 and MRP2 in ovarian cancer cell lines using the EXPRESS One-Step SYBR GreenER™ Kit and real-time cycler Mx3000P™ Stratagen (Stratagen, USA). The primers had the following sequences: MRP1: 5′-GTGTTTCTGGTCAGCC CAACT-3′ (forward) and 5′-TTGGATCTCAGGATGG CAGG-3′ (reverse); MRP2, 5′-AGCAGCCATAGAGCT GGCCCTT-3′ (forward) and 5′-AGCAAAACCAGGA GCCATGTGCC-3′ (reverse); β-actin: 5′-TCATGAAG

TGTGACGTGGACATC-3′ (forward) and 5′-CAGGA GGAGCAATGATCTTGATCT-3′ (reverse). Reactions were performed with an initial cDNA synthesis step at 50 °C for 5 min, followed by the denaturation step at 95 °C for 2 min and PCR amplification cycles (40 cycles at 95 °C for 15 s, 60 °C for 1 min). Relative expression levels for MRP1 or MRP2 were normalized to the β-actin by the MxPro-Mx3000P system. The relative expressions of MRP genes were reported as the target/reference ratio of the treated samples divided by the target/reference ratio of the untreated control sample.

Statistical analysis

Results (mean ± SD) were reported in three independent stages. Statistical analyses were performed by SPSS version 16.0 using ANOVA, with the Tukey's post-hoc to

show significant differences between the data and p values < 0.05 were considered significant.

Results

Effect of crocin on the proliferation rate of A2780 cancer cell lines

To investigate the effects of crocin on the cell survival of ovarian cancer cells, A2780 cells were incubated in the presence or absence of various concentrations of crocin (0–100 μM) for 4, 24, 48 and 72 h and then subjected to MTT cytotoxicity assay. Crocin showed inhibitory effects on the cell growth rate of A2780 cells in a concentration and time-dependent manner (Fig. 1a). Crocin exhibited a similar inhibitory pattern with less potency in A2780/RCIS (Fig. 1b), in which treatment with 60–100 μM and 80–100 μM of crocin significantly reduced the survival of A2780 and A2780/RCIS, respectively ($P < 0.05$ vs. control).

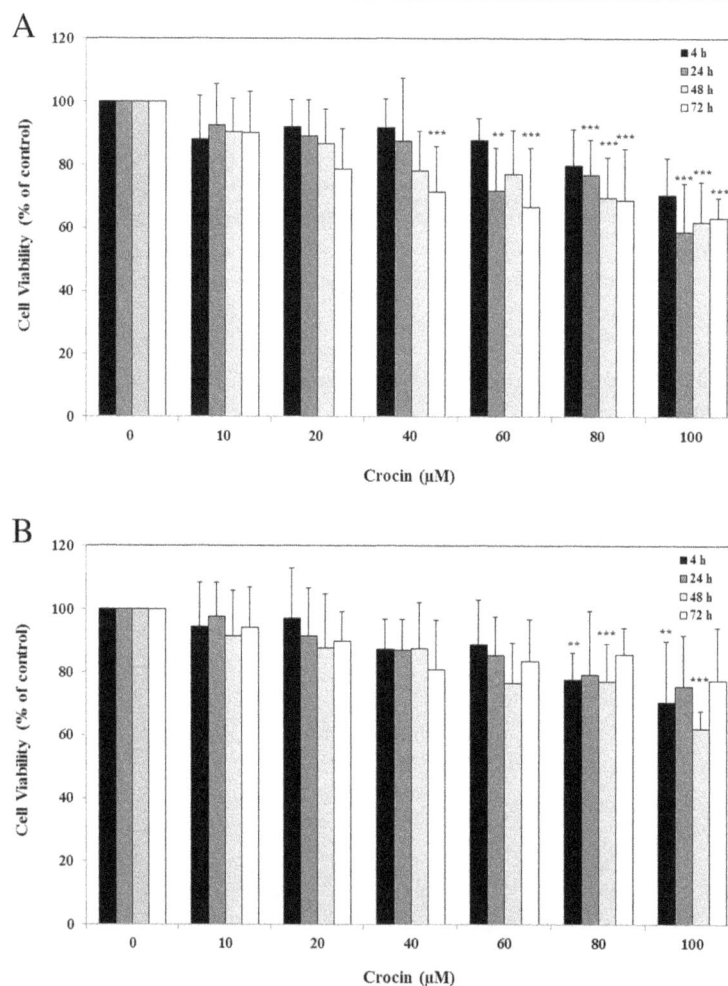

Fig. 1 The effects of crocin on cell viability of A2780 (a) and A2780/RCIS (b) cell lines. The cells were incubated with various concentrations of crocin at 37 °C for 4, 24, 48 and 72 h. Cell viability was measured by the MTT assay. Each experiment was repeated independently three times in triplicate tests and data are shown as mean ± SD. *$P \le 0.05$; **$P \le 0.01$; ***$P \le 0.001$

Expression of MRP1 and MRP2 in A2780 cell lines

Real-time RT-PCR was used to assess the basic level of the mRNA expression of MRP1 and MRP2 in cisplatin-resistant A2780/RCIS cells and sensitive parental A2780 cell line. As shown in Fig. 2a, the MRP1 mRNA level in the A2780/RCIS cell line was 1.29 times more than its expression level in A2780 cells. Also, the results showed that the expression level of MRP2 mRNA in the resistant cell line A2780/RCIS was about 13 times more than the MRP2 mRNA level in parental A2780 cells (Fig. 2b).

Effect of crocin on MRP1 and MRP2 gene expression

To evaluate the expression of MRP1 and MRP2 mRNA after treatment with crocin, the cells were treated with different concentrations of crocin (0–100 µM) for 4 and 48 h. Expression of MRP transporters was studied using Real-time RT-PCR. The results showed that crocin significantly reduced the expression level of MRP1 (up to about 50 %) in A2780/RCIS cells at 48 h (Fig. 3a). Similarly, crocin could significantly reduce MRP2 mRNA expression (up to 60 %) in cisplatin-resistant A2780/RCIS cells in a time dependent manner in compared with the control level (Fig. 3b).

Effect of crocin on multi-drug resistance protein activity

In order to evaluate the effects of crocin on MRP transporters activity, sensitivity of tested cell lines to doxorubicin in the presence or absence of crocin were studied. At first it was necessary to find the IC$_{50}$ of doxorubicin on A2780 and A2780/RCIS cells. For this purpose, cells were treated with different concentrations of doxorubicin (0–500 nM) for 4, 24, 48, and 72 h. Doxorubicin significantly reduced the proliferation rate

of A2780 (Fig. 4a) and A2780/RCIS cells (Fig. 4b) in a concentration and time-dependent manner. These anti-proliferative effects of doxorubicin were with a higher intensity in the parental cisplatin-sensitive cell line A2780 in comparison with the resistant cell line A2780/RCIS.

To test the combining effects of crocin and doxorubicin on the cell survival of A2780 cell lines, 30 different combinations (0–100 µM of crocin with 0–500 nM of doxorubicin) were evaluated using MTT assay. The combinatorial effects on cell survival were analyzed after 4, 24, 48, and 72 h incubation. There were no significant differences in A2780 cell viabilities between all crocin + doxorubicin concentrations and controls with the same amount of doxorubicin (data not shown). On the other hand, different concentrations of crocin could increase the percentage of doxorubicin cytotoxicity in A2780/RCIS, almost all in a time and concentration-dependent manner (Table 1). While crocin could not change the A2780/RCIS cell sensitivity to doxorubicin in 4 h, there were significant differences between the IC$_{50}$ of samples that were treated with crocin + doxorubicin and IC$_{50}$ of controls that were with the same amount of doxorubicin after 48 h (144 nM vs. 349 nM, $P < 0.001$) and 72 (162 nM vs. 326 nm, $P < 0.01$).

Discussion

Multidrug resistance (MDR) is one of the most important reasons for the insufficient effectiveness of chemotherapy drugs in cancer treatment. A major mechanism involved in MDR, is the presence of some of the ATP-binding cassette transporters (ABC) like Multidrug resistance-associated proteins 1 and 2 (MRP1 and MRP2),

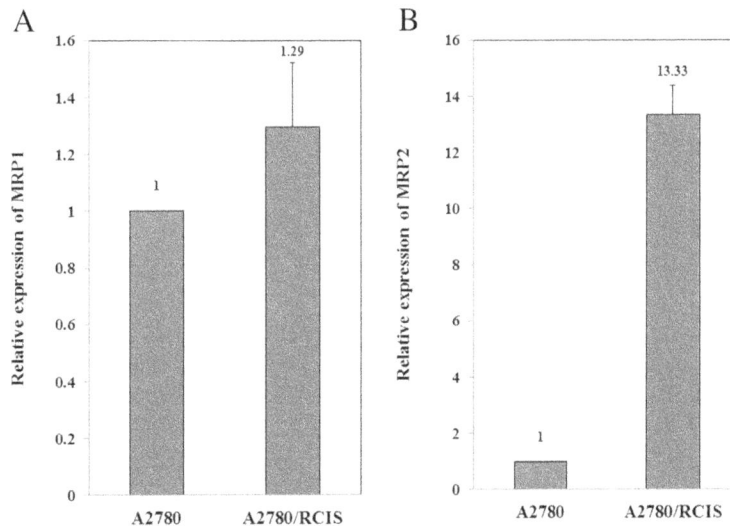

Fig. 2 Basal expressions of MRP1 (**a**) and MRP2 (**b**) mRNA in ovarian cancer cell lines were studied by real-time RT-PCR. The MRP mRNA level is compared with the drug-resistant cell line A2780/RCIS and parental drug-sensitive cell line A2780. Real-time RT-PCR analysis was performed on total RNA extracted from cells. Values were normalized to the β-actin content of samples and expressed as mean ± SD (n = 3).

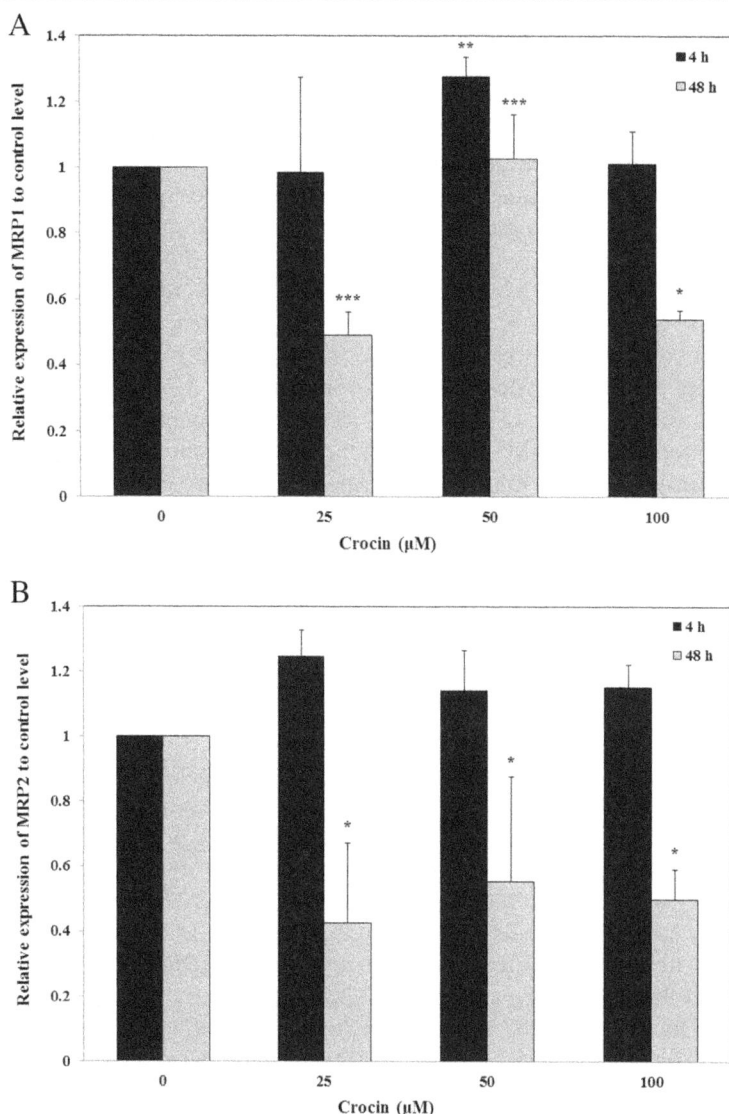

Fig. 3 The effects of crocin on the levels of MRP1 (**a**) and (**b**) mRNA in the A2780/RCIS cell line. Cells were treated for 4 and 48 h with crocin (0–100 μM), and MRP1 and MRP2 mRNA expressions were measured by real-time RT-PCR using total RNA extracted from control and treated cells. Values were normalized to the β-actin content of the samples. The results were expressed as the target/reference ratio of the treated samples divided by the target/reference ratio of the untreated control sample and expressed as mean ± SD ($n = 3$); *, $p < 0.05$; **, $p < 0.01$; ***, $p < 0.001$

which are expressed on the surface of cells and pumps chemotherapy drugs out of the cell. In recent years, scientists have tried to find efficient inhibitors of special ABC transporters to overcome MDR phenomenon [27]. Crocin, a major constitute of saffron [10], has shown anticancer activities against several cancer cell lines [19–23], and could be used clinically for the prevention and treatment of cancer in the near future. In this study, we evaluated the effects of crocin on the expression and function of MRP1 and MRP2 in the human ovarian carcinoma cell line A2780 and MRP2-overexpressing cell line A2780/RCIS.

It has been previously shown that induction of the MRP2 expression in human cancer cell lines enhances the resistance to doxorubicin [28], while down regulation of MRP2 enhances cell sensitivity to doxorubicin [29]. Based on these studies and similar studies for MRP1, doxorubicin has been introduced as a substrate of MRP1 and MRP2 transporters [30]. The results of the present study have shown that the MRP1 and MRP2 expression level in the cisplatin-resistant A2780/RCIS cell line was 1.29 and 13 times more than its expression level in its parental sensitive cell line A2780, respectively. On the other hand, doxorubicin had anti-proliferative effects

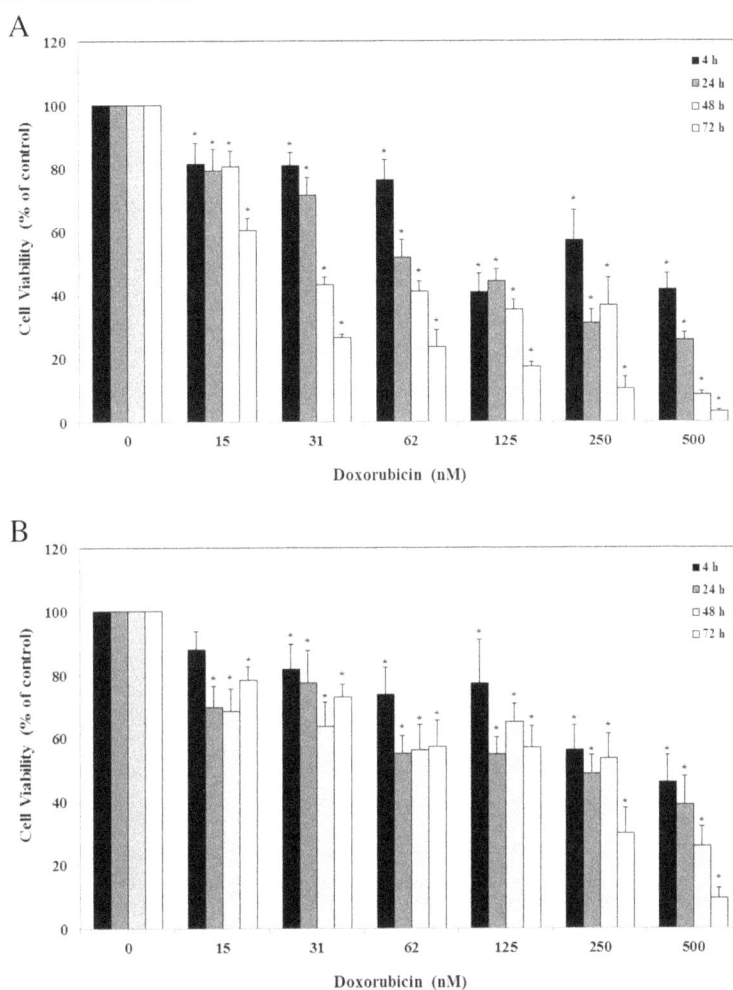

Fig. 4 The effects of doxorubicin on cell viability of A2780 (**a**) and A2780/RCIS (**b**) cell lines. The cells were incubated with different concentrations of doxorubicin (0–500 nM) for 4, 24, 48 and 72 h. Cell viability was measured by the MTT assay. Each experiment was repeated independently three times in triplicate tests and data are shown as mean ± SD. *$P \leq 0.001$

on the A2780 cells with higher intensity when compared with the A2780/RCIS cell line. These results indicated that the higher expression of MRP transporters in A2780/RCIS was accountable for the higher efflux of doxorubicin that resulted to its lower intracellular concentration and lower anti-proliferative activity in this drug-resistant cell line. Interestingly, crocin has shown a similar inhibitory pattern on cell growth of tested cell lines in which its anti-proliferative activity had less potency in A2780/RCIS in compared with the parental sensitive cell line. Totally, these results suggest that crocin could be a substrate of MRP transporters.

Several studies have investigated the molecular mechanism of anticancer activities of crocin against different human cancer cell lines. In one study, the differentially expressed gene of the bladder cancer T24 cell line after treatment with or without crocin has been evaluated using the cDNA microarray. The results showed that

under crocin treatment, 836 genes were up-regulated or down-regulated, which were replication factor or were involved in cell cycle controlling and DNA cell apoptosis [31]. Similarly, other studies have shown that crocin could arrest the tumor cell cycle and induce apoptosis by inhibition of the expression of Bcl-2, survivin, cyclin D1, and lactate dehydrogenase A (LDHA) or by up-regulation the expression and activity of Bax and nuclear factor erythroid 2-related factor 2 (Nrf2), and by inhibition of the telomerase activity [10, 19, 20, 32, 33]. The investigation of cellular targets of crocin using proteomic screening showed that crocin physically binds to a wide range of cellular proteins such as membrane transporters and enzymes involved in ATP and redox homeostasis [34]. In another study, researchers investigated the inhibition ability of a selection of carotenoids including β-carotene, crocin, retinoic acid, canthaxanthin, and fucoxanthin on the P-glycoprotein (P-gp; MDR1). These

Table 1 The effects of different concentrations of crocin on the cell survival percentages of A2780/RCIS cell lines under treatment with doxorubicin (mean ± SEM)

Time (h)	Dox (nM)	Crocin (µM)			
		0	25	50	100
4 h	16	97.04 ± 2.18	97.39 ± 10.06	95.88 ± 3.49	98.77 ± 3.05
	62	92.19 ± 4.94	96.51 ± 2.36	92.57 ± 0.70	95.91 ± 1.34
	125	91.52 ± 3.92	95.35 ± 0.91	91.77 ± 4.48	92.74 ± 2.33
	250	93.56 ± 2.70	95.13 ± 4.03	83.37 ± 5.05	84.1 ± 2.48
	500	77.64 ± 4.70	91.01 ± 9.06	80.95 ± 4.23	86.59 ± 3.93
24 h	16	95.54 ± 2.16	88.37 ± 1.55	96.30 ± 1.78	87.02 ± 6.36
	62	96.98 ± 2.80	95.83 ± 2.48	96.94 ± 1.63	93.58 ± 1.41
	125	96.95 ± 1.31	92.23 ± 0.51	96.33 ± 3.51	75.37 ± 5.73
	250	94.75 ± 2.33	75.84 ± 4.77	51.68 ± 4.70[***]	73.80 ± 5.33
	500	51.08 ± 1.17	26.58 ± 4.38[***]	35.35 ± 8.88[***]	23.06 ± 7.58[***]
48 h	16	99.39 ± 2.57	85.17 ± 3.68	80.87 ± 5.94[*]	53.66 ± 8.40[***]
	62	95.07 ± 3.99	73.01 ± 3.41[***]	60.60 ± 2.85[***]	54.96 ± 4.94[***]
	125	83.10 ± 2.02	71.49 ± 2.09	31.12 ± 8.98[***]	44.45 ± 6.49[***]
	250	53.04 ± 1.34	53.86 ± 1.73	25.77 ± 5.78[***]	7.219 ± 0.14[***]
	500	32.68 ± 3.40	19.11 ± 1.95	8.149 ± 3.16[***]	3.85 ± 0.29[***]
72 h	16	96.68 ± 3.55	84.31 ± 2.84	63.00 ± 1.68	63.29 ± 3.29[**]
	62	79.20 ± 3.88	65.62 ± 2.16	54.11 ± 5.12[***]	55.52 ± 1.85[***]
	125	60.52 ± 2.88	53.58 ± 1.63	47.77 ± 4.52[***]	34.41 ± 3.53[***]
	250	50.13 ± 2.80	33.17 ± 2.96[**]	34.49 ± 3.05[***]	28.09 ± 2.30[***]
	500	36.55 ± 2.82	22.21 ± 1.16	22.66 ± 1.71	9.27 ± 0.93[***]

Note: The results of the LSD test, which compared the effects of all crocin concentrations on the toxicity of each of the various concentrations of doxorubicin during 4, 24, 48, and 72 h. *, $p < 0.05$; **, $p < 0.01$; ***, $p < 0.001$

carotenoids decreased P-gp mRNA expression levels; increased accumulation of cytotoxic agents which are P-gp substrates that cause to enhance their cytotoxicity effects. Totally, they concluded that carotenoids could be used as adjuvants which are chemosensitizer in chemotherapy [35].

In this study, we aimed to evaluate the effects of crocin on MRP transporter expression and function. For this purpose the sensitivity of tested cell lines to doxorubicin in the presence or absence of non-toxic concentrations of crocin were studied. The MRP activity assay has been designed in two ways, short time exposure with crocin to evaluate the direct interaction between crocin and existing active transporters, and longtime exposure with crocin to evaluate the indirect effect of crocin on the transporter activity as a result of its modifications on the expression level. Interestingly, crocin could not change the A2780/RCIS cell sensitivity to doxorubicin in 4 h, while it significantly increased doxorubicin cytotoxicity after 48 and 72 h in a concentration-dependent manner in the drug-resistant A2780/RCIS cell line, but not in parental drug-sensitive A2780 cells. On the other hand, the real-time PCR results showed that crocin significantly reduced the

mRNA expression level of MRP1 and MRP2 in A2780/RCIS cells. Totally, these results indicated that crocin could suppress drug resistance via down regulation of MRP gene expression in the human ovarian cancer resistance cell line.

Conclusion

In this study we aimed to investigate the ability of crocin on inhibiting multidrug resistance in human ovarian cancer cells by interfering with MRP 1 and MRP2 transporters. The results showed that crocin could decrease the gene expression of MRP1 and MRP2 and exert MDR reversal, and enhance the cytotoxicity of doxorubicin in the human MRP2 overexpressing cell line A2780/RCIS. This study suggests that the application of crocin in combination with chemotherapeutics in cancer treatment could be an effective method to improve the efficacy of chemotherapy and moderate the impact of MDR.

Abbreviations

ABC, ATP-binding Cassette Transporters; DMSO, Dimethyl Sulfoxide; FBS, Fetal Bovine Serum; LDHA, Lactate Dehydrogenase A; LPS, Lipopolysaccharides; MDR, Multidrug Resistance; MRP, Multidrug Resistance-associated Protein; MTT, 3-(4, 5-dimethylthiazol-2-yl)-2, 5-diphenyl tetrazolium bromide; Nrf2,

Nuclear Erythroid 2-related Factor 2; RCIS, Cisplatin-Resistant Derivative; Real-time RT-PCR, Real-rime Reverse Transcription Polymerase Chain Reaction; ROS, Reactive Oxygen Species; PBS, Phosphate-Buffered Saline; P-gp, P-glycoprotein

Acknowledgments
The authors are indebted to the Research Council of Mashhad University of Medical Sciences, Iran, for approval and financial support of this project.

Authors' contributions
FK conceived of the study, designed the study, and coordination and helped to statistical analysis and draft the manuscript. SM carried out the molecular studies, performed the statistical analysis and drafted the manuscript. SA participated in molecular studies. GK, JB and HL conceived of the study and participated in its design. All authors read and approved the final manuscript.

Competing interests
The authors declare that they have no competing interests.

Author details
[1]Department of Cell and Molecular Biology, Kish International Campus, University of Tehran, Kish, Iran. [2]Medical Toxicology Research Center, School of Pharmacy, Mashhad University of Medical Sciences, Mashhad, Iran. [3]Biotechnology Research Center, School of Pharmacy, Mashhad University of Medical Sciences, P. O. Box 91775-1365, Mashhad, Iran. [4]Department of Pharmaceutical Biotechnology, School of Pharmacy, Mashhad University of Medical Sciences, Mashhad, Iran. [5]Institute of Pathology, Charite University, Campus Mitte, Humboldt, Berlin, Germany. [6]Medical Genetic Research Center, Mashhad University of Medical Sciences, Mashhad, Iran.

References
1. Ferlay J, Soerjomataram I, Dikshit R, Eser S, Mathers C, Rebelo M, et al. Cancer incidence and mortality worldwide: sources, methods and major patterns in GLOBOCAN 2012. Int J Cancer. 2015;136(5):E359–86.
2. Mitchison D. How drug resistance emerges as a result of poor compliance during short course chemotherapy for tuberculosis [Counterpoint]. Int J Tuberc Lung Dis. 1998;2(1):10–5.
3. Krishna R, Mayer LD. Multidrug resistance (MDR) in cancer: mechanisms, reversal using modulators of MDR and the role of MDR modulators in influencing the pharmacokinetics of anticancer drugs. Eur J Pharm Sci. 2000; 11(4):265–83.
4. Choi C-H. ABC transporters as multidrug resistance mechanisms and the development of chemosensitizers for their reversal. Cancer Cell Int. 2005; 5(1):30.
5. Eckford PD, Sharom FJ. ABC efflux pump-based resistance to chemotherapy drugs. Chem Rev. 2009;109(7):2989–3011.
6. Staud F, Pavek P. Breast cancer resistance protein (BCRP/ABCG2). Int J Biochem Cell Biol. 2005;37(4):720–5.
7. Bemis DLCJ, Costello JE, Vorys GC, Katz AE, Buttyan R. The use of herbal and over-the-counter dietary supplements for the prevention of prostate cancer. Curr Urol Rep. 2006;7(3):166–74.
8. Hemalswarya SDM. Potential synergism of natural products in the treatment of cancer. Phytother Res. 2006;20(4):239–49.
9. Abdullaev FIE-AJ. Biomedical properties of saffron and its potential use in cancer therapy and chemoprevention trials. Cancer Detect Prev. 2004;6(28):426–32.
10. Kim SH, Lee JM, Kim SC, Park CB, Lee PC. Proposed cytotoxic mechanisms of the saffron carotenoids crocin and crocetin on cancer cell lines. Biochem Cell Biol. 2014;92(2):105–11.
11. Wu Y, Pan R, Geng P. The effect of Crocin against hypoxia damage of myocardial cell and its mechanism. Chinese J Appl Physiol. 2010;26(4):453–7.
12. Asdaq SM, Inamdar MN. Potential of Crocus sativus (saffron) and its constituent, crocin, as hypolipidemic and antioxidant in rats. Appl Biochem Biotechnol. 2010;162(2):358–72.
13. Ordoudi SA, Befani CD, Nenadis N, Koliakos GG, Tsimidou MZ. Further examination of antiradical properties of Crocus sativus stigmas extract rich in crocins. J Agric Food Chem. 2009;57(8):3080–6.
14. Xu GL, Yu SQ, Gong ZN, Zhang SQ. Study of the effect of crocin on rat experimental hyperlipemia and the underlying mechanisms. Zhongguo Zhong Yao Za Zhi. 2005;30(5):369–72.
15. He SY, Qian ZY, Tang FT, Wen N, Xu GL, Sheng L. Effect of crocin on experimental atherosclerosis in quails and its mechanisms. Life Sci. 2005; 77(8):907–21.
16. Wang Y, Han T, Zhu Y, Zheng CJ, Ming QL, Rahman K, et al. Antidepressant properties of bioactive fractions from the extract of Crocus sativus L. J Nat Med. 2010;64(1):24–30.
17. Nam KN, Park YM, Jung HJ, Lee JY, Min BD, Park SU, et al. Anti-inflammatory effects of crocin and crocetin in rat brain microglial cells. Eur J Pharmacol. 2010;648(1–3):110–6.
18. Xu GL, Li G, Ma HP, Zhong H, Liu F, Ao GZ. Preventive effect of crocin in inflamed animals and in LPS-challenged RAW 264.7 cells. J Agric Food Chem. 2009;57(18):8325–30.
19. Zhao P, Luo CL, Wu XH, Hu HB, Lv CF, Ji HY. Proliferation apoptotic influence of crocin on human bladder cancer T24 cell line. Zhongguo Zhong Yao Za Zhi. 2008;33(15):1869–73.
20. Xu HJ, Zhong R, Zhao YX, Li XR, Lu Y, Song AQ, et al. Proliferative inhibition and apoptotic induction effects of crocin on human leukemia HL-60 cells and their mechanisms. Zhongguo Shi Yan Xue Ye Xue Za Zhi. 2010;18(4):887–92.
21. Chryssanthi DG, Lamari FN, Iatrou G, Pylara A, Karamanos NK, Cordopatis P. Inhibition of breast cancer cell proliferation by style constituents of different Crocus species. Anticancer Res. 2007;27(1A):357–62.
22. Aung HH, Wang CZ, Ni M, Fishbein A, Mehendale SR, Xie JT, et al. Crocin from Crocus sativus possesses significant anti-proliferation effects on human colorectal cancer cells. Exp Oncol. 2007;29(3):175–80.
23. Garcia-Olmo DC, Riese HH, Escribano J, Ontanon J, Fernandez JA, Atienzar M, et al. Effects of long-term treatment of colon adenocarcinoma with crocin, a carotenoid from saffron (Crocus sativus L.): an experimental study in the rat. Nutr Cancer. 1999;35(2):120–6.
24. Mosaffa F, Lage H, Afshari JT, Behravan J. Interleukin-1 beta and tumor necrosis factor-alpha increase ABCG2 expression in MCF-7 breast carcinoma cell line and its mitoxantrone-resistant derivative, MCF-7/MX. Inflamm Res. 2009;58(10):669–76.
25. Tatebe S, Sinicrope FA, Kuo MT. Induction of multidrug resistance proteins MRP1 and MRP3 and gamma-glutamylcysteine synthetase gene expression by nonsteroidal anti-inflammatory drugs in human colon cancer cells. Biochem Biophys Res Commun. 2002;290(5):1427–33.
26. Hadizadeh F, Mohajeri SA, Seifi M. Extraction and purification of crocin from saffron stigmas employing a simple and efficient crystallization method. PJBS. 2010;13(14):691–8.
27. Ozben T. Mechanisms and strategies to overcome multiple drug resistance in cancer. FEBS Lett. 2006;580(12):2903–9.
28. Cui Y, Konig J, Buchholz JK, Spring H, Leier I, Keppler D. Drug resistance and ATP-dependent conjugate transport mediated by the apical multidrug resistance protein, MRP2, permanently expressed in human and canine cells. Mol Pharm. 1999;55(5):929–37.
29. Koike K, Kawabe T, Tanaka T, Toh S, Uchiumi T, Wada M, et al. A canalicular multispecific organic anion transporter (cMOAT) antisense cDNA enhances drug sensitivity in human hepatic cancer cells. Cancer Res. 1997;57(24):5475–9.
30. Borst P, Evers R, Kool M, Wijnholds J. A family of drug transporters: the multidrug resistance-associated proteins. J Natl Cancer Inst. 2000;92(16):1295–302.
31. Lv CF, Luo CL, Ji HY, Zhao P. Influence of crocin on gene expression profile of human bladder cancer cell lines T24. Zhongguo Zhong Yao Za Zhi. 2008; 33(13):1612–7.
32. D'Alessandro AM, Mancini A, Lizzi AR, De Simone A, Marroccella CE, Gravina GL, et al. Crocus sativus stigma extract and its major constituent crocin possess significant antiproliferative properties against human prostate cancer. Nutr Cancer. 2013;65(6):930–42.
33. Noureini SK, Wink M. Antiproliferative effects of crocin in HepG2 cells by telomerase inhibition and hTERT down-regulation. APJCP. 2012;13(5):2305–9.
34. Hosseinzadeh H, Mehri S, Heshmati A, Ramezani M, Sahebkar A, Abnous K. Proteomic screening of molecular targets of crocin. Daru. 2014;22(1):5.
35. Eid SY, El-Readi MZ, Wink M. Carotenoids reverse multidrug resistance in cancer cells by interfering with ABC-transporters. Phytomedicine. 2012; 19(11):977–87.

3

Computational investigation of inhibitory mechanism of flavonoids as bovine serum albumin anti-glycation agents

Anahita Johari[1,2], Ali Akbar Moosavi-Movahedi[2] and Massoud Amanlou[1*]

Abstract

Background: Glycation of serum albumin and its consequence products were considered as an important factor in drug distribution and diabetic complications, therefore finding the glycation inhibitors and their inhibitory mechanisms became a valuable field of study. In this work, bovine serum albumin (BSA) became a subject as a model protein for analyzing the inhibitory mechanism of flavonoids, known as natural BSA glycation inhibitors in the early stage of glycation.

Methods: Firstly, for theoretical study, the three-dimensional model of BSA structure was generated by homology modeling and refined through molecular dynamic simulation. Secondly, several validation methods (statistical assessment methods and also neural network methods) by simultaneous docking study were employed for insurance about accuracy of our simulation. Then docking studies were performed for visualizing the relation between flavonoids' binding sites and BSA glycation sites besides, the correlation analyzes between calculated binding energy and reported experimental inhibitory IC_{50} values of the flavonoids set, was considered to explore their molecular inhibitory mechanism.

Results: The quality assessment methods and simultaneous docking studies on interaction of quercetin (as the most studied flavonoids) with BSA and Human serum albumin (HAS), confirm the accuracy of simulation and the second stage of docking results which were in close agreement with experimental observations, suggest that the potential residues in flavonoids binding sites (which were place neighbor of tryptophan 212 within 5Å) cannot be considered as one of glycation sites.

Conclusions: Based on the results, flavonoids don't participate in inhibitory interference mechanism, and also, the differentiation between complexes of flavonoids with BSA and HSA could destroy the speculation of using them as an exchangeable model protein in study of serum albumin and flavonoids interactions.

Keywords: Homology modeling, Molecular dynamics simulation, Correlation analyzes, Glycation sites, Flavonoids, BSA

Background

Diabetes is considered as one of the main threat to human health, according to WHO report, it is predicted that diabetes will exceed to 300 million in the years of 2025. Diabetes has a devastating effect on almost every organ in body. The hyperglycemia in diabetic conditions causes non-enzymatic glycation of proteins [1]. This reaction initiates the formation of reversible Schiff base between glucose and ε-amino group of lysine residues in proteins which by consequent intermolecular rearrangements leading to a formation of ketamine adduct. Then, the potent precursors of protein cross-linkers such as glucosone, 5-hydroxymethyl-2-furaldehyde, and 3-deoxyglucosone are formed due to the initial reaction. Next, those intermediates are oxidized, and cross linked, and fluorescent heterogeneous group of protein-bound moieties (called advanced glycated end products or AGEs) are detected in the last stage of glycation [2,3]. With body of evidence, formation and accumulation of advanced glycation products can be considered as a major factor

* Correspondence: amanlou@tums.ac.ir
[1]Department of Medicinal Chemistry, Faculty of Pharmacy and Pharmaceutical Sciences Research Center, Tehran University of Medical Sciences, Tehran, Iran
Full list of author information is available at the end of the article

in development of diabetic complication, Alzheimer's disease, and normal aging process. Therefore, the considerable efforts have been made to propose and discover inhibitors of glycation for therapeutic application in treatment of diseases that advanced glycation end product could be responsible for their pathogenesis [4].

Serum albumin is the most abundant protein in body which has a tremendous interest for binding to various natural or synthetic small-molecules such as glucose and related compounds. In diabetic condition, serum albumin undergoes glycation [5]. This character, continually expose serum albumin to altering factors which can participate in serum albumin modifications and biological compound formation that can be considered as a causative agent for some diseases [6]. Among the wide variety of interaction, the none-enzymatic interaction of serum albumin with glucose is one of the most important underlying modification factors, which are in associated with various alterations of albumin's structure and functions [7,8].

Among the glycation inhibitors' which were examined on bovine serum albumin (BSA) as a model protein, specific considerations were given to dietary natural products such as several phenolic compounds [9,10]. Researches on a limited number of flavonoids compounds indicated their ability to prevention both stage of glycation reaction [7]. In the late stage, the inhibition mechanisms of flavonoids are that, they may act as a both metal chelator and radical scavenger [11,12]. However, the inhibitory mechanism of flavonoids in the early stage completely remains unclear [7]. For some anti-glycation agent such as α-lipoate or non-steroidal anti-inflammatory drugs such as diclofenac and aspirin, hydrophobic hindrance or binding near the glycation site was considered as possible mechanism of anti-glycation activity [9,13]. Although we have no evidence that flavonoids react with the glycation site [7], in the present study, the attentions are drawn to binding behavior of flavonoids to clarifying the inhibition mechanism of them for the early stage of glycation.

Since, docking simulation results can be used to understanding the molecular interaction and analyze biological presses, rapidly and efficiently [2], in the present study, we explored the series of flavonoids' binding behavior with BSA through docking studies.

However, in the case of BSA which was considered here as a model protein (such as studies mentioned above by Morimitsu, Y., et al. and Matsuda, H., et al. [3,12]). When this study was started nobody has succeeded in obtaining crystals of intact BSA [14]. However, simultaneous with our study the importance of this protein draws the other researchers' attention to solving the tertiary structure of BSA. However, the new crystals also haven't been at high resolution (<2 Å resolution limit) [15], which can be satisfactory resolution for using in docking simulation. In this study, simulation, homology

modeling was employed. While, it is generally recognized that homology modeling of proteins could be considered as accurate methods for 3D structure prediction while a model and related template sharing high sequence identity [16,17].

In present work, the model was refined with energy minimization and molecular dynamic simulation. Then, different assessment tools were adapted for checking the proper folding of constructed BSA 3D structure.

Consequently, by docking methods the validity of the model protein was examined and for getting better insight into the flavonoids' inhibitory mechanism. Firstly, the predicted binding affinity and reported IC_{50} [12] was subjected to correlation analyzes and secondly, the flavonoids binding location was studied for tracing the relation among participated amino acids in the flavonoids' binding site with ones proposed as the glycation site of BSA [18].

In addition, according to docking results, the comparison is made between obtained 3D structure of BSA and crystallographic structure of HSA for understanding their specificity in flavonoids binding location and the verification of using BSA and HSA as an exchangeable mode protein for the same case of investigation.

Methods

Amino acid sequence alignment and homology modeling of bovine serum albumin

In the first step, Amino acid sequence of BSA (UniProt ID: P02769) was retrieved from Swiss-Prot (http://www.uniprot.org/uniprot). And then, Blastp matrix blosum62 against PDB database was used to find out the best homologous structure with a known 3D structure, for applying as a template in homology modeling. Finally, among the HSA structures, the structure with a highest resolution at 1.9 Å [19] that belong to HSA (PDB ID: 1N5U) was adopted as the final target.

Sequence alignment was generated using 2d alignment function of MODELLER 9v8 program (www.salilab.org/modeller). Align 2d is based on a dynamic programming algorithm, considering the template structural information for constructing an alignment, this advantages is more significant as the similarity between the sequences decrease and the number of gaps increase [20]. After alignment, the 3D structure of fifty models were calculated completely automatically with MODELLER 9v8 [21].

Refinement of homology model by minimization and MD simulation

Molecular dynamic simulation were carried out using the parallel version of GROMACS 4.5.3 [22] In the AMBER99SB force field [23] to monitor stability and conformation of the selected model. The starting coordinates were taken from the best model that was retrieved from MODELLER and for prediction of non-standard ionization state of residues PROPKA 2.0 was applied [24]. Among the whole residues that may be adapted standard ionization state, lysine 219 was deprotonated and six histidine residues (histidine 16, histidine 37, histidine 143, histidine 239, histidine 335, and histidine 332) were completely protonated.

After assigning charge state, the protein was put into a suitable sized simulation cubic box and immersed in 41760 simple point charges (SPC) water model. Then, appropriate number of Na^+ ions were added to neutralize the charge of the system. The first energy minimization, which targeted water molecules and ions alone while configuration of protein was kept, fixed, followed by 20 ps MD simulation which again, the protein was kept fixed and the water molecules and ions were allowed to evolve. The second minimization step began with 1000 steepest descent and conjugate gradient of 9000 steps afterward. For equilibrating further the system v-rescale thermostat [25] was applied by using coupling constant (τ_t) of 0.1 ps to keep the system at the constant temperature in 100 ps at 100 K and 200 K respectively. While the pressure of the system maintained at 1 atm by using the Berendsen weak coupling algorithm [26] with coupling constant (τ_p) of 0.5 ps. For obtaining the stable system at 300 K and 1 atm, the same aforementioned parameters were determined for heating the system.

In this simulation, the non-bonded interactions were calculated by applying a 14 Å cut off and periodic boundary conditions were also applied in all directions. The Electrostatic interactions were calculated using the Particle Mesh Ewald (PME) [27]. During simulation, the frame was stored at every 1.000 ps.

Subsequently, all the analysis was performed by taking advantage of Gromacs tools and the structure which was retrieved after system stabilization was subject to evaluate the protein geometry.

Assessment of the homology model
To verify the quality of the model after molecular dynamic refinement, using different tools, which include: PRoQ, as a neural network based predictor [28], verify 3D, which analyzes the compatibility of an atomic model (3D) with its own amino acid sequence (1D) [29], PROSA program, which evaluate the energy of using a distance based pair potential [30] as well PROCHECK for checking the detailed stereochemical properties [31].

Docking analysis
Autodock 4.0 [32] was used for docking studies and for adding charges and active torsions to the ligands and assign Kollman charges to protein AutoDockTools (ADT) was employed. The rectangular lattice ($100 \times 100 \times 100$) with points separated by 0.375 Å was built by AutoGrid that was superposed on subdomin IIA of serum albumin

(proposed as a primarily binding site of flavonoids) [33]. The Lamarckian genetic algorithm (LGA) was used with 100 runs for docking simulation, while an initial population size of 100, and the maximum number of 2500000 energy evaluations. All other parameters were set to default values, and the results were ranked according to Autodock scoring function and the final conformation of each structure was selected based on the highest dock score.

The chemical structures of interested flavonoids were optimized at MM+ level of molecular mechanic methods using HYPERCHEM software program (version 8.0.3 Hypercube, Inc) [34]. The geometry optimization was preceded by Polak-Ribiere algorithm to reach the 0.01 root mean square gradient. Then all these refinement structures were subject to docking simulations.

MD simulation after docking
All MD simulations were performed using the Gromacs 4.5.3 program together with the 43a2 force field [35-37] for each simulation to study the complex of BSA-quercetin, while the topology of quercetin was generated by the PRODRG 2.5 beta server [38].

Then, the protein was solvated by simple point charge water molecule in the cubic box with minimal distance of protein from its wall being 1.0 nm and the system was neutralized by adding appropriate counter ions. After performing energy minimization of the entire system, it was equilibrated under NVT ensemble for 100 ps and the periodic boundary conditions were used in tree-coordinate direction, whereas, position restrains were placed on ligand using force restraint of 1000 kcal/mol. NVT equilibration is followed by isothermal–isobaric (NPT) which was performed for 100 ps. The pressure of the system was regulated by Berendsen barostat with a relaxation time (τp) of 2.0 ps. The position restraints and simulation parameter which was applied in the NPT ensemble was the same as the ones which have been used during NPT equilibration. After convergence had been reached, the protein-ligand and water-ions groups were coupled in separate temperature baths, and v-rescale thermostat was used to keep the temperature constant at 300 k during the 2 ns simulation. Lennard-Jones interactions were calculated within a cut-off distance of 1.0 nm, and electrostatic interactions were treated with the particle mesh Ewald's method. Ultimately, from 2 ns MD simulation, the structure with low RMSD value was selected for analyzing the local conformational changes of BSA- quercetin complex.

Computational resources
The computational studies were performed on computer cluster 4 HP Prolient ML370-G5 Tower servers equipped with 2 Quad Core Intel Xeon processors E5355, 2.66 GHz and 4GB of RAM on a Linux platform.

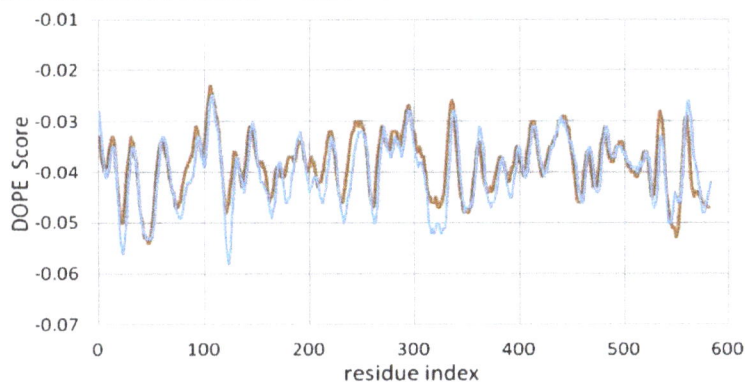

Figure 1 Analysis of DOPE score profile (obtained from Modeller). The Blue line indicates, energy profile of HSA (PDB ID: 1N5U) which used as a model and the red line indicates energy profile of target, which constructed by Modeller.

Results

Sequence alignment and modeling building

Based on the highest similarity and the lowest D-value, human serum albumin (HSA) can be considered the best homologues structure for BSA. The Sequence alignment of BSA (UniProt ID: P02769) and HSA (UniProt ID: P02768) which was generated by ClustalX program shows 76% identity between them [39]. The precursor proteins of BSA and HSA have 603 and 607 amino acid in length, respectively. Though all the crystallographic structures of HSA which were reported, only consist of 583 amino

acids. This can be referred to the fact that during a secretion and maturation process of serum albumins, the 25 N-terminal amino acids were cleaved [40]. Therefore, the 25 N –terminal amino acids, which are placed out of the chain, were separated from the HSA amino acids sequence and the rest of them used as a target for homology modeling.

After alignment, the 3D structure of fifty models was calculated completely automatically with modeler 9v8. In this process, the population of the constructed model was increased for improving the DOPE energy assessment

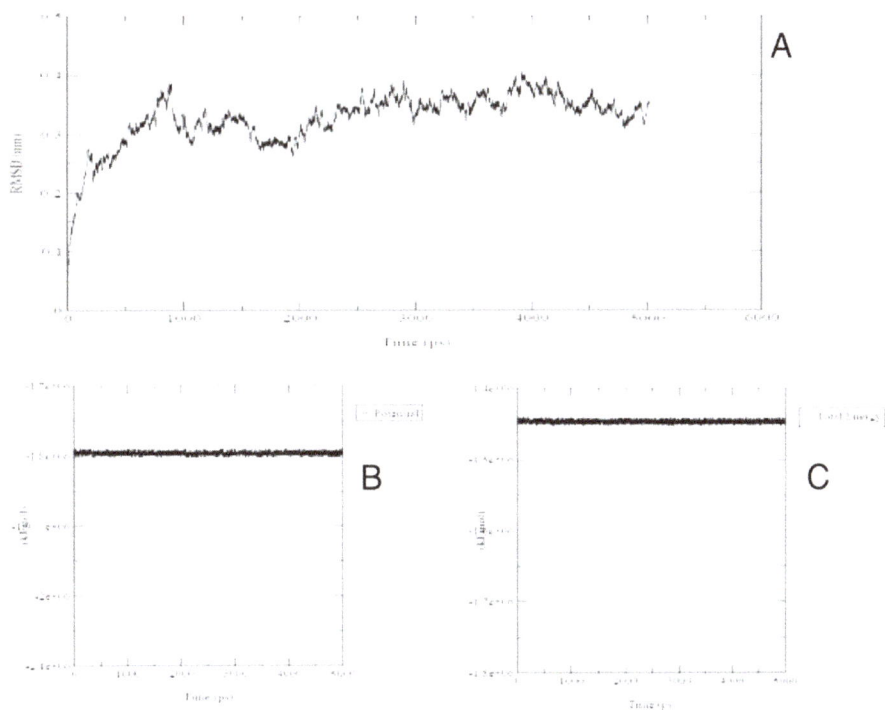

Figure 2 Analysis of a molecular dynamics simulation trajectory during 5ns generated by Gromacs. (A) The backbone root mean square deviation (RMSD) plot of the model, during 5ns simulation. **(B)** The variation of potential around constant value. **(C)** The fluctuation of total energy.

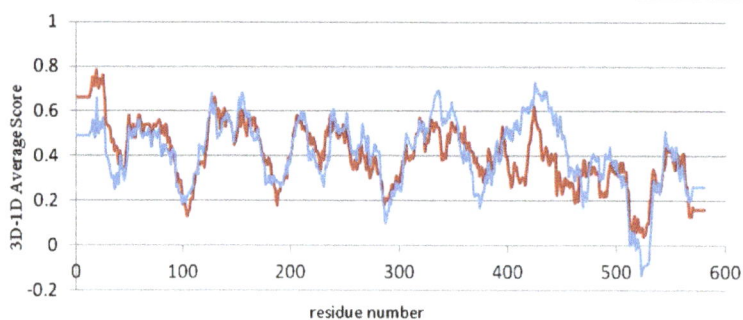

Figure 3 The Verify-3D analysis is shown for all residues. The blue line belongs to molecular structure after MD, and red one belongs to model that constructed by the Modeller. The refinement model after MD was validated by positive scores of Verify-3D.

and MODELLER objective function calculation and then the best model was selected based on the lowest DOPE score. Next, for gave an idea about the quality of input alignment the DOPE score profile (Figure 1) was calculated with "assess_dope" function of MODELLER. It can be seen in Figure 1, that in the whole range of residues, the DOPE score of both proteins converges and the results aren't showing any problematic regions.

Analysis the trajectory of the molecular dynamics simulation

During 5 ns MD simulation, the system was analyzed for its stability. The deviation plot of potential, and root mean square deviation (Figure 2) were derived from the respective trajectory by Gromacs software output. The low degree of RMSD fluctuation during last 2 ns indicates

that the system tends to be converging and therefore, it is become stable. According to what illustrated in Figure 2, the total energy of the complex was observed within the range from −1.4 to −1.5 kJ/mol, which can be a reasonable value.

Assess the validity of generated model after MD

In present work two statistical approaches such as verify3D and PROSA confirm a reliability of the constructed model.

In the first approach, the Verify 3D profile (Figure 3) represents that 3D-1D average score of the most residues in the model proteins both before and after MD, given a score over 0.2 except the ones rage 514–532. In the model protein that refined after MD, the whole residues have a positive score, whereas in the model that constructed by the modeler the amino acids in the range of 518–530 have a negative score. Therefore, based on these results, the sign of model folding improvement after molecular dynamic simulation is traceable.

The second statistical assessment method was processed with ProSA program. The Normalized Z-score calculation indicates standard deviation value is found in the range of native conformation of crystallographic structure and also according to Figure 4, ProSA score, which was calculated interaction energy per residues, has a negative score across the most of the residues' length.

After performing those earlier methodologies based on statistical approaches (Verify3D, ProSA), the PRoQ was applied to compare the validity of the model before and after MD simulation. This program is based on a neural

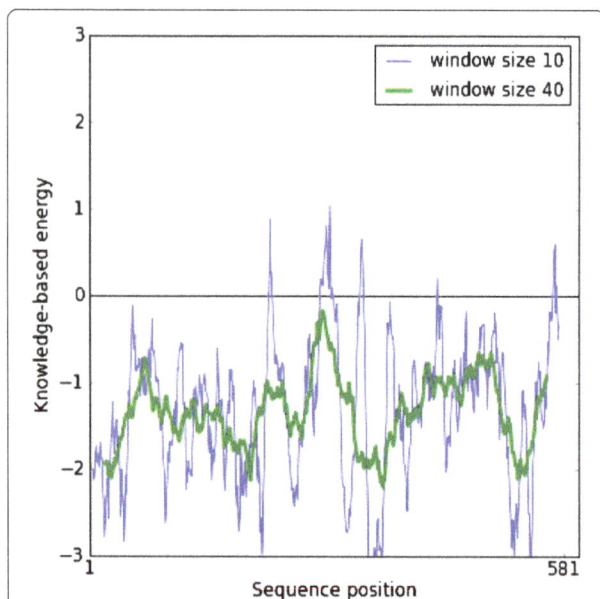

Figure 4 Energy plot from ProSA program, all residues have negative ProSA energies which confirms the reliability of the model.

Table 1 Ramachandran plot statistics

% residues in most favored regions	90.8%
% residues in additional allowed regions	8.8%
% residues in generously allowed regions	0.4%
% residues in disallowed regions	0.0%
% Num. of non-glycine and non-proline residues	100.0%

Table 2 Main chain parameters plot statistics

Stereochemical parameter	No. of data pts	Parameter value	Comparison values Typical value	Comparison values Band width	No. of band widths from mean	
%-tage residues in A,B,L	535	90.8	84.9	10.0	0.6	Inside
Omega angle Std. dev.	380	7.0	6.0	3.0	0.3	Inside
Bad contacts/100 residues	0	0.0	3.3	10.0	−0.3	Inside
Zeta angle Std. dev.	565	1.3	3.1	1.6	−1.1	Better
H-bond energy Std. dev.	400	0.7	0.8	0.2	0.5	Inside
Overall G-factor	581	0.0	−0.3	0.3	1.0	Better

network that by considering the Wallner and Elofsson's study it is indeed superior to statistics-based methods [41]. In this method two quality measures are predicted, LG score and MaxSub score. Based on their range of qualities; predicted LG score and MaxSub score of the model after MD is 4.14 (which is within the range of a 'extremely good') and 0.45(which are within the range of 'good'), while values of 2.915 and 0.304 were obtained for LG score and MaxSub score, respectively in the model before MD simulation. These scores indicate the refinement of the model after MD simulation.

Ultimately, the validity of the model was evaluated by PROCHECK, and stereochemical properties of protein structure were listed in Tables 1 and 2 [31,42]. In the Figure 5, phi and psi distribution of Ramachandran plot indicate that 100% of residues were present in favored and allowed regions, which confirm that the structure is comparable with good homology model [43]. Also the main chain parameters which consist of six properties plotted are all well within the established limit of reliable structures (Table 2).

In brief, according to all applied evaluated methods, it can be concluded that obtained 3.D structural model has an acceptable geometry for further study by docking approach.

Docking studies

With the interest of comparability of docking result with experimental data (which studied the interaction among flavonoids and BSA), and also shedding the light at an ambiguous point of experimental observation in molecular level, with respect to Dufour and Dangles work [33] one stage of docking simulation was designed. Therefore, the binding interaction of quercetin (as the most studied flavonoid) and warfarin (as a site marker of subdomain IIA HSA) was subject to docking simulation.

First of all, in this process, the accuracy of applied docking protocol was examined. So, warfarin as a probe of HSA (whose high affinity binding site was known as a subdomain IIA) was docked into HSA (PDB ID: 1H9Z), which co-crystallized with it. Docking results demonstrates that the warfarin docks back into the experimental binding location which was retrieved based on the crystallographic study (Figure 6).Therefore; this protocol was confirmed and consequently, applied in docking simulation for complexes of quercetin with HSA and BSA.

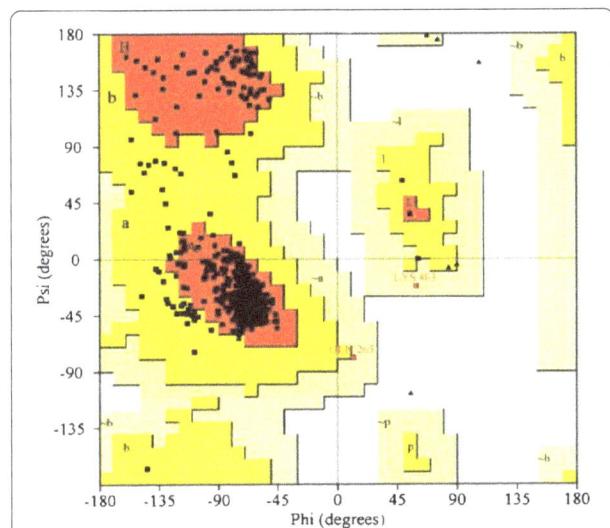

Figure 5 Ramachandran plot for 3D structural model of bovine serum albumin.

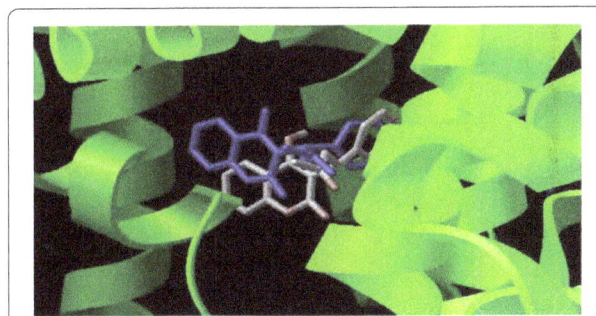

Figure 6 The docking conformation and location of warfarin on the Human serum albumin (PDB ID: 1H9Z). The conformation of warfarin after docking indicates with DG colored sketch (David Goodsell's scheme) and what was retrieved from the crystallographic study indicate as a blue sketch.

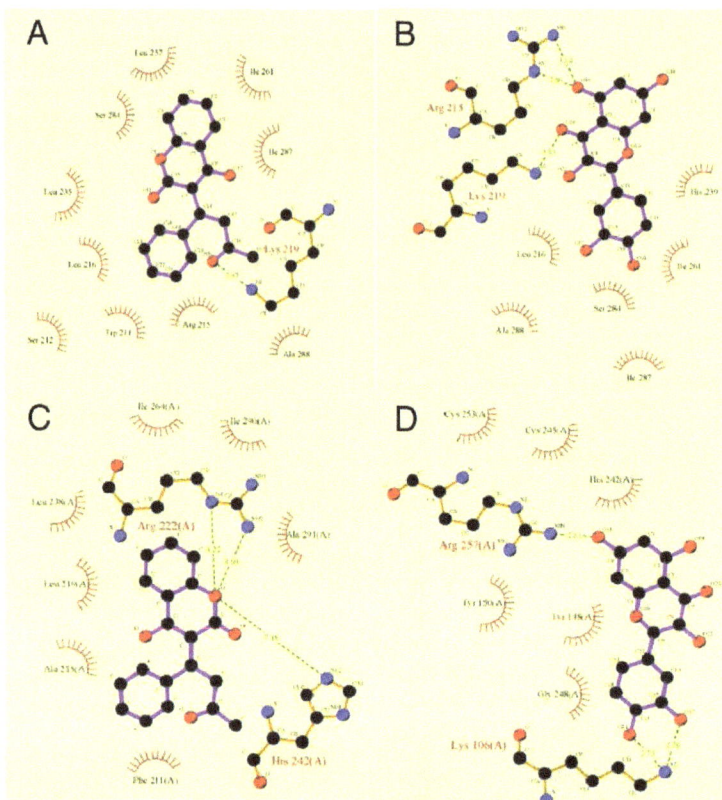

Figure 7 The structure of bovine serum albumin complexes with warfarin and quercetin (A, B), consequently (C) The structure of human serum albumin complexes with warfarin and quercetin, (D) was analyzed using the Ligplot 4.22 program. The hydrogen bonds are shown as dash lines and hydrophobic contacts are indicated with half-moon.

For analyzing the specific contact and indicating the participated amino acids in biding sites the Ligplot program was employed [44]. It is indicated in Figure 7, That in the binding site of bovine serum albumin, serine 284, isoleucine 261 and 287, alanine 288 involve in hydrophobic interaction with quercetin and warfarin, and also arginine 219 contribute in a hydrogen bond with both,

this means that in the case of BSA, the warfarin and quercetin binding sites completely overlap, while these ligands are bonded in different location in HSA.

The Dufour and Dangles fluorescence spectroscopy study had shown that fluorescence of BSA-quercetin complex (protein/marker molar ratio of 1) is affected by constant concentration of warfarin (site marker of subdomain IIA),

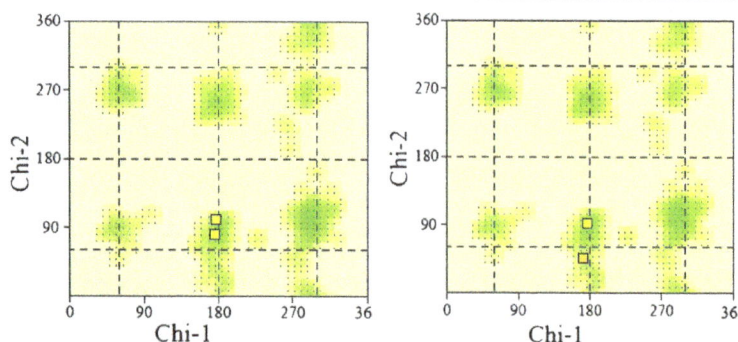

Figure 8 The χ_1/χ_2 plots are obtained from PROCHECK program. Each square represents one residue. The color coding of the squares is corresponding the range of yellow to red which is reflects the degree to which the orientation is favored; therefore, yellow indicate the residue is in a favored and red indicate the residue is an unflavored region. Two tryptophan of bovine serum albumin was indicated in both plots. The left plot indicate χ_1/χ_2 coordinate of tryptophans before MD (Left). The right plot indicates the χ_1/χ_2 coordinates of tryptophans after MD (Right). How it is shown, trp 134 remains constant while the χ_1/χ_2 coordinates of trp 212 is changed and located in unflavored region.

but fluorescence of HSA-quercetin complex is independent of warfarin presence [33].

For better understanding of the relation between experimental observations and what was retrieved from docking calculations. The more investigations were taken to visualization the effect of BSA-flavonoids interaction on local conformational changes, which leads to fluorescence quenching.

First notable issue which was considered is that the amino acids lining in the common binding site of quercetin and warfarin, are neighbors of tryptophan 212 within 5Å. This is important because the intrinsic fluorescence of BSA with excitation at 295 nm is due to the tryptophan residues (BSA has two tryptophan, tryptophan 212 and tryptophan 134) and quercetin actually promoted a strong quenching of the tryptophan emission at 340 nm

Table 3 The free energy of binding between, 12 Flavones, 12 Flavonols, 3 Flavanones, 2 Flavan-3-ols and bovine serum albumin obtained from docking study, and their AGEs inhibitions' IC$_{50}$ (in regard to Matsuda, H., et al. [12])

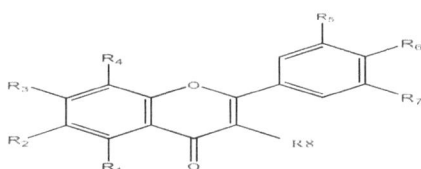

Num	Name	R^1	R^2	R^3	R^4	R^5	R^6	R^7	R^8	ΔG (Kcal/mol)	AGEs inhibition IC$_{50}$ (% in 200 µM)
1	Flavone	H	H	H	H	H	H	H	H	−7.09	5%
2	7-Hydroxyflavone	H	H	OH	H	H	H	H	H	−6.96	27%
3	Chrysin	OH	H	OH	H	H	H	H	H	−7.56	43%
4	4,7-Dihydroxyflavone	H	H	OH	H	H	OH	H	H	−7.0	44%
5	3,4,7-Trihydroxyflavone	H	H	OH	H	OH	OH	H	H	−7.53	44%
6	Apigenin	OH	H	OH	H	H	OH	H	H	−7.52	53%
7	Luteolin	OH	H	OH	H	OH	OH	H	H	−7.53	64%
8	Diosmetin	OH	H	OH	H	OH	OCH$_3$	H	H	−7.05	27%
9	Pilloin	OH	H	OCH$_3$	H	OH	OCH$_3$	H	H	−7.9	29%
10	10 F	OH	H	OCH$_3$	H	OCH$_3$	OCH$_3$	H	H	−7.0	29%
11	Wogonin	OH	H	OH	OCH$_3$	H	H	H	H	−7.03	50%
12	Baicalin	OH	OH	OH	H	H	H	H	H	−7.75	79%
13	3-Hydroxyflavone	H	H	H	H	H	H	H	OH	−7.1	3%
14	Kaempferol	OH	H	OH	H	H	OH	H	OH	−7.47	46%
15	Quercetin	OH	H	OH	H	OH	OH	H	OH	−7.67	57%
16	Rhamnetin	OH	H	OCH$_3$	H	OH	OH	H	OH	−7.57	55%
17	Tamarixetin	OH	H	OH	H	OH	OCH$_3$	H	OH	−7.89	45%
18	F18	OH	H	OCH$_3$	H	OH	OH	H	OCH$_3$	−7.4	57%
19	Ombuine	OH	H	OCH$_3$	H	OH	OCH$_3$	H	OH	−7.66	27%
20	Ayanin	OH	H	OCH$_3$	H	OH	OCH$_3$	H	OCH$_3$	−7.66	40%
21	21 F	OH	H	OCH$_3$	H	OCH$_3$	OCH$_3$	H	OH	−7.69	13%
22	Myricetin	H	H	H	H	H	H	H	OH	−7.48	61%
23	Mearnsetin	H	H	H	H	H	CH3	H	OH	−7.51	10%
24	24 F	H	H	CH$_3$	H	H	H	H	OH	- 7.81	42%
25	Liquiritigenin	H	H	OH	H	H	OH	H	H	−7.16	40%
26	26 F	H	H	OCH$_3$	H	H	OH	H	H	−6.74	44%
27	Eriodictyol	OH	H	OH	H	OH	OH	H	H	−7.46	46%
28	(+)-Catechin	OH	H	OH	H	OH	OH	H	β-OH	−7.74	69%
29	(−)-Epigallocatechin	OH	H	OH	H	OH	OH	OH	α-OH	−7.06	4%

[33]. These observations lead to further study of checking the tryptophan flexibility after interaction between the quercetin and BSA complex.

So, the complex of BSA model and quercetin (best conformation after docking) was subjected to molecular dynamic simulation for 2 ns. After the stability of the system, for describing the side chain conformational changes the dihedral angles of our interested aromatic residue, χ_1 / χ_2 plot was provided by PROCHECK program [31]. The results represent the significant shuffling between side-chain conformations of tryptophan 212 before and after the refinement of BSA-quercetin complex with molecular dynamic simulation. Figure 8 indicates that the BSA residues which were involved in interaction with quercetin, pushing the tryptophan 212 side chain conformations to unflavored regions.

Discussion

In present work, based on docking calculation and molecular dynamic simulation, the detailed understanding was obtained about the interaction of quercetin (as a typical flavonoids) and BSA, which is in consistence with previous experimental data [33]. In addition, these calculations in molecular levels demonstrate its ability to providing the interpretation for experimental observation.

The first-stage docking results confirm on one hand the reliability of obtained 3D structural model, and on the other hand, by showing the significant specificity between high homologous BSA and HSA proteins, indicate the necessity of constructing BSA model's for analyzing the interaction flavonoids with it.

According to visualization of the predicted binding site of quercetin, any interventions are not observed between the quercetin binding site and reported glycation site of BSA [18]. However, for the more reliable conclusion, a number of flavonoids which introduced as an inhibitor of BSA glycation [3,12] were employed for the further docking studies.

By the speculation that the radical scavenging activity in physiological condition could inhibit oxidative fragmentation of Amadori rearrangement product and subsequently prevented the AGEs formation, the number of flavonoids was studied to find a correlation between the experimental anti glycation activity and radical scavenging activity of them [12]. In the present investigation with respect to their works, interested flavonoids was selected and by considering an interference reaction in the glycation site as the possible inhibitory mechanism [9,45,46], the theoretical binding energies of flavonoids in the complex with BSA were calculated by docking methods(calculated free energy of binding were listed in Tables 3 and 4). Then, analytical methods were performed by SPSS software (version 15). The correlation analyzes between the experimental activity (IC$_{50}$) and predicted binding energy reveal that there is no significant correlation between these values (p > 0.3).

Besides the statistical analyzes, the AutoDockTools (ADT) was used for visualization the relationship between the predicted flavonoids' binding site and the reported glycation site on BSA. Interestingly, despite the structural differentiations which exist among these flavonoids, the most likely conformation of each one of them, were placed in the same binding site (consist of lysine 219, arginine 215, isoleucine 287, and serine 284) (Figure 9) which can't be considered as any glycation sites of BSA (in respect to aforementioned Hinton and Ames study). Therefore, by considering these results, maybe it can be concluded that the hydrophobic hindrances in the glycation site can't be considered as an inhibitory mechanism for flavonoids.

Conclusion

In previous experimental studies, the high homology between BSA and HSA has invoked speculation that they have a similar structure and so share similar capability in some of their properties like ligands binding [45]. However, simulating the quercetin (as the most studied flavonoids) interactions with both BSA and HSA show significant differences between them, which confirms our speculation about the necessity of providing the affordable BSA 3D structural model for analyzing its specific

Table 4 The free energy of binding between 3 isoflavones and bovine Serum albumin obtained from docking study, and their AGEs inhibitions' IC$_{50}$

Num.	Name	R^1	R^2	R^3	R^4	R^5	ΔG (Kcal/mol)	AGEs inhibition IC$_{50}$ (% in 200 μM)
30	Daidzein	H	H	OH	H	OH	−7.05	33%
31	Genistein	OH	H	OH	H	OH	−6.44	34%
32	Biochanin A	OH	H	OH	H	OCH$_3$	−7.68	36%

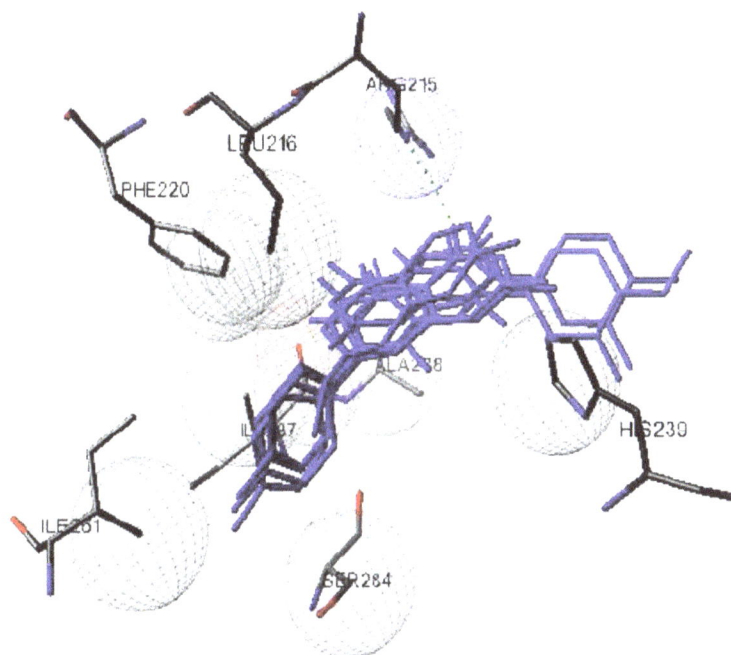

Figure 9 The superimposition of docked complex. The most likely conformation of representative flavonoids of under study groups (Flavones, flavonols, flavanones, flavan-3-ols, isoflavones), is represented in their binding site.

binding location and binding affinity for our interested ligands.

Interestingly, in the present study, the consistency between docking results and experimental data not only indicate the validity of our simulation but also become helpful in interpreting about experimental observation in molecular levels [33].

Thus different aspect of results was considered, on one hand the visualization of quercetin binding site leads to find the relationship between the binding site residues and tryptophan 212, and also by employing the MD simulation it is revealed that participated residues in flavonoids interaction site affect on tryptophan local conformational change, which at last is observed as fluorescence quenching.

On the other hand, according to our obtained results, the possibility of relation between the flavonoids binding site and glycation sites was investigated, while the correlation analyzes was adopted between binding affinity of flavonoids to BSA and IC_{50} of AGE inhibition. How was mentioned before based on the results, the flavonoids can't be considered as an intervention agent for glycation site and therefore, the possibility of this inhibitory mechanism is unacceptable in the case of flavonoids.

Ultimately, the other interesting outcome of this study is laid beneath the final examination. Coincident with our study the crystallographic structure of bovine serum albumin was determined [15]. Therefore, the comparison has been made between our calculated 3D structural models of BSA with the reported model which retrieved

from crystallographic technique to get insight into their distinctive difference. These two structures were superimposed with Swiss PDB viewer software (Figure 10) [47]. And strong correlation (RMSD: 1.9) between them shades a light in the hypothesis that applied methods in this study are accurate and reliable.

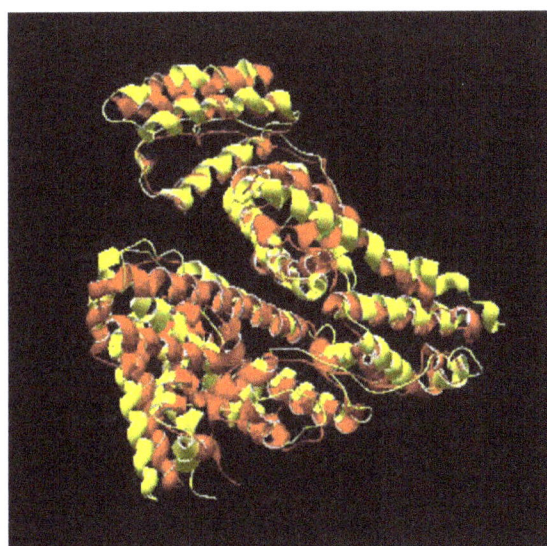

Figure 10 The superimposition between crystallographic structure of bovine serum albumin (PDB ID: 4F5S) (orange) and calculated 3D structure model (yellow), obtained with Swiss PDB viewer software.

Competing interests

The authors declare that they have no competing interests.

Authors' contributions

All authors contributed to the concept and design of study. AJ and MA performed all computational experiments and analyzed the data. MA is responsible for the study registration, financial and administrative support. AJ, MA and AAMM wrote the manuscript and all authors read and approved the final manuscript.

Acknowledgements

This work was financially supported by grants from Research Council of Tehran University of Medical Science and UNESCO Chair on Interdisciplinary Research in Diabetes, University of Tehran, Iran.

Author details

[1]Department of Medicinal Chemistry, Faculty of Pharmacy and Pharmaceutical Sciences Research Center, Tehran University of Medical Sciences, Tehran, Iran. [2]Institute of Biochemistry and Biophysics, University of Tehran, Tehran, Iran.

References

1. Nawale RB, Mourya VK, Bhise SB: Non-enzymatic glycation of proteins: a cause for complications in diabetes. *Indian J Biochem Biophys* 2006, **43**:337–344.
2. Iberg N, Fluckiger R: Nonenzymatic glycosylation of albumin in vivo. identification of multiple glycosylated sites. *J Biol Chem* 1986, **261**:13542–13545.
3. Morimitsu Y, Yoshida K, Esaki S, Hirota A: Protein glycation inhibitors from thyme (*Thymus vulgaris*). *Biosci Biotechnol Biochem* 1995, **59**:2018–2021.
4. Rahbar S, Figarola JL: Novel inhibitors of advanced glycation endproducts. *Arch Biochem Biophys* 2003, **419**:63–79.
5. Deeb O, Rosales-Hernández MC, Gómez-Castro C, Garduño-Juárez R, Correa-Basurto J: Exploration of human serum albumin binding sites by docking and molecular dynamics flexible ligand–protein interactions. *Biopolymers* 2010, **93**:161–170.
6. Crdova J, Ryan JD, Boonyaratanakornkit BB, Clark DS: Esterase activity of bovine serum albumin up to 160°C: a new benchmark for biocatalysis. *Enzyme Microb Techno* 2008, **42**:278–283.
7. Rondeau P, Bourdon E: The glycation of albumin: structural and functional impacts. *Biochimie* 2011, **93**:645–658.
8. Bousova I, Vukasovic D, Juretic D, Palicka V, Drsata J: Enzyme activity and AGE formation in a model of AST glycoxidation by D-fructose in vitro. *Acta Pharm* 2005, **55**:107–114.
9. Kawabata T, Packer L: [alpha]-lipoate can protect against glycation of serum albumin, but not low-density lipoprotein. *Biochem Biophys Res Commun* 1994, **203**:99–104.
10. Gutiérrez RMP, Diaz SL, Reyese IC, Gonzalez AMN: Anti-glycation effect of spices and chilies uses in traditional mexican cuisine. *J Nat Prod* 2010, **3**:95–102.
11. Bors W, Heller W, Michel C, Saran M: Flavonoids as antioxidants: determination of radical-scavenging efficiencies. *Methods Enzymol* 1990, **186**:343–355.
12. Matsuda H, Wang T, Managi H, Yoshikawa M: Structural requirements of flavonoids for inhibition of protein glycation and radical scavenging activities. *Bioorg Med Chem* 2003, **11**:5317–5323.
13. Van Boekel MA, van den Bergh PJ, Honders HJ: Glycation of human serum albumin: inhibition by Diclofenac. *Biochim Biophys Acta* 1992, **1120**:201–204.
14. Tai HC: *X-ray Crystallographic Studies of Bovine Serum Albumin and Helicobacter Pylori Thioredoxin-2*. Saskatoon, Canada: Thesis, University of Saskatchewan; 2004.
15. Bujacz A: Structures of bovine, equine and leporine serum albumin. *Acta Crystallogr Sect D Biol Crystallogr* 2012, **68**:1278–1289.
16. Ginalski K: Comparative modeling for protein structure prediction. *Curr Opin Struct Biol* 2006, **16**:172–177.
17. Azizian H, Bahrami H, Pasalar P, Amanlou M: Molecular modeling of Helicobacter pylori arginase and the inhibitor coordination interactions. *J Mol Graph Model* 2010, **28**:626–635.
18. Hinton DJS, Ames JM: Site specificity of glycation and carboxymethylation of bovine serum albumin by fructose. *Amino Acids* 2006, **30**:425–434.
19. Wardell M, Wang Z, Ho JX, Robert J, Ruker F, Ruble J, Carter DC: The atomic structure of human methemalbumin at 1.9 A. *Biochem Biophys Res Commun* 2002, **291**:813–819.
20. Sali A, Blundell TL: Comparative protein modelling by satisfaction of spatial restraints. *J Mol Biol* 1993, **234**:779–815.
21. Laurie AT, Jackson RM: Q-SiteFinder: an energy-based method for the prediction of protein-ligand binding sites. *Bioinformatics* 2005, **21**:1908–1916.
22. Hess B, Kutzner C, van der Spoel D, Lindahl E: GROMACS 4: algorithms for highly efficient, load-balanced, and scalable molecular simulation. *J Chem Theory Comput* 2008, **4**:435–447.
23. Hornak V, Abel R, Okur A, Strockbine B, Roitberg A, Simmerling C: Comparison of multiple Amber force fields and development of improved protein backbone parameters. *Proteins* 2006, **65**:712–725.
24. Bas DC, Rogers DM, Jensen JH: Very fast prediction and rationalization of pKa values for protein–ligand complexes. *Proteins Struct Funct Bioinf* 2008, **73**:765–783.
25. Bussi G, Donadio D, Parrinello M: Canonical sampling through velocity rescaling. *J Chem Phys* 2007, **126**:014101.
26. Berendsen H, Postma J, van Gunsteren W, DiNola A, Haak J: Molecular dynamics with coupling to an external bath. *J Chem Phys* 1984, **81**:3684–3690.
27. Essmann U, Perera L, Berkowitz ML, Darden T, Lee H, Pedersen LG: A smooth particle mesh ewald method. *J Chem Phys* 1995, **103**:8577–8593.
28. Wallner B, Elofsson A: Can correct protein models be identified? *Protein Sci* 2003, **12**:1073–1086.
29. Luthy R, Bowie JU, Eisenberg D: Assessment of protein models with three-dimensional profiles. *Nature* 1992, **356**:83–85.
30. Wiederstein M, Sippl MJ: ProSA-web: interactive web service for the recognition of errors in three-dimensional structures of proteins. *Nucleic Acids Res* 2007, **35**:W407–W410.
31. Laskowski RA, MacArthur MW, Moss DS, Thornton JM: PROCHECK: a program to check the stereochemical quality of protein structures. *J Appl Crystallogr* 1993, **26**:283–291.
32. Morris GM, Goodsell DS, Halliday RS, Huey R, Hart WE, Belew RK, Olson AJ: Automated docking using a Lamarckian genetic algorithm and an empirical binding free energy function. *J Comput Chem* 1998, **19**:1639–1662.
33. Dufour C, Dangles O: Flavonoid-serum albumin complexation: determination of binding constants and binding sites by fluorescence spectroscopy. *Biochim Biophys Acta* 2005, **1721**:164–173.
34. Froimowitz M: HyperChem: a software package for computational chemistry and molecular modeling. *Biotechniques* 1993, **14**:1010–1013.
35. Bekker H, Berendsen H, Dijkstra E, Achterop S, van Drunen R: Gromacs method of virial calculation using a single sum. In *Physics Computing*. 1993:257-26.
36. Lindahl E, Hess B, van der Spoel D: GROMACS 3.0: a package for molecular simulation and trajectory analysis. *J Mol Mod* 2001, **7**:306–317.
37. Berendsen H, van der Spoel D, van Drunen R: GROMACS: a message-passing parallel molecular dynamics implementation. *Comp Phys Comm* 1995, **91**:43–56.
38. Schuttelkopf AW, Van Aalten DM: PRODRG: a tool for high-throughput crystallography of protein-ligand complexes. *Acta Crystallogr Sect D Biol Crystallogr* 2004, **60**:1355–1363.
39. Thompson JD, Gibson TJ, Plewniak F, Jeanmougin F, Higgins DG: The CLUSTAL_X windows interface: flexible strategies for multiple sequence alignment aided by quality analysis tools. *Nucleic Acids Res* 1997, **25**:4876–4882.
40. Hirayama K, Akashi S, Furuya M, Fukuhara K: Rapid confirmation and revision of the primary structure of bovine serum albumin by ESIMS and Frit-FAB LC/MS. *Biochem Biophys Res Commun* 1990, **14**:639–646.
41. Fasnacht M, Zhu J, Honig B: Local quality assessment in homology models using statistical potentials and support vector machines. *Protein Sci* 2007, **16**:1557–1568.
42. Sakkiah S, Thangapandian S, John S, Lee KW: Identification of critical chemical features for Aurora kinase-B inhibitors using Hip-Hop, virtual screening and molecular docking. *J Mol Struct* 2011, **985**:14–26.

43. Xu Y, Colletier JP, Weik M, Jiang H, Moult J, Silman I, Sussman JL: Flexibility of aromatic residues in the active-site gorge of acetylcholinesterase: X-ray versus molecular dynamics. *Biophys J* 2008, **95**:2500–2511.

44. Wallace AC, Laskowski RA, Thornton JM: L{IGPLOT}: a program to generate schematic diagrams of protein-ligand interactions. *Protein Eng* 1995, **8**:127–134.

45. Hosseinzadeh R, Maleki R, Matin AA: Interaction of diclofenac with bovine serum albumin investigated by diclofenac-selective electrode. *Acta Chim Slov* 2007, **54**:126–130.

46. Hamilton JA1, Era S, Bhamidipati SP, Reed RG: Locations of the three primary binding sites for long-chain fatty acids on bovine serum albumin. *Proc Natl Acad Sci* 1991, **88**:2051–2054.

47. Guex N, Peitsch MC: SWISS-MODEL and the Swiss-Pdb viewer: an environment for comparative protein modeling. *Electrophoresis* 1997, **18**:2714–2723.

4

Improved anticancer delivery of paclitaxel by albumin surface modification of PLGA nanoparticles

Mehdi Esfandyari-Manesh[1,2], Seyed Hossein Mostafavi[2,3,4], Reza Faridi Majidi[4], Mona Noori Koopaei[2], Nazanin Shabani Ravari[1,2], Mohsen Amini[5], Behrad Darvishi[1,4], Seyed Nasser Ostad[6], Fatemeh Atyabi[1,2] and Rassoul Dinarvand[1,2]*

Abstract

Background: Nanoparticles (NPs) play an important role in anticancer delivery systems. Surface modified NPs with hydrophilic polymers such as human serum albumin (HSA) have long half-life in the blood circulation system.

Methods: The method of modified nanoprecipitation was utilized for encapsulation of paclitaxel (PTX) in poly (lactic-co-glycolic acid) (PLGA). Para-maleimide benzoic hydrazide was conjugated to PLGA for the surface modifications of PLGA NPs, and then HSA was attached on the surface of prepared NPs by maleimide attachment to thiol groups (cysteines) of albumin. The application of HSA provides for the longer blood circulation of stealth NPs due to their escape from reticuloendothelial system (RES). Then the physicochemical properties of NPs like surface morphology, size, zeta potential, and in-vitro drug release were analyzed.

Results: The particle size of NPs ranged from 170 to 190 nm and increased about 20–30 nm after HSA conjugation. The zeta potential was about -6 mV and it decreased further after HSA conjugation. The HSA conjugation in prepared NPs was proved by Fourier transform infrared (FT-IR) spectroscopy, faster degradation of HSA in Differential scanning calorimetry (DSC) characterization, and other evidences such as the increasing in size and the decreasing in zeta potential. The PTX released in a biphasic mode for all colloidal suspensions. A sustained release profile for approximately 33 days was detected after a burst effect of the loaded drug. The in vitro cytotoxicity evaluation also indicated that the HSA NPs are more cytotoxic than plain NPs.

Conclusions: HSA decoration of PLGA NPs may be a suitable method for longer blood circulation of NPs.

Keywords: PLGA, Surface modified nanoparticles, Drug delivery, Albumin, Paclitaxel

Background

Different scientists including pharmaceutics, chemists, biologist, and nanotechnologist have been working indefatigably to defeat cancer. A major interest in this area is to improve drug targeting towards tumor cells and decrease the unwilling effects of chemotherapeutics [1-3]. Nanotechnology is very promising in this field and increases the efficacy of targeting by introducing passive and active targeting [4,5].

* Correspondence: dinarvand@tums.ac.ir
[1]Nanotechnology Research Centre, Faculty of Pharmacy, Tehran University of Medical Sciences, Tehran, Iran
[2]Novel Drug Delivery Lab, Department of Pharmaceutics, Faculty of Pharmacy, Tehran University of Medical Sciences, Tehran, Iran
Full list of author information is available at the end of the article

The interest on utilizing NPs formulated from biodegradable and biocompatible polymers such as the most commonly used PLGA are rising rapidly [6]. These NPs are broadly studied as anticancer delivery systems since it has special characteristics such as controlled release and biocompatibility [6].

A new approach to evade the short half-life of the conventional drug and allow targeted delivery to tumor cells is drug targeting achieved by size engineering and surface modification [7,8]. Vasculatures in tumor presents several irregularities in contrast with normal vessels resulting in enhanced permeation and retention (EPR) effect [9,10] and this will cause the nanoparticles with diameters less than 100 nm being selectively taken up by tumor Vasculatures [8,11]. However, the drug bio-distribution profile of the cytotoxic drugs change massively while they are incorporated with NPs, because the modified particles are swiftly opsonised and massively cleared by mono nuclear phagocytes system (MPS) [10-12]. Surface modification of particles with hydrophilic polymers like polyethylene glycol (PEG) and albumin leading to the development of long-circulating and stealth particles for delivery of anticancer drugs [13,14]. Furthermore, the lack of lymph vessels and higher interstitial fluid pressure in the most tumors than normal ones causes inefficient removal of interstitial fluid and soluble macromolecules [15]. Therefore, the NPs mount up in the interstitium which retards their uptake (EPR effect), unless those particles are degraded [16,17].

The HSA coated NPs were prepared in two ways. First, non-covalent interactions where HSA molecules only saturate the surface without any covalent linkage [11] and second, albumin conjugated particles were synthesised via reaction between ξ-amino groups of lysine residues and the protein ligand with aldehyde functional or carboxylic acid [18,19]. The second method is more common.

Accordingly, we have developed a novel strategy that benefit from high efficiency and selectivity of the thiol. In this study we did a site-specific conjugation on the HSA that in spite of the fact that it minimize a loss in biological activity of it but meanwhile decrease immunogenicity. It happens because reagents that specifically react with the thiol group of cysteines, and the number of free cysteines on the surface of a protein is much less [15]. HSA conjugation to surface of NPs was done through the disulphide bonds between the HSA and the paramaleimido benzoic hydrazid (PMBH) derivative of PLGA. The encapsulation efficiency (EE), drug release, and morphology of nanoparticles were then investigated. At last cyto-toxicity of PTX loaded NPs was studied using 3-(4,5-dimethyathiazol-2-yl)-2,5-diphenyltetrazoliumbromide (MTT) assay.

Materials and methods
Materials
PLGA (50:50, M_W: 48000 g/mol) with carboxyl end group and HSA were purchased from Sigma company. N, N'-dicyclohexylcarbodiimide (DCC), N–hydroxysuccinimide (NHS), and 3-(4,5-dimethyathiazol-2-yl)-2,5-diphenyltetrazoliumbromide (MTT) were purchased from Sigma-Aldrich (St. Louis, MO, USA). PMBH, Na_3PO_4, NaH_2PO_4, NaOH, sodium bicarbonate and also NaCl was obtained from Merck. PTX purchased from Cipla Company. Dulbecco's modified eagle's medium (DMEM), penicillin, streptomycin antibiotic mixture and fetal bovine serum (FBS) were obtained from Life technologies (grand Island, NY, USA). Polyvinyl alcohol (PVA) was acquired from Acros (Geel, Belgium). 2-(N-morpholino

ethane sulfonic acid) (MES) was purchased from Fluka (St. Louis, MO, USA). All other solvents and reagents which are not stated were from Merck (Darmstadt, Germany).

Methods
Synthesis of PLGA with functional group of maleimide
Maleimide-functionalized copolymer PLGA was synthesized using the conjugation between paramaleimido benzoic hydrazid (PMBH) and PLGA–COOH. PLGA–COOH (5 g, 0.1 mmol) in 10 ml of methylene chloride was changed to PLGA–NHS with surfeit of N-hydroxysuccinimide (NHS, 135 mg, 1.1 mmol) in the presence of N, N'-dicyclohexylcarbodiimide (230 mg, 1.1 mmol). Then, 0.42 mol PMBH was added to the solution of activated PLGA and the reaction was allowed to proceed overnight on magnetic stirrer. The mixture was evaporated using rotary evaporator and the prepared film of PLGA-PMBH polymer was washed properly using de-ionized water and dried naturally for about two weeks. The synthesized polymer was assessed using H-NMR and FT-IR spectroscopy.

Preparation of PTX-loaded NPs
The method of modified nanoprecipitation was utilized for the preparation of drug encapsulated into particles of PLGA-PMBH [20-22]. In brief, 20 mg of polymer and 1.4 mg of PTX were dissolved in 4 ml of acetone and then injected (rate = 0.5 ml/min) into 16 ml of aqueous phase containing 0.5% PVA as surfactant and emulsified by probe sonication (Misonix, USA) for 5 min with amplitude of 10. Subsequently, the organic solution was evaporated gently on magnetic stirrer (600 rpm) for 9 hours. The NPs were washed and recovered using centrifuge process 25,000 rpm for 30 min (Sigma 3K30, Germany) and then lyophilized at − 40°C for 48 h (Christ Alpha 1–4; Germany). It should be mentioned that during the procedure, Several parameters in NPs preparation such as surfactant concentration, ratio of organic to aqueous, ratio of drug to polymer, and applied external energy witch have critical effects on the eventual size of NPs and drug loading were assessed in this experiment to obtain optimize situation.

HSA conjugation on the surface of PLGA NPs
5 mg of NPs was dispersed in 4 ml of degassed deionized water using bubbling nitrogen. HSA (10 mg/ml) were dissolved in 5 ml of degassed deionized water which have NaCl 0.15 M (pH 6.2–6.5) instantly before injecting it into the suspension. 1 ml of degassed solution contained ethylene diamine tetra acetic acid (EDTA) 4 mM and NaCl 0.3 M (pH 6.2–6.5) then were added to the suspension under the nitrogen pressure. The mixture was put a side overnight for the conjugation to perform

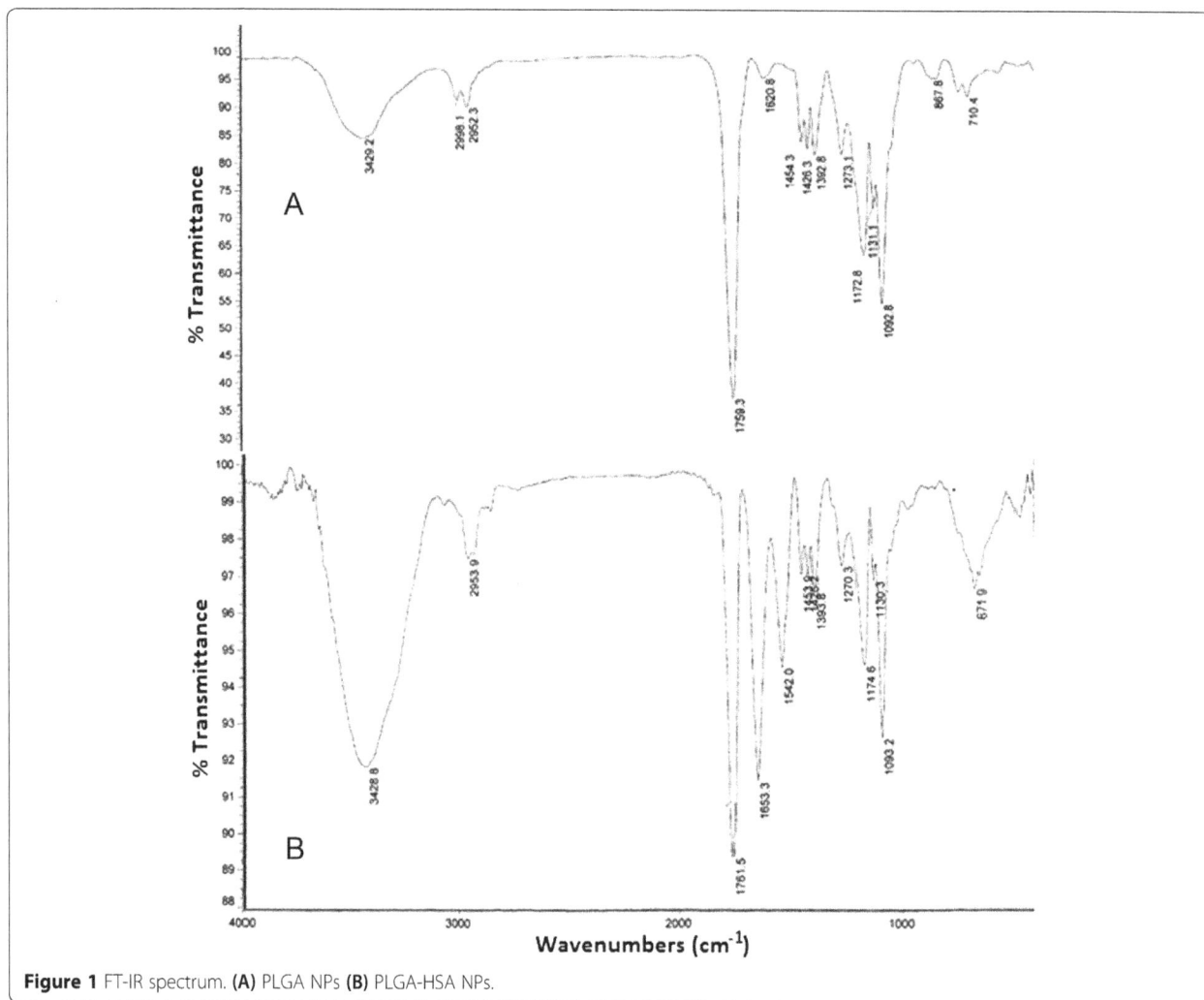

Figure 1 FT-IR spectrum. **(A)** PLGA NPs **(B)** PLGA-HSA NPs.

on the stirrer. The HSA conjugated PLGA NPs was purified and the unreacted HSA was removed using centrifuge (18000 rpm, 30 min, 3 times).

Measurement of size and zeta potential of NPs
Nearly 1 mg of NPs was suspended in 2 ml deionized
water using bath sonicator. Mean size and polydispersity
index (PDI) of NPs were evaluated using dynamic light
scattering (DLS) instrument (Nano ZS, Malvern Instruments, UK). Afterward, samples were placed in an electrophoretic cell and zeta potential was determined.

Surface morphology
Scanning electron microscopy (SEM, Philips XL 30,
Philips, The Netherlands) was used to determine the
shape and surface morphology of the produced NPs.
NPs were coated with gold under vacuum before scan-
ning electron microscopy.

FT-IR analysis
To examine the conjugation was done correctly IR analysis. To perform this procedure we prepared a uniform
mixture of lyophilized PLGA and PLGA-HSA NPs (separately) and KBr.

Differential scanning calorimetry (DSC)
Different ratio of physical mixture of raw materials included
PLGA, HSA, PTX and also PLGA NPs and PLGA-HSA
NPs were weighted equivalently (7 mg) and then sealed in
standard aluminum pans. The experiment carried out using

**Table 1 Particle size, zeta potential, encapsulation, and
loading of NPs before and after conjugation**

NPs	Size (nm)	Zeta (mV)	Encapsulation %	Loading
PLGA	187.0 ± 10.0	-6.7 ± 1.5	80.1 ± 11.0	10.7 ± 2.6
PLGA-HSA	207.0 ± 5.2	-13.6 ± 1.4	75.4 ± 12.0	8.2 ± 1.3

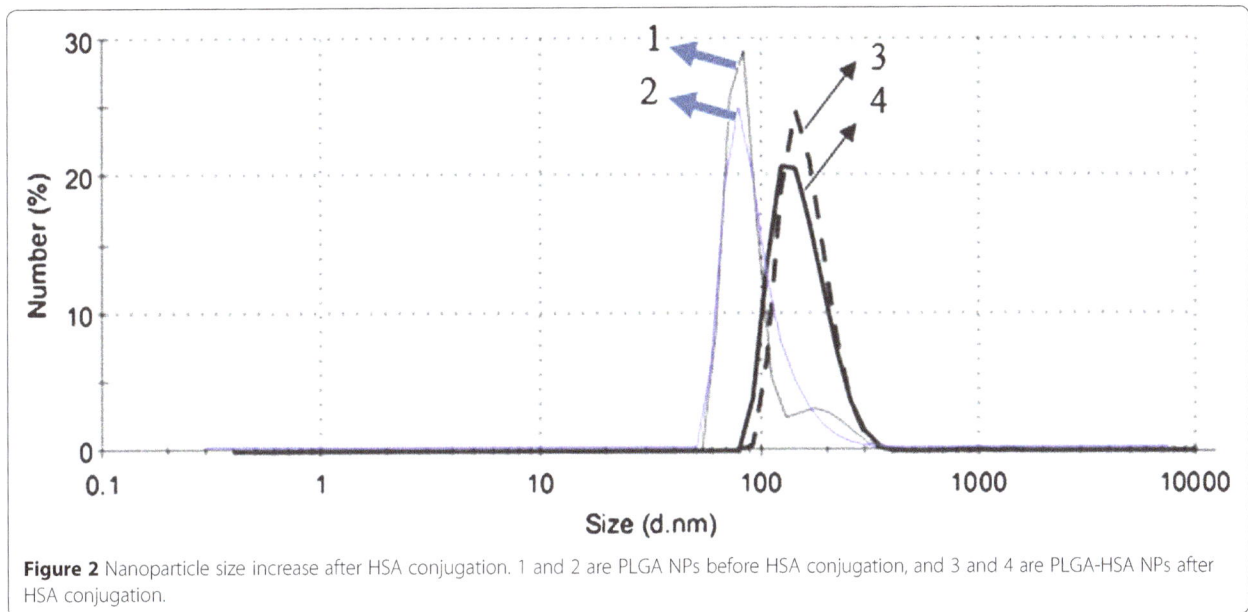

Figure 2 Nanoparticle size increase after HSA conjugation. 1 and 2 are PLGA NPs before HSA conjugation, and 3 and 4 are PLGA-HSA NPs after HSA conjugation.

(Mettler Toledo, GmbH, Switzerland) in ascending mode (10°C min/min) started from 40°C to 600°C.

Drug loading and encapsulation efficiency

To determine the drug loading and encapsulation efficiency, PTX entrapped in the NPs was measured by HPLC (Agilent LC1100, Agilent, Tokyo, Japan) at room temperature. The column was C18 column (25 cm × 0.46 cm internal diameter, pore size 5 µm; Teknokroma, Barcelona, Spain). The mobile phase consisted of aceto-nitrile/water (1/1 v/v). Lyophilized NPs (2.5 mg) were dissolved in acetonitrile (1 ml) (a common solvent for PLGA and drug) and shaken lightly followed by sonication for 6 min. Then, 2 ml of methanol was added to precipitate the polymer. The sample was filtered and drug quantity in filterant was determined by HPLC analysis.

$$Drug\ Loading\ \% = \left(\frac{weight\ of\ drug\ in\ NPs}{weight\ of\ NPs}\right) \times 100$$

$$Encapsulation\ Efficiency\ \% = \left(\frac{weight\ of\ drug\ in\ NPs}{weight\ of\ feed\ NPs}\right) \times 100$$

In vitro drug release

In order to evaluate in vitro release profile of PTX from PLGA and PLGA-HSA NPs, 2.5 mg of lyophilized samples were dispersed in 5 ml phosphate buffer saline solution (PBS, 0.01 M) containing 5% w/v of sodium dodecyl sulphate (SDS) with different pH (5 and 7.4) [21]. Afterward, suspensions poured into dialysis bags (cut off molecular weight 12000 g/mol) and immersed into the 50 ml of PBS with similar pH to the PBS in the bags. Subsequently, beakers placed on a shaker pre-set its temperature on 37°C

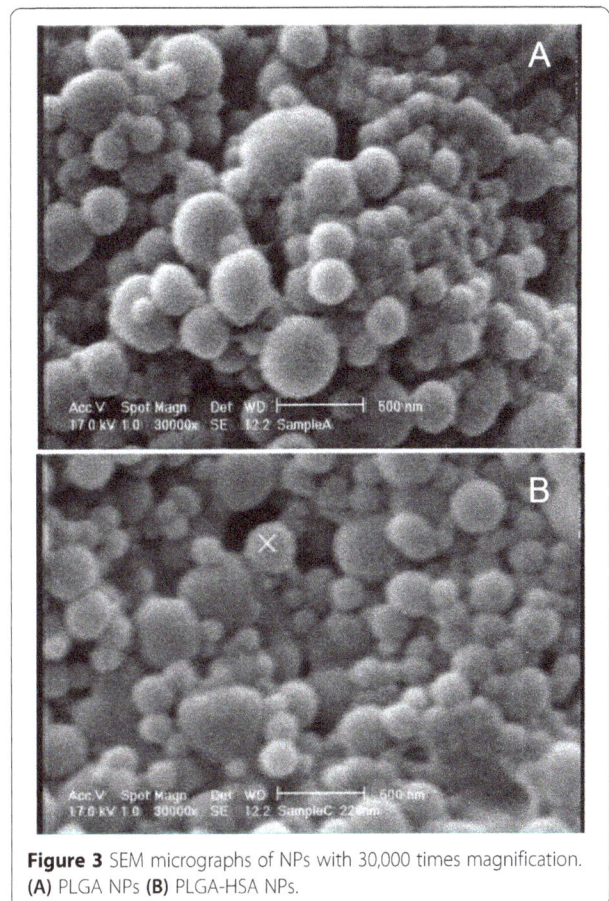

Figure 3 SEM micrographs of NPs with 30,000 times magnification. **(A)** PLGA NPs **(B)** PLGA-HSA NPs.

and 100 cycles per minute for during 33 days because of slow degradation proses of PLGA. For further assessments, all 50 ml of media (PBS) replaced with a same amount of new PBS at predetermined time intervals. The amount of released PTX was determined by HPLC in wavelength of 228 nm.

In vitro cell viability

MTT test was used to study the in vitro cytotoxicity of the subsequent PTX formulations on cell line of T47D: PTX loaded PLGA-HSA NPs, PTX loaded PLGA NPs, free PTX, and unloaded NPs.

T47D cells were seeded at the density of 1×10^4 viable cells/well in 96-well plates (Costar, Chicago, IL) and it is also incubated for 24 hours to providing enough time for cell attachments. Then the formulation (100 µL, 1–200 nM, and 48 h) was used to substitute the medium. A stock solution made in dimethyl sulfoxide (1 mg/ml PTX) for PTX. The concentration of dimethyl sulfoxide kept under 0.5% since at this concentration it has no effect on proliferation of cells and RPMI-1640 culture medium was used as diluents for preparing the working solution of free PTX drug and NPs. 20 µl MTT (5 mg/ml in phosphate-buffered saline) was added at specified periods of time to each well, and after 3 – 4 hours the culture medium containing MTT solution was eliminated. Then, micro plate reader (570 nm)

used to read it after dissolve of formazan crystals in dimethyl sulfoxide (100 µL). At last following equation used to evaluate cell viability:

$$\text{Cell viability } (\%) = (\text{Ints}/\text{Intcontrol}) \times 100$$

In this equation Ints equal to the colorimetric intensity of cells which is incubated with the samples, and Intcontrol is the colorimetric intensity of cells that incubated with the phosphate-buffered saline only as positive control.

Results and discussion
Synthesis of polymer

PLGA functionalized with maleimide group was synthesized and characterized. 1H-NMR and FT-IR analysis was used for confirmation of the primary chemical structure of PMBH–PLGA.

There was overlapping doublets at 1.6 ppm which are a confirmation for the methyl groups of the lactic acid. The multiples peaks at 4.8 ppm and 5.2 ppm correspond to the $-CH_2$ of glycolic acid and -CH of lactic acid, respectively. The high complexity of the peaks at 4.8 ppm and 5.2 ppm resulting from different sequences of glycolic acid and lactic in the backbone of polymer. There are also some detectable proton signals from maleimide and phenyl groups. Peaks which were present the hydrogens of linker are very weak compered to peaks present

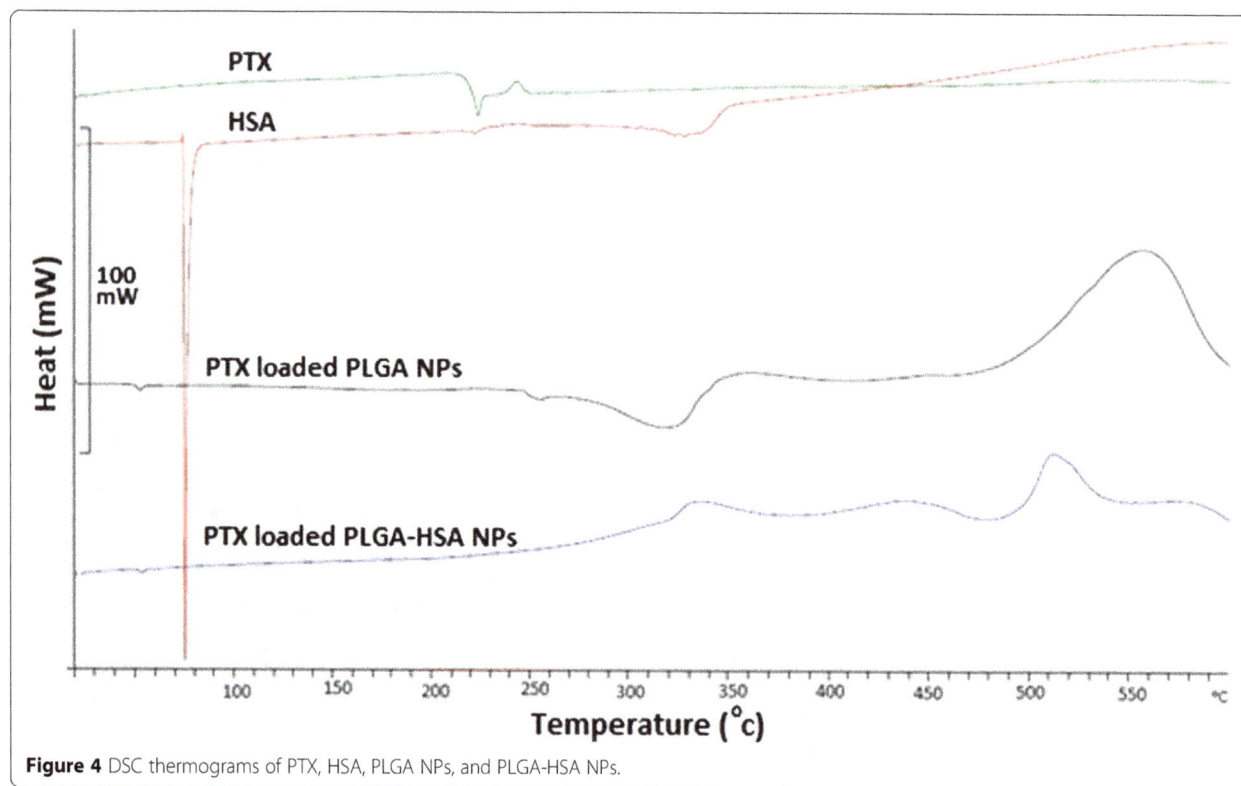

Figure 4 DSC thermograms of PTX, HSA, PLGA NPs, and PLGA-HSA NPs.

PLGA hydrogens because of the small ratio of linker to PLGA. A triplet peak on 7.2- 7.4 can be interoperating as benzoic hydrogens and a small peak found on 6.6 ppm shows the maleimide's hydrogens [22].

Conjugation of PLGA-PMBH was shown by FT-IR assessment (Figure 1). Formation of amide bonds are one of the most important reactions in synthesis of PLGA-PMBH. FTIR spectrum of synthesised polymer verified the amide group formation by some peaks, more specifically; the weak bands at 1620 cm^{-1} were assigned to amide bonds. These results verified the formation of PLGA-PMBH was done successfully.

Nanoparticles characterization

In the current study the modified nanoprecipitation method was chosen for NPs preparation. Several parameters in NPs preparation such as surfactant concentration, ratio of organic to aqueous, ratio of drug to polymer, and applied external energy have crucial effects on the eventual size of NPs and drug loading, so all of these parameters effects were assessed and the optimized formulations were used to prepare NPs to obtain optimized size [23]. Zeta potential, drug loading, and size of NPs were assessed using DLS and HPLC, respectively (Table 1). The evaluation of NPs size by DLS instrument revealed that the mean particle size of NPs was 190 ± 10 nm and when it was conjugated with HSA it increased about 20–30 nm and reached the mean size of 210 ± 10 nm. Theoretically if HSA with axial ratio of 2.66 nm and hydrodynamic radius of 3.7 nm conjugates in high amount around the surface of NPs, it should increase the size of each NPs roughly 19.7 nm and DLS assessment shows the predicted growth in dimension of each NPs (Figure 2). This phenomenon is clearly observed in SEM pictures that are shown in Figure 3. SEM pictures evaluation shows that NPs have spherical shape and mostly have monodispersed size distribution. The nanoparticle's zeta potential assessed by DLS display that PLGA NPs have negative charge (-6 mV) and the zeta potential reaches to -13 mV after HSA conjugation in PLGA-HSA NPs. HSA is also is a negative protein and conjugation will reduce the NPs charge [24].

DSC thermograms of pure PTX, pure HSA, and PTX loaded PLGA NPs and PTX loaded PLGA-HSA NPs demonstrated in Figure 4. In the drug diagram an endothermic peak observed around 220°C and the absence of that in NPs calorimetric curves proposes the lack of crystallinity after NPs preparation; this suggests that during NPs formation polymer hinders crystallization of PTX and the drug exist in the amorphous state. Other verifications, the differences between PLGA NPs and PLGA-HSA NPs peaks show the conjugation of HSA because of the faster degradation of HSA in PLGA-HSA NPs compared to PLGA NPs [25].

HSA conjugation

The infrared spectra of PLGA NPs and PLGA-HSA NPs were recorded by using the KBr pellet method (Figure 1). A very sharp peak at 1650 cm^{-1} in PLGA-HSA NPs that obviously point towards amide bonds existed in amino acids in HSA proved the conjugation take place correctly. FT-IR spectrum, faster degradation of HSA in DSC characterization, increasing the size of NPs, and decreasing the zeta potential are reasons which were proved the conjugation of HSA to PLGA-PMBH.

Drug release profile

In vitro drug release was evaluated in PBS with 2 different pH including 5.5 and 7.4 to assess how the different pH may affect the release profile. Acidic pH was chosen to simulate drug release behavior in the cancer cells. It also was examined before and after conjugation of HSA. In all NPs, 80% of loaded PTX released continuously in a sustained manner during 33 days when assessed in pH of 5.5 and about 70% drug released when experiment was carried out in neutral medium. This phenomena

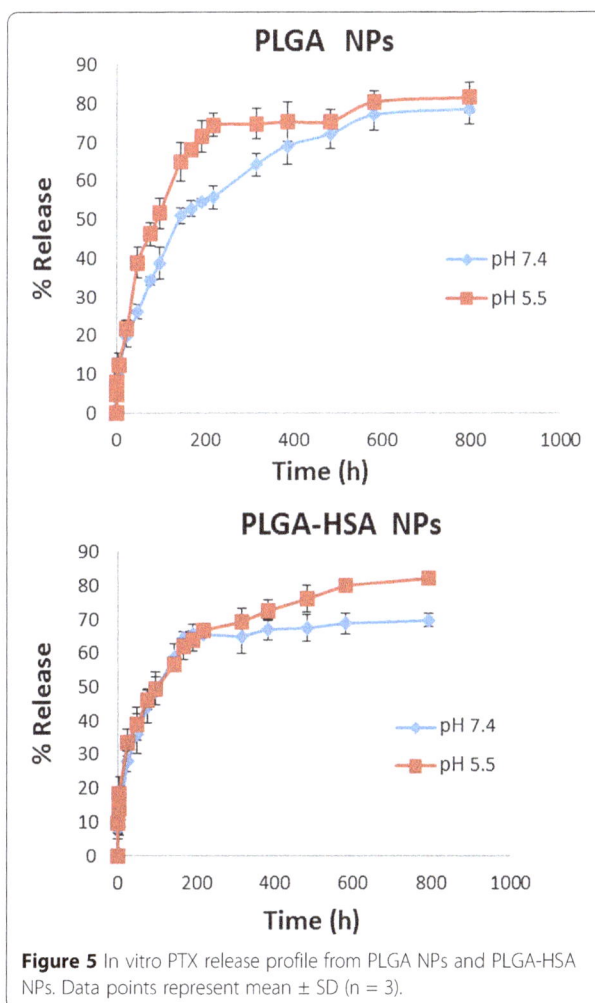

Figure 5 In vitro PTX release profile from PLGA NPs and PLGA-HSA NPs. Data points represent mean ± SD (n = 3).

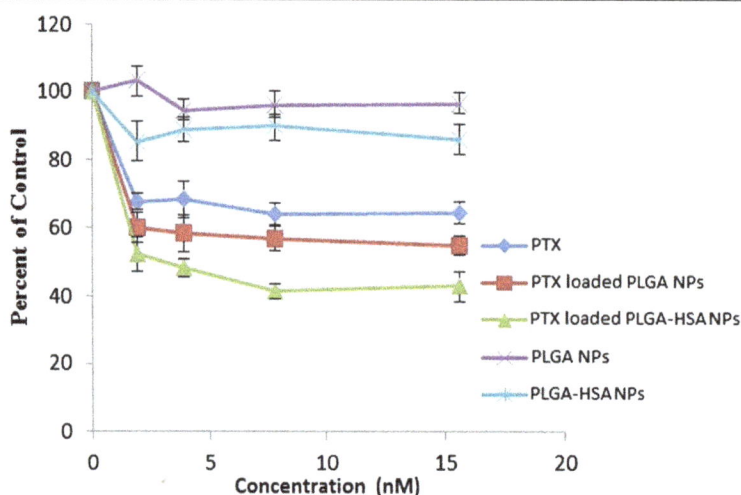

Figure 6 The in vitro cytotoxicity of free PTX, PTX loaded PLGA NPs, and PTX loaded PLGA-HSA NPs with different amount of PTX on T47D breast cancer cells. Data points represent mean ± SD (n = 3).

shows that drug disperse uniformly inside particles and it comes out of it by diffusion. Figure 5 shows that the drug release in acidic environment is faster than neutral ones for all NPs. Hence, this carrier can release drug faster in acidic surroundings of tumors. Acidic pH enhances hydrolization of ester linkage in PLGA and help encapsulated drug to release in control and sustain manner [24-27].

In vitro cytotoxicity

Figure 6 shows the in vitro cytotoxicity of free PTX, PTX loaded PLGA NPs, and PTX loaded PLGA-HSA NPs with different amount of PTX on breast cancer cells (T47D). Figure 6 illustrate that the cytotoxicity of PTX loaded PLGA-HSA NPs was significantly higher than the free PTX and PTX loaded PLGA NPs. Moreover, PTX loaded PLGA NPs have significantly more cytotoxic effect than free PTX. The percent viability of free PTX, PTX loaded PLGA NPs, and PTX loaded PLGA-HSA NPs were 64%, 54%, and 43% in 15 nM concentration, respectively. The enhancement of antitumor activity of PLGA-HSA NPs may be caused by gp60 (albondin) receptor and caveolar transport which both help these particles to increased transendothelial cell transportation of HSA [23,24]. First, HSA molecules bind to gp60 receptors and this binding activates caveolin. After caveolin configuration, HSA and other plasma constituents transfer transversely the endothelial cell to the interstitial space. Improved intratumor delivery of PTX may also other reason for the increased antitumor activity of PLGA-HSA NPs. Activated gp60 receptors which are specific for HSA help transportation of this molecule into tumor tissues by bypassing blood vessel wall barriers [25]. Unloaded NPs tested to evaluate the effect of polymerization and conjugation on cell viability

and statistical analysis proved that these parameters do not affect cell viability.

Conclusions

Preparation of the PTX loaded PLGA NPs were done by modified nanoprecipitation method. The hydrophobic PLGA NPs were decorated by hydrophilic HSA as novel anticancer delivery system. The PMBH was used as linker for the conjugation of HSA on the surface of PLGA NPs. The drug loading and encapsulation efficiency were 13% and 80%, respectively. Our results demonstrated that by using PMBH as linker and this method of nanoprecipitation, HSA conjugated NPs would be obtained with desired size, morphological, and drug loading properties. The in vitro cytotoxicity also showed that the HSA decorated NPs are more cytotoxic when compared with plain NPs and free anticancer agent, so these NPs can be used successfully in drug delivery of anticancer agents.

Competing interests
The authors declare that they have no competing interests.

Authors' contributions
MEM conceived the study and drafted the manuscript. SHM carried out the experiments and assisted in preparation of the manuscript. RFM and MNK supervised the synthesis and characterization of nanoparticles. NSR reviewed and revised the manuscript, MA supervised the synthesis and characterization of nanoparticles, BD helped with the characterization tests. SNO supervised the cell culture study, FA co-supervised the study, and RD supervised and coordinated the study and is the corresponding author of the manuscript. All authors read and approved the final manuscript.

Authors' information
Mehdi Esfandyari-Manesh and Seyed Hossein Mostafavi are considered as first author with equal responsibility and rights.

Author details
[1]Nanotechnology Research Centre, Faculty of Pharmacy, Tehran University of Medical Sciences, Tehran, Iran. [2]Novel Drug Delivery Lab, Department of Pharmaceutics, Faculty of Pharmacy, Tehran University of Medical Sciences,

Tehran, Iran. [3]Department of Bioengineering, University of California, Riverside, CA, USA. [4]Medical Nanotechnology Department, School of Advanced Technologies in Medicine, Tehran University of Medical Sciences, Tehran, Iran. [5]Department of Medicinal Chemistry, Faculty of Pharmacy, Tehran University of Medical Sciences, Tehran, Iran. [6]Department of Toxicology and Pharmacology, Faculty of Pharmacy, Tehran University of Medical Science, Tehran, Iran.

References

1. Soppimath KS, Aminabhavi TM, Kulkarni AR, Rudzinski WE. Biodegradable polymeric nanoparticles as drug delivery devices. J Control Release. 2001;70:1–20.
2. Langer R. Drug delivery and targeting. Nature. 1998;392:5–10.
3. Koopaei MN, Khoshayand MR, Mostafavi SH, Amini M, Khorramizadeh MR, Jeddi Tehrani M, et al. Docetaxel loaded PEG-PLGA nanoparticles: optimized drug loading, in-vitro Cytotoxicity and in-vivo Antitumor Effect. Iran J Pharm Res. 2014;13:819–33.
4. Koo OM, Rubinstein I, Onyuksel H. Role of nanotechnology in targeted drug delivery and imaging: a concise review. Nanomed Nanotechnol, Biol Med. 2005;1:193–212.
5. Koopaei MN, Maghazei MS, Mostafavi SH, Jamalifar H, Samadi N, Amini M, et al. Enhanced antibacterial activity of roxithromycin loaded pegylated poly lactide-co-glycolide nanoparticles. Daru. 2012;20:92–9.
6. Sourabhan S, Kaladhar K, Chandra PS. Method to enhance the encapsulation of biologically active molecules in PLGA nanoparticles. Trends Biomater Artif Organs. 2009;22:211–5.
7. Mostafavi SH, Aghajani M, Amani A, Darvishi B, Noori Koopaei M, Pashazadeh AM, et al. Optimization of paclitaxel-loaded poly (D, l-lactide-co-glycolide-N-p-maleimido benzoic hydrazide) nanoparticles size using artificial neural networks. Pharm Dev Technol. 2014;1:1–9.
8. Danhier F, Feron O, Preat V. To exploit the tumor microenvironment: passive and active tumor targeting of nanocarriers for anti-cancer drug delivery. J Control Release. 2012;148:135–46.
9. Park K. Questions on the role of the EPR effect in tumor targeting. J Control Release. 2013;172:391.
10. Fang J, Sawa T, Maeda H. Factors and mechanism of "EPR" effect and the enhanced antitumor effects of macromolecular drugs including SMANCS. Adv Exp Med Biol. 2003;519:29–49.
11. Maeda H, Sawa T, Konno T. Mechanism of tumor-targeted delivery of macromolecular drugs, including the EPR effect in solid tumor and clinical overview of the prototype polymeric drug SMANCS. J Control Release. 2001;74:47–61.
12. Hirsjarvi S, Passirani C, Benoit JP. Passive and active tumour targeting with nanocarriers. Curr Drug Discov Technol. 2011;8:188–96.
13. Okamura Y, Fujie T, Maruyama H, Handa M, Ikeda Y, Takeoka S. Prolonged hemostatic ability of polyethylene glycol-modified polymerized albumin particles carrying fibrinogen gamma-chain dodecapeptide. Transfusion. 2007;47:1254–62.
14. Moghimi SM, Hunter AC, Murray JC. Long-circulating and target-specific nanoparticles: theory to practice. Pharmacol Rev. 2001;53:283–318.
15. He X, Ma J, Mercado AE, Xu W, Jabbari E. Cytotoxicity of Paclitaxel in biodegradable self-assembled core-shell poly (lactide-co-glycolide ethylene oxide fumarate) nanoparticles. Pharm Res. 2008;25:1552–62.
16. Marcucci F, Lefoulon FO. Active targeting with particulate drug carriers in tumor therapy: fundamentals and recent progress. Drug Discov Today. 2004;9:219–28.
17. Stylianopoulos T. EPR-effect: utilizing size-dependent nanoparticle delivery to solid tumors. Ther Deliv. 2013;4:421–3.
18. Manjappa AS, Chaudhari KR, Venkataraju MP, Dantuluri P, Nanda B, Sidda C, et al. Antibody derivatization and conjugation strategies: application in preparation of stealth immunoliposome to target chemotherapeutics to tumor. J Control Release. 2010;150:2–22.
19. Weber C, Reiss S, Langer K. Preparation of surface modified protein nanoparticles by introduction of sulfhydryl groups. Int J Pharm. 2000;211:67–78.
20. Fonseca C, Simões S, Gaspar R. Paclitaxel-loaded PLGA nanoparticles: preparation, physicochemical characterization and in vitro anti-tumoral activity. J Control Release. 2002;83:273–86.
21. Wang YM, Sato H, Adachi I, Horikoshi I. Preparation and characterization of poly (lactic-co-glycolic acid) microspheres for targeted delivery of a novel anticancer agent, Taxol. Chem Pharm Bull. 1996;44:1935–40.
22. Fessi H, Puisieux F, Devissaguet JP, Ammoury N, Benita S. Nanocapsule formation by interfacial polymer deposition following solvent displacement. Int J Pharm. 1989;55:R1–4.
23. Liu J, Meisner D, Kwong E, Wu XY, Johnston MR. A novel trans-lymphatic drug delivery system: Implantable gelatin sponge impregnated with PLGA "paclitaxel microspheres. Biomaterials. 2007;28:3236–44.
24. Tessmar J, Mikos A, Gopferich A. The use of poly (ethylene glycol)-block-poly (lactic acid) derived copolymers for the rapid creation of biomimetic surfaces. Biomaterials. 2003;24:4475–86.
25. Manchanda R, Fernandez-Fernandez A, Nagesetti A, McGoron AJ. Preparation and characterization of a polymeric (PLGA) nanoparticulate drug delivery system with simultaneous incorporation of chemotherapeutic and thermo-optical agents. Colloids Surf B: Biointerfaces. 2009;75:260–7.
26. Musumeci T, Ventura CA, Giannone I, Ruozi B, Montenegro L, Pignatello R, et al. PLA/PLGA nanoparticles for sustained release of docetaxel. Int J Pharm. 2006;325:172–9.
27. Gindy ME, Ji S, Hoye TR, Panagiotopoulos AZ, Prud'homme RK. Preparation of poly (ethylene glycol) protected nanoparticles with variable bioconjugate ligand density. Biomacromolecules. 2008;9:2705–11.

5

Women-only drug treatment services and needs in Iran

Zahra Alam-mehrjerdi[1], Reza Daneshmand[2*], Mercedeh Samiei[3], Roya Samadi[4], Mohammad Abdollahi[5] and Kate Dolan[1]

Abstract

Background: Iran (Persia) has a women-only drug treatment system. However, literature is not documented. The current study aimed to review the development of women-only drug treatment and harm reduction services (WODTHRS) and the factors associated with treatment entry and outcomes in Iran. The review was based on a comprehensive search for all literature focusing on WODTHRS in Iran.

Methods: Data were collected by conducting systematic searching of scientific English and Persian databases and grey literature. This was done in line with Cochrane Guideline for conducting systematic reviews. Overall, 19,929 studies were found. But, only 19 original studies were included after excluding non-relevant studies.

Results: The review findings indicate how WODTHRS have been developed in the past 15 years. The review findings underscore the roles of numerous factors in treatment entry such as the side effects of illicit drug use. In addition, cognitive-behavioral interventions, methadone treatment and some factors outside drug treatment such as family support increase positive treatment outcomes among women.
In contrast, financial problems as well as other factors such as insufficient medical, psychiatric and social work services hamper treatment entry and positive treatment outcomes.

Conclusions: The review results highlight that eliminating barriers to treatment entry and positive treatment outcomes should be addressed. Conducting randomized controlled trials is needed to evaluate the effectiveness of WODTHRS. This issue should address the factors influencing service utilization to incorporate the best practice for women. The evaluation of the long-term efficacy of WODTHRS is a critical research gap which should be addressed in future studies.

Keywords: Women, Iran, Drug, Methadone, Persian Gulf

Background

The origins of illicit drug use

Smoking opium has a long history in Iran which dates back hundreds of years before the tribal Arab invasion to Iran. At the time of Zoroaster, the Persian prophet, the use of some plants with euphoric effects was the main part of religious ceremonies among the Persians.

Persian physicians such as Zakariya-al-Razi and Avicenna were among the first scientists who used opium for surgery. Iran has remained a transit and consumer country for opiates because of Afghanistan, the main opium producer through the centuries [1].

The current prevalence of illicit drug use

The total number of regular and recreational substance users is estimated to be between four and seven million [1]. It is estimated that 1,200,000-2,000,000 people are dependent on illicit drugs mainly inexpensive Afghan opium, heroin and/or methamphetamine [1, 2]. The main route of drug use is smoking [1, 2]. Other main types of illicit drugs include opium residues, hashish, tramadol and prescription opioids [1, 3, 4].

* Correspondence: prof.reza.daneshmand@gmail.com; re.daneshmand@uswr.ac.ir
[2]Substance Abuse and Dependence Research Center, University of Social Welfare and Rehabilitation Sciences, Tehran, Iran
Full list of author information is available at the end of the article

Illicit drug use among women

According to the Ministry of Health and Medical Education (MoHME), almost ten percent of drug-dependents are women [5]. MoHME (2014) reported that there was one drug-using woman per eight drug-using men in the country. According to the report, illicit drug use is a health concern among some women [5].

In general, women are opiate smokers or poly-smokers of opiates and methamphetamine. But drug injection among women is rare because of stigma [6–10]. In addition, women with illicit drug use problem have poorer education and employment than men [11]. Women initiate illicit drug use later than men or are raised in poor environments with drug use problem [12].

Study objectives

The provision of a drug response has been addressed for women in Iran [11, 13–15]. But, there is no previous systematic review of how women-only drug treatment and harm reduction services (WODTHRS) have been developed. Furthermore, the motivations and barriers associated with facilitating or hampering treatment entry and positive treatment outcomes among this group have not been documented. The current review aimed to address this gap in literature.

Methods

Searching procedure

The review procedure was prepared in compliance with Cochrane Guideline for conducting systematic reviews [16]. Data regarding the evidence of WODTHRS and the associated motivations and barriers were collected through a systematic literature search.

To be included in the review, years 1980–2015 were selected for searching because of a paucity of studies of illicit drug use before 1980. Studies were included if they emphasized drug treatment and/or harm reduction services for women only and their motivations and barriers for treatment. The term "motivations" refers to reasons that women report specialized for using drug treatment and/or harms reduction services. The term "barriers" refers to reasons that women do not report specialized for using drug treatment and/or harm reduction services. Studies were excluded if they were not women-only research studies.

Medical Subject Headings (MeSH) of 'women-only drug services' and 'women-only harm reduction services' were employed. MeSH subtitle headings were 'Iran', 'development', 'treatment entry', and 'treatment outcomes'. Keywords added to the search parameters were 'motivations', 'barriers', 'utilization', and 'access'. Searches in Google Scholar employed the phrases 'drug treatment in Iran', 'harm reduction in Iran', 'women-only

drug treatment services in Iran', and 'access to drug treatment and harm reduction for women in Iran'.

Based on the Guideline, English publications were retrieved through searching Web of Sciences, Medline, EMBASE, PubMed citation indexes, CINHAL, Scopus and Google Scholar. In addition, scientific Persian databases including Scientific Information Database, Magiran, Iran Medex and the website of the conference papers of Iran were searched.

Based on the Guideline, part of the searching included grey literature. This included the regional reports of the United Nations Office on Drugs and Crime, the conference abstract books of Harm Reduction Association, the National Institute on Drug Abuse and the College on Problems of Drug Dependence. The reports of MoHME and the Persian Welfare Organization were also searched.

Search findings

Systematic searching resulted in finding 19,929 English and Persian articles, reports and conference papers. Overall, 19 relevant studies were included. Most of the studies were related to English papers indexed in Pub Med or grey literature. Seven studies were related to the development of WODTHRS. Overall, 12 studies were related to treatment motivations and barriers. Duplicates such as editorials were excluded from the final searching (See Fig. 1).

Results

The development of drug treatment services

Gender-mixed drug treatment clinics were established for the first time between 1974 and 1977 that provided methadone treatment. Over the same time, 30,000 heroin and opium-dependents were on methadone program. But, because of Islamic views, illicit drug use was considered as a criminal activity between 1979 and 2000. Therefore, methadone treatment was not provided [1, 17, 18].

The western health policy of drug treatment was re-approved by the government in 2000 [1]. This was the result of considering illicit drug use as a health concern and the collaboration of the medical sector with the government. According to a recent MoHME report, more than 500,000 clients have received medication-assisted treatment (MAT) programs at 3,373 drug treatment centers [13].

The development of women-only services

According to a recent report from the Welfare Organization, almost ten percent of people seeking treatment at drug treatment centers are women [19]. Women' needs for drug treatment motivated some health policy makers to approve women-only drug services in the community [19].

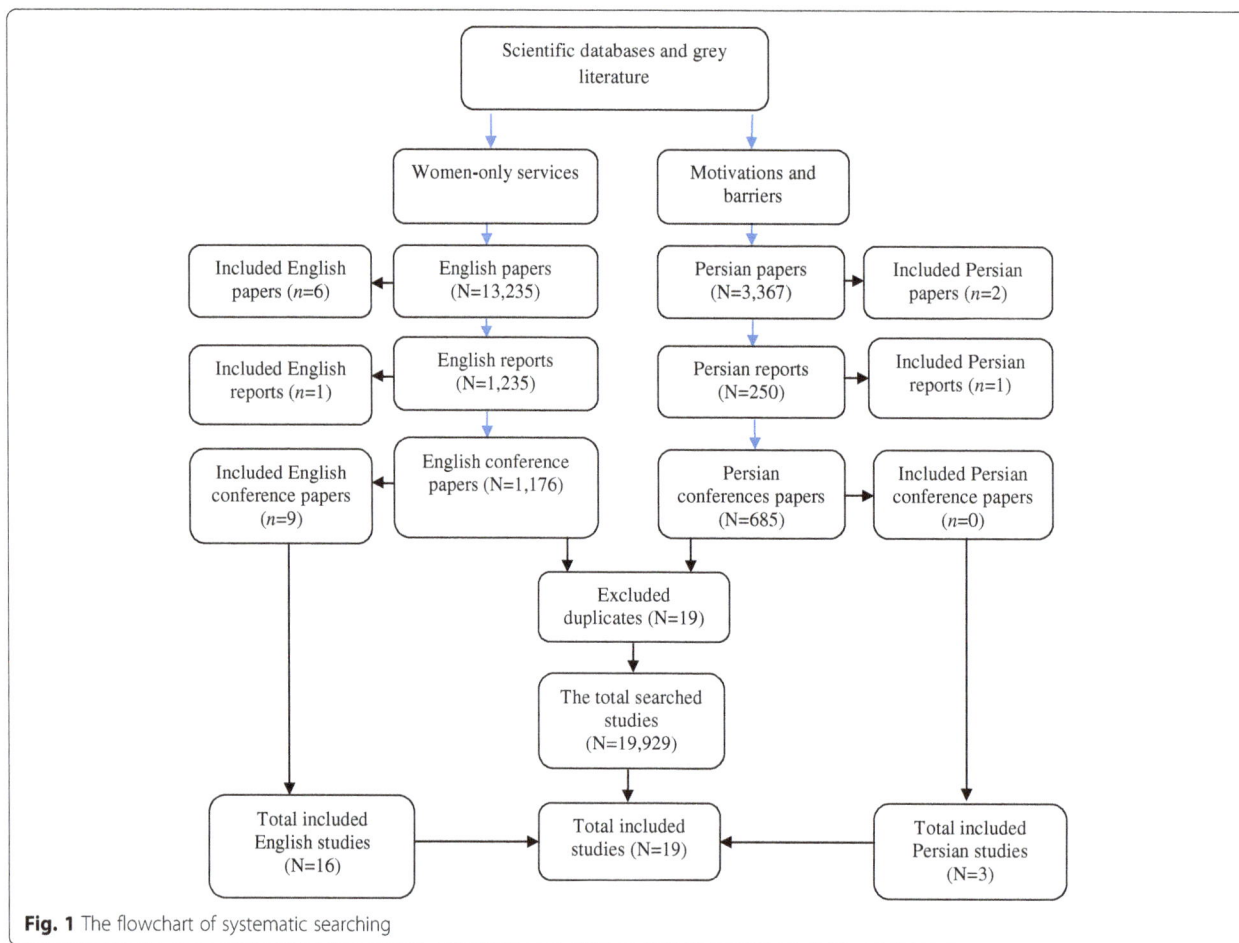

Fig. 1 The flowchart of systematic searching

The presence of some at-risk women in the community was also a motivation to approve WODTHRS. Stigma was another motivation to develop such services. A survey at eight main methadone clinics in Tehran found that only four percent of the clients were women [20]. Some women reported unwillingness to seek professional help at methadone treatment centers because of social stigma [20].

The idea of developing WODTHRS was initiated in Shiraz city near the Persian Gulf in 2001. This issue was supported by the Welfare Organization and the government [5]. The first women-only residential center was established by Rebirth Society (NGO) in the same city in 2002. The treatment program included 12-step meetings and a faith-based intervention. Over the same time period, "Chitgar" therapeutic community center was established by Rebirth Society in Tehran to admit women from all-over Iran [1].

In addition, "Khaneye khorshid" drop in center was established in Tehran in 2006. The center provides methadone maintenance treatment and free harm reduction services for women [1]. The first women-only

methadone clinic (i.e., Persepolis clinic) was established in Tehran in 2007 [8]. Two studies at the same clinic found that only 20 % of the women reported lifetime drug treatment [9] and they needed methadone treatment [10].

Over the same time, some women especially in low socio-economic areas reported opiate dependence. This issue necessitated more opiate treatment. Therefore, some women-only therapeutic community and MAT programs were developed throughout the country after 2007 [11–13, 21],

Illicit drug use also led to engagements with high risk behaviors among some women which necessitated a specific response. Therefore, harm reduction services have been provided for at-risk women at women-only centers since 2007. Some of these centers include Atabak, Parniyan, Nader, Navid-e-Hamrazi-e-Iranians and Mikhak clinics in Tehran and other cities. The services have been based on the simultaneous provision of drug treatment and harm reduction programs [5].

The success of these centers in admitting women and the provision of WODTHRS encouraged some health

Table 1 Provided services at the centers

Clients	Harm reduction		STI[a] management		Counseling		Referral for VCT[b]	
	n	%	n	%	n	%	n	%
Spouses of IDUs[c]	50.9	21.7	21	4.2	52	2.4	21	4.4
Spouses of prisoners	51	2.2	57	11.5	154	7.2	66	13.7
Spouses with high risk sex	10	0.4	19	3.8	394	15.8	333	6.8
Spouses of NIDUs[d]	52	2.2	55	11.1	149	7.0	55	11.4
IDUs	1366	58.1	51	10.3	130	6.1	61	12.7
NIDUs	201	8.5	142	28.6	245	11.5	120	24.9
Clients with high risk sex	134	5.7	123	24.8	948	44.6	83	17.2
Clients with recent imprisonment problem	28	1.2	28	5.6	54	2.5	43	8.9

Reference: Fahimfar et al. (2013) [14]
[a]Sexually transmitted infections
[b]Voluntary counseling and testing
[c]Injecting drug users
[d]Non-injecting drug users

policy makers to develop similar centers. Therefore, a center for at-risk women was established in Shiraz and Esfahan near the Persian Gulf of Iran in 2007. A study found that most of the women at the center were smokers of opiates. Women needed regular visits by infectious diseases specialists and methadone treatment. Women needed other treatment services such as an increase in the duration of receiving women-only services [21].

Furthermore, the government attempted to provide more free services for at-risk women. Therefore, five women-only harm reduction centers were established in five provinces between 2007 and 2008. Specific groups of women such as female injecting drug users were admitted at the centers [14] (See Table 1).

A survey found that 442 women were admitted at the centers by March 2008. Overall, 27.1 % of them reported high risk sexual behaviors. Overall, 11.3 % of them were injecting drug users. Methadone maintenance treatment, harm reduction programs such as HIV education and condom promotion were the most provided services. Overall, more than 5,000 drug treatment and harm reduction services were provided for the clients [14] (See Fig. 2).

There were 29 registered women-only centers in the main cities by the end of April 2014. More than 6,000 women were voluntarily admitted at the centers between 2007 and 2014. A national survey found that 2,100 women were admitted at least once at the centers to receive free WODTHRS by the end of April 2014 [14, 15].

Approximately, 45 % of women were maintained on methadone program. Counselling sessions were provided for all women. In addition, outreach teams distributed 22,000 condoms and 7,500 syringes among 3,500 at-risk women in the community. Overall, 1,762

syringes, 38,000 male condoms and 2,500 female condoms were distributed among women and their partners [14] (See Table 2).

Motivation for treatment entry and positive treatment outcomes

Drug treatment entry and positive treatment outcomes may be increased by specific motivations among women. In contrast, low rates of drug treatment entry and positive treatment outcomes may emphasize specific barriers among women. Recent women-only studies in Iran found that the encouragement of others, an individual need to take methadone and poor satisfaction with some drug treatments were strong motivations for treatment entry [7].

A study found that the side effects of drug use, anxiety, depression and familial problems [22] were strong motivations for treatment entry. Two studies found that adequate methadone dose, as well as psychological services, drug education [23], motivational interviewing and life skills training [24] facilitated positive treatment

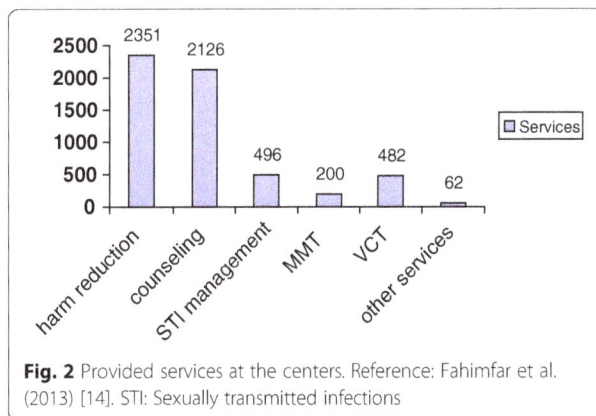

Fig. 2 Provided services at the centers. Reference: Fahimfar et al. (2013) [14]. STI: Sexually transmitted infections

Table 2 Studies related to the development of women-only services, drug treatment entry and outcomes

Study citation	Year	Sample	Study site	Main drugs	Study outcomes
Ministry of Health and Medical Education. 2014 [5]	2007–2014	All women (i.e., 10 % of illicit drug users)	Main cities	Any type of illicit drug especially opiates	Women-only residential centers and drop in centers such as Chitgar center and Khaneye khorshid were established for female drug users and at-risk women such as female sex workers and female injecting drug users.
Dolan et al. 2011a [8]	2007	78	The first women-only methadone clinic, Tehran	Opiates and poly use of opiates and methamphetamine	The first methadone clinic was established for women.
Dolan et al. 2011b [9]	2007–2008	78	The first women-only methadone clinic, Tehran	Opiates and poly use of opiates and methamphetamine	Only 20 % of women reported lifetime drug treatment. Women reported poor social functioning, depression, poor general health and stigma.
Dolan et al. 2012 [10]	2007–2008	78	The first women-only methadone clinic, Tehran	Opiates and poly use of opiates and methamphetamine	Women who had attended the clinic between 2007 and 2008 were followed in 2009–2010. Of the 78 women recruited, 40 women were followed seven months later. There was a significant reduction in heroin use at follow-up. Women needed continued methadone treatment.
Radfar. 2013 [21]	2007	15	The first two centers for health promotion among at-risk women, Shiraz and Esfahan, The Persian Gulf region	Opiates and poly use of opiates and methamphetamine	Women needed women-only medical, psychiatric, social and psychological services for drug treatment.
Fahimfar et al. 2013 -[14]	2007–2008	442	The first five harm reduction centers, five provinces	Opiates and poly use of opiates and methamphetamine	Women received drug treatment and harm reduction services at the centers.
Fahimfar et al. 2014 [15]	2007–2014	6,000	Five provinces	Opiates and poly use of opiates and methamphetamine	Women received free drug treatment and harm reduction services such as methadone, sterile syringes and condoms.
					Treatment motivations
Babakhanian et al. 2013 [7]	2010	69	Sixteen methadone clinics, Tehran	Opiates	Receiving information from informant sources in the community such as mass-media, treatment success of relatives and friends, the encouragement of healthy family members, the need for keeping family and children, an individual need to take methadone to relieve the side effects of opiate use and poor satisfaction with other drug treatments such as therapeutic community program increased treatment entry.
Ahmadan-Panah et al. 2014 [22]	2012	59	Ten drug treatment centers, Hamadan, western Iran	Opiates, illicit methadone and hashish	Drug withdrawal, depression, anxiety, familial problems and headaches increased treatment entry.
Alam-mehrjerdi et al. 2013b [23]	2008–2009	62	Ten methadone clinics, Tehran	Opiates	Adequate methadone dose to substitute with opiate use, counseling sessions, group therapy, individual psychological sessions, family therapy and drug education on methadone program increased positive treatment outcomes such as treatment retention, relapse prevention and the improvement of general health.
Ghasemi-Arganeh et al. 2014 [24]	2012	32	A women-only therapeutic community center, Isfahan	Opiates	Group motivational interviewing and life skills training increased positive treatment outcomes including the reduction of drug relapse, anxiety, depression and increased mental health.
Daneshmand et al. 2014a [25]	2011–2012	500	Chitgar women-only therapeutic community center, Tehran	Methamphetamine	Family support, employment, counseling and psychological services, having an ongoing program for daily activities, learning motivations to change, strategies to cope with craving, dealing with lapse, refusal skills and relapse prevention increased treatment

Table 2 Studies related to the development of women-only services, drug treatment entry and outcomes *(Continued)*

					outcomes including the improvement of general health and the provision of drug-free urine specimens.
Tafaoli-Masooleh. 2010 [26]	2009	70	Chitgar women-only therapeutic community center, Tehran	Methamphetamine	Cognitive-behavioral therapy (CBT) increased treatment outcomes including treatment retention and the provision of drug-free urine specimens in treatment.
Dehghani-Firooz-Abadi et al. 2013 [27]	2012	30	Ayandenh- Roshan women-only therapeutic community center, Esfahan	Opiates	CBT increased positive treatment outcomes including the provision of drug-free urine specimens and the improvement of general health.
Hadadi et al. 2014 [28]	2013	43	Four drug treatment centers and clinics, Tehran	Methamphetamine	The Matrix Model of Intensive Outpatient Treatment (CBT) increased positive treatment outcomes including treatment retention, the provision of drug-free urine specimens and the improvement of general health and psychiatric comorbidities (i.e., depression and anxiety). Treatment barriers
Ebrahimi et al. 2014 [29]	2012	409	Eight districts, Esfahan, central Iran	Opium	Poor treatment motivations, insufficient information and misconceptions about drug use treatment were strong barriers to treatment entry.
Shaditalab et al. 2014 [30]	2011	48	Khaneye Khorshid women drop in center, Chitgar and Congress 60 [1] centers, Tehran	Poly use of opiates and methamphetamine	Unemployment, low income, unstable accommodation and poor vocational training, poor physical and psychological health and poor education were barriers to achieving positive treatment outcomes. Service providers emphasized the necessity of providing social and financial supports and health insurance for increasing positive treatment outcomes such as relapse prevention.
Rahimi-Movaghar et al. 2011 [31]	2011	62	Chitgar center and Khaneye khorshid center, Tehran	Opiates and poly use of opiates and methamphetamine	Social stigma, poor family acceptance and low economic status were barriers to achieving treatment retention. Insufficient numbers of female medical doctors and a paucity of health counseling and educational services, living in drug-using environments and inadequate medical and social work services were barriers to achieving positive treatment outcomes such as treatment retention, relapse prevention and reduced psychiatric comorbidities.
Daneshmand et al. 2014b [32]	2010–2011	150	A central women-only drop in center, Tehran	Poly use of opiates and methamphetamine	Long duration of poly use of opiates and methamphetamine, poor family support, poor motivations to change methamphetamine use, poor participation in psychological and counseling sessions, depression, an inability to cope with everyday life pressures and inadequate skills to cope with methamphetamine craving and relapse were barriers to achieving positive treatment outcomes such as treatment compliance and the improved general health.

[1]Congress 60: a chain non-governmental organization that officially provides drug treatment and harm reduction services

outcomes. One study found that positive treatment outcomes were increased by having family support, employment and a program for daily activities [25]. Furthermore, three studies found that cognitive-behavioral interventions increased positive treatment outcomes [26–28] (See Table 2).

Barriers to treatment entry and positive treatment outcomes

Women with poor treatment motivations or misinformation about drug treatment experience barriers to treatment entry and positive outcomes during treatment [29]. Only one study found that poor treatment motivation and lack of sufficient information about drug use were barriers to treatment entry [29]. Three studies found that financial problems as well as other factors such as insufficient women-only services were barriers to achieving positive treatment outcomes [30–32] (See Table 2).

Discussion

Studies in western countries show that relatively low proportions of women enter drug treatment and harm reduction centers [33, 34]. WODTHRS create a unique environment that focuses on women's issues and provides a comfortable setting in which women can discuss sensitive issues such as sex work and drug injection. Such services support women because drug treatment and harm reduction services traditionally tend to target men' needs [35, 36].

Studies of women and drug treatment have remained undeveloped in the region that Iran has been situated [37–40]. However, Iran has initiated research on women and drug use in recent decades [41]. It should be noted that the recent development of WODTHRS in Iran is not because of the segregation of women from men [14, 15]. WODTHRS in Iran aim to address women-only needs for drug treatment [14, 15].

Gender may not be solely the predictor of treatment entry and positive treatment outcomes. However, certain drug treatment and harm reduction services may have differential impacts on treatment entry and outcomes by gender. As the numbers of female drug users may increase in Iran [14, 15], studies attempt to understand motivations and barriers associated with treatment entry and outcomes are needed in order to provide the most effective drug treatment services.

The current review findings underscore the roles of numerous factors in treatment entry. Furthermore, the review underscores that cognitive-behavioral interventions, adequate methadone dose as well as some factors outside treatment such as employment and family support increase positive treatment outcomes. In contrast, the review findings highlight that financial problems in combination with some factors such as stigma hamper treatment entry and positive treatment outcomes. Studies in the United Sates indicate that drug treatment entry and positive treatment outcomes among women are influenced by numerous individual and social factors such as social stigma, poor motivations to change and unemployment [42–44].

The highlighted role of cognitive-behavioral interventions may be related to the necessity of learning essential skills to manage drug craving and relapse. Furthermore, studies show that drug treatment is more likely to be successful if it includes both methadone and psychological services [44]. Considering the facilitating factors related to treatment entry and positive

treatment outcomes, as well as the provision of CBT should be considered by health policy makers in Iran. The professional provision of cognitive-behavioral interventions is suggested to increase positive treatment outcomes. Mass-media and families should encourage women for drug treatment entry and utilizing harm reduction services in the community.

In contrast, the review results indicate that individual and social factors such as poor motivations to change hamper treatment entry and positive treatment outcomes. Studies in the United States indicate that women may encounter some barriers to treatment entry and engaging with treatment such as poor education about drug treatment or poor motivation to change drug use behaviors [34, 42–44]. The elimination of the barriers to treatment entry and positive treatment outcomes should be targeted by health policy makers in Iran.

It should be noted that programs with good treatment outcomes are those programs that can keep clients in treatment for long time periods [34, 44]. In addition, longer drug treatment episodes are related to positive treatment outcomes. Funded ancillary psychiatric, medical and social work services are needed to increase positive treatment outcomes among women in Iran. In addition, such programs are needed to address special needs of at-risk women such as trauma, rape or poly drug use [45, 46].

Conclusion

The current review has a main limitation. The study is only based on reviewing the development of WODTHRS with an emphasis on treatment entry and outcomes in general. Conducting further reviews with an emphasis on cultural, social and ethnic barriers to drug treatment especially among women in rural areas is primarily required.

WODTHRS in Iran have been developed to address women' needs. But, the development of similar services for women is still required. Enriching women-only services with enhancements such as psychiatric and employment services may increase treatment entry and positive treatment outcomes. The evaluation of the efficacy of WODTHRS versus gender-mixed services is primarily suggested. The main research gap is the long-term efficacy of WODTHRS which should be addressed with conducting more studies in future. Such evaluations are needed to recruit representative samples of women with longitudinal follow-ups.

Abbreviations
CBT: cognitive-behavioral therapy; IDUs: injecting drug users; MeSH: Medical Subject Headings; MoHME: Ministry of Health and Medical Education; NIDUs: non-injecting drug users; STI: sexually transmitted infections; VCT: voluntary counseling and testing; WODTHRS: women-only drug treatment and harm reduction services.

Competing interests
The authors declare that they have no competing interests.

Authors' contributions
ZAM designed the review. ZAM, RD, MS and RS contributed to data collection. ZAM wrote the manuscript. MA and KD contributed to editing the final darft of the paper and provided technical advice for conducting the review. All authors read and approved the final manuscript.

Author details
[1]Program of International Research and Training, National Drug and Alcohol Research Centre, Faculty of Public Health and Community Medicine,, University of New South Wales, Sydney, Australia. [2]Substance Abuse and Dependence Research Center, University of Social Welfare and Rehabilitation Sciences, Tehran, Iran. [3]Department of Psychiatry, School of Behavior Sciences, University of Social Welfare and Rehabilitation Sciences, Tehran, Iran. [4]Psychiatry and Behavioral Sciences Research Center, Department of Psychiatry, Mashhad University of Medical Sciences, Mashhad, Iran. [5]Department of Toxicology and Pharmacology, Faculty of Pharmacy and Pharmaceutical Sciences Research Center, Tehran University of Medical Sciences, Tehran, Iran.

References
1. Alam-mehrjerdi Z, Abdollahi M, Higgs P, Dolan K. Drug use treatment and harm reduction programs in Iran: a unique model of health in the most populated Persian Gulf country. Asian J Psychiatr. 2015;16:78–83.
2. Alam-mehrjerdi Z, Mokri A, Dolan K. Methamphetamine use and treatment in Iran: a systematic review from the most populated Persian Gulf country. Asian J Psychiatr. 2015;16:17–25.
3. Sahebi L, Asghari-Jafar-Aabadi M, Mousavi SH, Khalili M, Seyedi M. Relationship between psychiatric distress and criminal history among intravenous drug abusers in Iran. Iran J Psychiatry Behav Sci. 2015;9:e838.
4. Razzaghi E, Nassirmanesh B, Afshar P, Ohiri K, Claeson M, Power R. HIV/AIDS harm reduction in Iran. Lancet. 2006;368:434–5.
5. Ministry of Health and Medical Education. AIDS progress report. Tehran: Iran. 2014. http://www.unaids.org/en/.../country-progress-reports/2014countries. Accessed12 /11/14.
6. Alam-mehrjerdi Z, Abarashi Z, Mansoori S, Deylamizadeh A, Salehi-Fadardi J, Noroozi A, et al. Methamphetamine use among Iranian heroin Kerack-dependent women: implications for treatment. Int J High Risk Behav Addict. 2013;2:15–21.
7. Babakhanian M, Alam-mehrjerdi Z, Sotodeh N, Shenaiy Y, Tavana S. A survey of motivational factors associated with entry to methadone maintenance treatment among women: a short report. J Rafsanjan Uni Med Sci [Persian]. 2013;12:667–72.
8. Dolan K, Salimi S, Nassirimanesh B, Mohsenifar S, Mokri A. The establishment of a methadone treatment clinic for women in Tehran, Iran. J Public Health Policy. 2011;32:219–30.
9. Dolan K, Salimi S, Nassirimanesh B, Mohsenifar S, Allsop D, Mokri A. Characteristics of Iranian women seeking drug treatment. J Women Health (Larchmt). 2011;20:1687–91.
10. Dolan K, Salimi S, Nassirimanesh B, Mohsenifar S, Allsop D, Mokri A. Six-month follow-up of Iranian women in methadone treatment: drug use, social functioning, crime, and HIV and HCV sero-incidence. J Subst Abuse Rehab. 2012;3:37–43.
11. Hajiabdobaghi M, Razani N, Karami N, Kheirandish P, Mohraz M, Rasoolinejad M, et al. Insights from a survey of sexual behaviour among a group of at-risk women in Tehran, Iran, 2006. AIDS Educ Prev. 2007;19:519–30.
12. Roshanfekr P, Noori R, Dejman M, Fathi Geshnigani Z, Rafiey H. Drug use and sex work among at-risk women: a qualitative study of initial factors. Iran J Psychiatry Behav Sci. 2015;9:e953.
13. Alam-mehrjerdi Z, Noori R, Dolan K. Opioid use, treatment and harm reduction service: the first report from the Persian Gulf region. J Subst Use. 2014; Early online:1–7. doi:10.3109/14659891.2014.966344
14. Fahimar N, Sedaghat A, Hatami H, Kamali K, Gooya MM. Counseling and harm reduction centers for vulnerable women to HIV/AIDS in Iran. Iran J Public Health. 2013;42:98–104.
15. Fahimfar N, Sedaghat A, Kamali K, Valipour A, Moghaddam MS, Gouya MM. Drug use in HIV vulnerable women attending to "HIV Sexual Harm Reduction Centers" in Iran. Tehran: Iran: 8th International Addiction Science Congress; 2014.
16. Langendam MW, Akl EA, Dahm P, Glasziou P, Guyatt G, Schunemann HJ. Assessing and presenting summaries of evidence in Cochrane reviews. Syst Rev. 2013;2:81.
17. Lawrinson P, Ali R, Buavirat A, Chiamwongpaet S, Dvoryak S, Habrat B, et al. Key findings from the WHO collaborative study on substitution therapy for opioid dependence and HIV/AIDS. Addiction. 2008;103:1484–92.
18. Moharreri MR. Out-patient treatment of opium addicts: report of a pilot project in Shiraz. Bull Narc. 1976;28:31–9.
19. Tavakoli M, Mohammadi L, Yamohammadi M, Farhoodian A, Jafari F, Farhadi MH. Status and trend of substance abuse and dependence among Iranian women. J Rehab [Persian]. 2014;14:30–7.
20. Shekarchizadeh H, Ekhtiari H, Khami MR, Virtanen JI. Patterns of pre-treatment drug abuse, drug treatment history and characteristics of addicts in methadone maintenance treatment in Iran. Harm Reduct J. 2012;9:18.
21. Radfar SR. Ways to increase coverage of harm reduction programs in women-friendly facilities in Iran: a qualitative study. California: USA: CPDD 75th annual meeting; 2013.
22. Ahmadan-Panah M, Ghaleiha A, Jahangard L, Mosavi S, Haghighi M. The process of substance abuse onset in women: a cross-sectional study in Hamedan, western Iran. Avicenna J Neuro-Psychol Physiol. 2014;1:e18090. doi:10.17795/ajnpp-18090.
23. Alam-mehrjerdi Z, Rezaei F, Arshad L, Noori M. Stability in methadone maintenance treatment among Iranian women: the first qualitative study of facilitating factors. Beirut: Lebanon. 2013b.
24. Ghasemi-Arganeh H, Heidari H, Ghasemi N, Dehghani SA. A study of the effectiveness of motivational interviewing in changing the life style of drug-dependent women in recovery. Quarter J Res Addict [Persian]. 2014;8:25–34.
25. Daneshmand R, Shishegar S, Alam-mehrjerdi Z, Fathy Z. Psychological problems of female co-users of opiates with methamphetamine: implications for longer treatment retention. Tehran: Iran: 8th International Addiction Science Congress; 2014.
26. Tafaoli-Masooleh K. The effectiveness of group cognitive-behavioral motivational interviewing in reducing psychological problems among methamphetamine-dependent Persian women. Tehran: Iran: Master's Thesis in psychology [Persian]; 2010.
27. Dehghani-Firooz-Abadi S, Ghasemi H, Safari S, Ebrahimi AK, Etemadi A. A study of the effectiveness of group sessions of motivational interviewing on increasing self- confidence and efficacy. Quarter J Res Addict [Persian]. 2013;7:145–58.
28. Hadadi H, Motlagh N, Kamali N, Mohammadi S, Keshavarz G, Bakht S. The effects of matrix model in the treatment of methamphetamine use. Quarter J Res Addict [Persian]. 2014;8:57–69.
29. Ebrahimi A, Agahi B, Asadi H. Study of the factors and barriers that affect women participation in drug use prevention. Tehran: Iran: 8th International Addiction Science Congress; 2014.
30. Shaditalab J, Ghafari S, Azizzadeh M, Khanjaninejad L. The need for gender responsive social support programs. Tehran: Iran: 8th International Addiction Science Congress; 2014.
31. Rahimi Movaghar A, Malayerikhah Langroodi Z, Delbarpour Ahmadi S, Amin Esmaeili M. A qualitative study of specific needs of women for treatment of addiction. Iran. J Psychiatr Clin Psychol [Persian]. 2011;17:116–25.
32. Daneshmand R, Arshad L, Alam-mehrjerdi Z, Ghenaatian Z. Treatment needs of women with methamphetamine use: implications for implementing cognitive-behavioral intervention. Tehran: Iran: 8th International Addiction Science Congress; 2014.
33. Murray CJ, Ortblad KF, Guinovart C, Lim SS, Wolock TM, Roberts DA, et al. Global, regional, and national incidence and mortality for HIV, tuberculosis, and malaria during 1990–2013: a systematic analysis for the global burden of disease study 2013. Lancet. 2014;384:1005–70.
34. Greenfield SF, Sudie E, Lawson BK, Brady KT. Substance abuse in women. Psychiatr Clin North Am. 2010;33:339–55.
35. Bozicevic I, Riedner G, Calleja JM. HIV surveillance in MENA: recent developments and results. Sex Transm Infect. 2013;89:iii11–6.
36. Springer SA, Larney S, Alam-mehrjerdi Z, Altice FL, Metzger D, Shoptaw S. Drug treatment as HIV prevention among women and girls who inject drugs from a global perspective: progress, gaps and future directions. J Acquir Immune Defic Syndr. 2015;69:S155–61.

37. Khajehkazemi R, Haghdoost A, Navadeh S, Setayesh H, Sajadi L, Osooli M, et al. Risk and vulnerability of key populations to HIV infection in Iran: knowledge, attitudes and practices of female sex workers, prison inmates and people who inject drugs. Sex Health. 2014;11:568–74.
38. Sajjadi L, Mirzazadeh A, Navadeh S, Osooli M, Khajehkazemi R, Gouya MM, et al. HIV prevalence and related risk behaviors among female sex workers in Iran: results of the national bio-behavioural survey, 2010. Sex Transm Infect. 2013;89:iii37–40.
39. Taghizadeh H, Taghizadeh F, Fathi M, Reihani P, Shirdel N, Rezaee SM. Drug use and high-risk sexual behaviors of women at a drop in center in Mazandaran province, Iran, 2014. Iran J Psychiatry Behav Sci. 2015;9:e1047.
40. Ahmadi K, Rezazade M, Nafarie M, Moazen B, Yarmohammadi-Vasel M, Assari S, et al. Unprotected sex with injecting drug users among Iranian female sex workers: unhide HIV risk study. AIDS Res Treat. 2012;65:1070.
41. Mumtaz GR, Weiss HA, Thomas SL, Riome S, Setayesh H, Riedner G, et al. HIV among people who inject drugs in the Middle East and North Africa: systematic review and data synthesis. PLoS Med. 2014;11:e1001663.
42. Lloyd JJ, Ricketts EP, Strathdee SA, Cornelius LJ, Bishai D, Huettner S, et al. Social contextual factors associated with entry into opiate agonist treatment among injection drug users. Am J Drug Alcohol Abuse. 2005;31:555–70.
43. Lal R, Deb KS, Kedia S. Substance use in women: current status and future directions. Indian J Psychiatr. 2010;57:S275–85.
44. Ashley OS, Marsden ME, Brady TM. Effectiveness of substance abuse treatment programming for women: a review. Am J Drug Alcohol Abuse. 2003;29:19–53.
45. Alam Mehrjerdi Z, Barr AM, Noroozi A. Methamphetamine-associated psychosis: a new health challenge in Iran. Daru. 2013;21:30.
46. Alam Mehrjerdi Z. Crystal in Iran: methamphetamine or heroin Kerack. Daru. 2013;15:21.

6

Pharmacological evaluation of the semi-purified fractions from the soft coral *Eunicella singularis* and isolation of pure compounds

Monia Deghrigue[1]*, Carmen Festa[2], Lotfi Ghribi[3], Maria Valeria D'auria[2], Simona de Marino[2], Hichem Ben Jannet[3], Rafik Ben Said[4] and Abderrahman Bouraoui[1]

Abstract

Background: Gorgonians of the genus *Eunicella* are known for possessing a wide range of pharmacological activities such as antiproliferative and antibacterial effect. The aim of this study was to evaluate the anti-inflammatory and gastroprotective effect of the organic extract and its semi-purified fractions from the white gorgonian *Eunicella singularis* and the isolation and identification of pure compound(s) from the more effective fraction.

Methods: Anti-inflammatory activity was evaluated, using the carrageenan-induced rat paw edema test and in comparison to the reference drug Acetylsalicylate of Lysine. The gastroprotective activity was determined using HCl/EtOH induced gastric ulcers in rats. The purification of compound(s) from the more effective fraction was done by two chromatographic methods (HPLC and MPLC). The structure elucidation was determined by extensive spectroscopic analysis (^{1}H and ^{13}C NMR, COSY, HMBC, HMQC and NOESY) and by comparison with data reported in the literature.

Results: The evaluation of the anti-inflammatory activity of different fractions from *Eunicella singularis* showed in a dependent dose manner an important anti-inflammatory activity of the ethanol fraction, the percentage of inhibition of edema, 3 h after carrageenan injection was 66.12%, more effective than the reference drug (56.32%). In addition, this ethanolic fraction showed an interesting gastroprotective effect compared to the reference drugs, ranitidine and omeprazole. The percentage of inhibition of gastric ulcer induced by HCl/ethanol in rats was 70.27%. The percentage of the reference drugs (ranitidine and omeprazol) were 65 and 87.53%, respectively. The purification and structure elucidation of compound(s) from this ethanolic fraction were leading to the isolation of five sterols: cholesterol (5α-cholest-5-en-3β-ol) **(1)**; ergosterol (ergosta-5,22-dien-3β-ol) **(2)**; stigmasterol (24-ethylcholesta-5, 22-dien-3b-ol) **(3)**; 5α,8α-epidioxyergosta 6,22-dien-3β-ol **(4)** and 3β-hydroxy-5α,8α-epidioxyergosta-6-ene **(5)**; and one diterpenoid: palmonine D **(6)**.

Conclusion: Based on data presented here, we concluded that diterpenoids and sterols detected in the ethanolic fraction can be responsible for its pharmacological activity.

Keywords: *Eunicella singularis*, Anti-inflammatory activity, Gastroprotective effect, Marine natural product, Diterpenoid, Sterols

* Correspondence: monia.deghrigue@laposte.net
[1]Laboratoire de développement chimique, galénique et pharmacologique des médicaments (LR12ES09). Equipe de Pharmacologie marine, Faculté de pharmacie de Monastir, Université de Monastir, Monastir, Tunisie
Full list of author information is available at the end of the article

Background

Nature has developed an enormous diversity during several billion years of evolution. The Mediterranean Area represents one of the world's major centers of animal diversity; with around 20 gorgonian species, four belong to the genus *Eunicella*: *E. verrucosa*, *E. filiformis*, *E. cavolini* and *E. singularis* [1].

Although natural compounds have been replaced by synthetic chemistry as the main source of new drugs, marine invertebrates remain an unequalled source of biochemical diversity. The studies on gorgonian have great importance in the research of marine resources of active compounds mainly by the pharmaceutical industry or for other uses. In fact, the gorgonians (Anthozoa, Gorgonacea) are known for possessing a wide range of pharmacologic and health promoting properties including antibacterial [2], antiviral [3], antiplasmodial [4], antifouling [5], antiproliferative [6], cytotoxic [7] and insecticidal [8] effects. The gorgonian of the genus *Eunicella* has been demonstrated to contain a wide variety of natural products as steroids and diterpenes [9,10]. These compounds posses anticancer, gastroprotective and anti-inflammatory activities [11]. For many years, our marine pharmacological group in Tunisia has been involved in an accurate research program on gorgonian constituents in order to define both their chemical composition and their biological activities. On the other hand, the use of non-steroidal anti-inflammatory drugs (NSAID) for the treatment of inflammatory diseases is associated with adverse effects as peptic ulcer [12]. Therefore, the research of potent anti-inflammatory drugs from natural sources and with fewer side effects had become necessary. This study has yielded the anti-inflammatory and gastroprotective effects of the organic extract and its semi-purified fractions of the white gorgonian *Eunicella singularis* (Esper, 1791). The structure elucidation of the isolated compounds from the active fraction was done by 1D and 2D NMR experiments and by comparison with literature data.

Methods
General procedures

HPLC was performed using a Waters model 510 pump equipped with Waters Rheodine injector and a differential refractometer, model 401. Medium pressure liquid chromatography (MPLC) was performed on a Buchi apparatus using a silica gel (230–400 mesh) column.

NMR spectra were obtained on Varian Inova 400 and Varian Inova 500 NMR spectrometers (^{1}H at 400 and 500 MHz, ^{13}C at 100 and 125 MHz, respectively) equipped with a Sun hardware, δ (ppm), *J* in hertz, and spectra referred to CD_3Cl_3 (δH=7.27; δC= 70.0) as internal standard. High-resolution ESIMS spectra were performed

with a Micromass QTOF Micro mass spectrometer. All reagents were commercially obtained (Aldrich, Fluka) at the highest commercial quality and used without further purification except where noted. All reactions were monitored by TLC on silica gel plates (Macherey–Nagel). Carrageenan (BDH Chemicals Ltd Poole England), Acetylsalicylate of Lysine (ASL) were purchased from Sigma Chemical (Berlin, Germany). Ranitidine was obtained from Medis (Tunis, Tunisia), omeprazole was obtained from AstraZeneca (Monts).

Collection and extraction

E. singularis was collected from the Mediterranean Sea in various areas of the coastal region of Tabarka (Tunisia), in June 2010, at a depth between 20 and 30 m. Identification of specimens was carried out in the National Institute of Marine Sciences and Technologies (Salamboo, Tunisia) where a voucher specimen of *E. singularis* was deposited under the following reference 1132. After maceration of 600 g of the powdered material with methanol and dichloromethane (1:1, v/v) for 48h three times, the organic extract (40 g) was purified, using C18 cartridges (Sep-pack, Supelco), by gradient elution with different organic solvents in the order of decreased polarity: ethanol, acetone and methanol/CH_2Cl_2 (1:1) to give three semi-purified fractions: ethanol (F-EtOH), acetone (F-Ac) and methanol/CH_2Cl_2 (F-MeOH/CH_2Cl_2) fractions. Organic solvents were removed from recuperated fractions using rotating evaporator at 40°C.

Purification, isolation and structure elucidation

F-EtOH (15 g) was fractionated according to the Kupchan partitioning procedure [13] as follow: the ethanolic fraction was dissolved in a mixture of MeOH/H_2O containing 10% H_2O and partitioned against *n*-hexane to give 10.3 g of the crude extract. The water content (% v/v) of the MeOH extract was adjusted to 30% and partitioned against $CHCl_3$ to give 3.9 g of the crude extract. The aqueous phase was concentrated to remove MeOH and then extracted with *n*-BuOH (268 mg of crude extract) (Figure 1). The *n*-hexane extract (5 g) was fractioned by silica gel MPLC using a solvent gradient system from CH_2Cl_2 to MeOH. Fraction eluted with CH_2Cl_2: MeOH 99:1 (307 mg) was purified by HPLC on a Nucleodur 100–5 C18 (5 μm; 10 mm i.d. × 250 mm) with 99% MeOH: H_2O as eluent (flow rate 3mL/min) to give 1.3 mg of 5α-cholest-5-en-3β-ol (**1**) (t_R=55 min) and 2.4 mg of 24-ethylcholesta-5, 22-dien-3β-ol (**3**) (t_R=83min) (Figure 1).

Fraction eluted with CH_2Cl_2:MeOH 95:5 (288 mg) was purified by HPLC on a Nucleodur 100–5 C18 (5 μ, 4.6 mm i.d. × 250 mm) with 95% MeOH:H_2O as eluent (flow rate 1 mL/min) to give 0.1 mg of ergosta-5,22-dien-3β-ol (**2**) (t_R=74 min) (Figure 1).

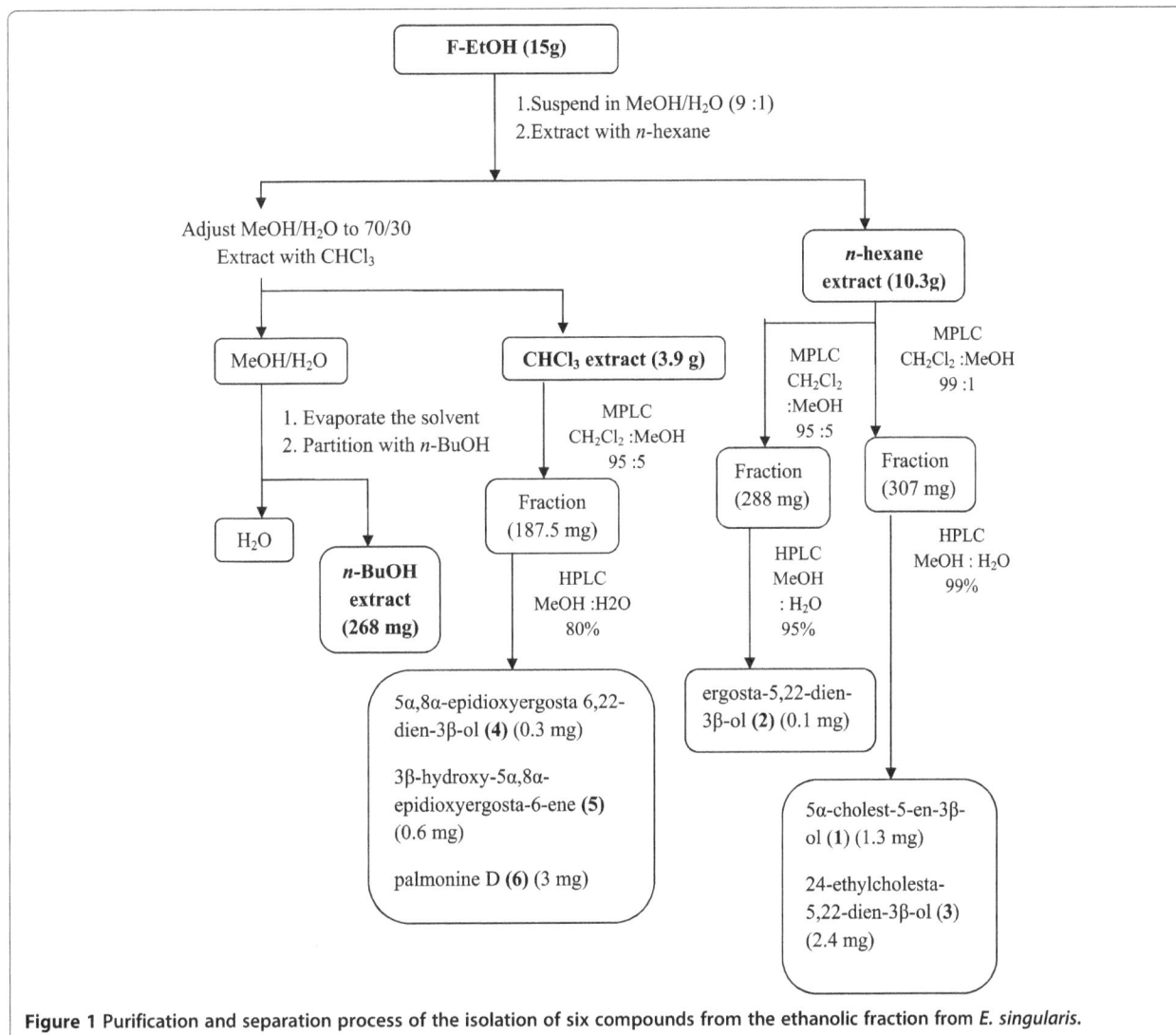

Figure 1 Purification and separation process of the isolation of six compounds from the ethanolic fraction from *E. singularis*.

The CHCl₃ extract (3.9 g) was chromatographed by silica gel MPLC using a solvent gradient system from CH₂Cl₂ to CH₂Cl₂: MeOH 1:1.

Fraction eluted with CH₂Cl₂: MeOH 95:5 (187.5 mg) was further purified by HPLC on a Nucleodur 100–5 C18 (5 μ, 4.6 mm i.d. × 250 mm) with 80% MeOH:H₂O as eluent (flow rate 1 mL/min) to give 0.3 mg of 5α,8α-epidioxyergosta 6,22-dien-3β-ol (4) (t_R=29 min), and 0.6 mg of 3β-hydroxy-5α,8α-epidioxyergosta-6-ene (5) (t_R=2 min) and 3 mg of palmonine D (6) (t_R=3 min) (Figure 1).

The purities of compounds were determined to be greater than 95% by HPLC and NMR. Furthermore, HPLC chromatograms and spectroscopic data of each compound were reported (Additional file 1).

Pharmacological evaluation
Animals
Wistar rats of either sex, weighing 150–200 g were obtained from Pasteur Institute (Tunis, Tunisia). Housing

conditions and *in vivo* experiments were approved according to the guidelines established by the European Union on Animal Care (CCE Council 86/609).

Carrageenan-Induced Rat Paw Edema
The anti-inflammatory activity of the organic extract and its semi-purified fractions on carrageenan-induced paw edema was determined according to Winter et al. [14]. The animals were divided into eleven groups of six rats each. The control group received an intraperitoneal (i.p.) dose of saline solution (NaCl 9g/L, 2.5 mL/kg), the reference group received Acetylsalicylate of Lysine (ASL) (300 mg/kg, i.p.), and the test groups received the organic extract of *E. singularis* (50, 100 and 200 mg/kg, i.p.) and its semi-purified fractions F-EtOH, F-Ac and F-MeOH/CH₂Cl₂ (25 and 50 mg/kg, i.p.). After 30 min, 0.05mL of a 1% carrageenan suspension was injected into the left hind paw. The paw volume up to the tibiotarsal articulation was measured using a plethysmometer (model

7150, Ugo Basile, Italy). The measures were determined at 0 h (V_0) (before carrageenan injection) and 1, 3 and 5 h later (V_T) (after carrageenan injection). Paw swelling was determined for each rat and the difference between V_T and V_0 was taken as the edema value. The percentages of inhibition were calculated according to the following formula:

$$\% \text{ inhibition} = \big[(V_T-V_0)_{control} - (V_T-V_0)_{treated\ group} / (V_T-V_0)_{control}\big] \times 100$$

Gastric lesions induced by HCl/ethanol
The gastroprotective activity of the organic extract of E. singularis and its semi-purified fractions F-EtOH, F-Ac and F-MeOH/CH$_2$Cl$_2$ was studied in 150 mM HCl/EtOH induced gastric ulcer [15]. Rats were divided into fifteen groups, fasted for 24 h prior receiving an intraperitoneal doses of vehicle (NaCl 9g/L, 2.5 mL/kg) for the control group, organic extract (50, 100 and 200 mg/kg, i.p.) and its semi-purified fractions F-EtOH, F-Ac and F-MeOH/CH$_2$Cl$_2$ (5, 10 and 25 mg/kg, i.p.) for the twelve test groups. Two other groups received ranitidine (60 mg/kg, i.p.) and omeprazole (30 mg/kg, i.p.) as reference drugs. After 30 min, all groups were orally treated with 1mL of 150 mM HCl/EtOH solution for gastric ulcer induction. Animals were killed 1 h after the administration of ulcerogenic agent, their stomachs were excised and opened along the great curvature, washed and stretched on cork plates. The surface was examined for the presence of lesions and the extent of the lesions was measured. The summative length of the lesions along the stomach was recorded (mm) as lesion index.

Statistical analysis
Data are presented as the mean±standard error (s.e.m). Statistical analysis was performed using Student's t-test. The significance of difference was considered to include values of $P<0.05$.

Results and discussion
The current study was carried out to determine the in vivo anti-inflammatory and gastroprotective activities of the organic extract of E. singularis and its semi-purified fractions. The chemical composition of the more effective fraction was determined by both 1D and 2D NMR experiments.

As shown in Figure 2, 1D and 2D NMR analysis of the ethanolic fraction (F-EtOH) from the gorgonian E. singularis resulted in the identification of six compounds.

Compound 1 was isolated as colorless powder. The molecular formula was determined to be C$_{27}$H$_{46}$O. Analysis of ^{1}H and ^{13}C NMR data evidenced a Δ^5 dihydroxysteroid structure with a saturated C8 cholestane side chain. Comparison with literature data allowed assigning the 5α-cholest-5-ene-3β-ol (cholesterol) structure [16].

Compound 2 has a molecular formula of C$_{28}$H$_{46}$O as determined by HRESIMS. Compound 2 was identified as ergosta-5,22-dien-3β-ol (ergosterol) [17] (Figure 2). This compound was also isolated from the soft coral Tubastraea coccinea and T. tagusensis [17].

Compound 3 was isolated as colorless powder. The molecular formula was determined to be C$_{28}$H$_{46}$O. Its identity was determined by 1D and 2D NMR data as 24-ethylcholesta-5,22-dien-3b-ol (stigmasterol) earlier isolated from the halophyte Salicornia herbacea [18] and then reported also from the plant Aglaia eximia [19].

Compound 4 was isolated as white powder. The molecular formula was determined to be C$_{28}$H$_{44}$O$_3$ by HRESIMS data. NMR data disclosed the 5α,8α-epidioxyergosta 6,22-dien-3β-ol structure. This compound was also isolated from the fungus Sporothrix schenckii [20] and the fungus Cryptoporus volvatus [21].

Compound 5 has a molecular formula of C$_{28}$H$_{46}$O$_3$ as determined by HRESIMS. ^{1}H and ^{13}C NMR indicated that compound 5 is the Δ^{22} derivative of compound 4. Therefore compound 5 was identified as 3β-hydroxy-5α,8α-epidioxyergosta-6-ene [21].

Compound 6 was isolated as colorless oil. The molecular formula was determined to be C$_{24}$H$_{36}$O$_6$ by HRESIMS. The analysis of ^{1}H NMR spectrum clearly revealed an eunicellin diterpenoid structure. The ^{13}C NMR spectrum revealed 24 carbon signals. ^{1}H- and ^{13}CNMR assignments were carried out with the aid of the detailed 2D analyses (COSY, HMQC, NOESY, and HMBC) and the resulting NMR evidence revealed 6 to be defined as palmonine D [22]. Three sterols named 5α, 8α-epidioxysterols, pregnanes and 9,11-secosterols were separated from E. cavolini, another specie of the genus Eunicella [10,11]. The five sterols identified in our study were isolated for the first time from E. singularis and were not yet found with another specie from this genus.

Palmonine D is also purified from E. labiata, another specie of the genus Eunicella [22]. Other researchers reported the isolation of five diterpenoids from the gorgonian E. labiata, labiatamide A, labiatamide B, labiatin A, labiatin B and labiatin C [23] but these compounds were not yet separated from E. singularis. Massileunicellin A, was obtained from E. cavolini [24] but also was not identified from E.singularis.

The results reported in Figures 3 and 4 showed the anti-inflammatory effects of organic extract and its semi-purified fractions from E. singularis administered intraperitoneally.

E. singularis organic extract presented a dose- related, statistically significant anti-inflammatory activity on carrageenan induced paw edema which was comparable with the reference drug, Acetylsalicylate of Lysine (ASL),

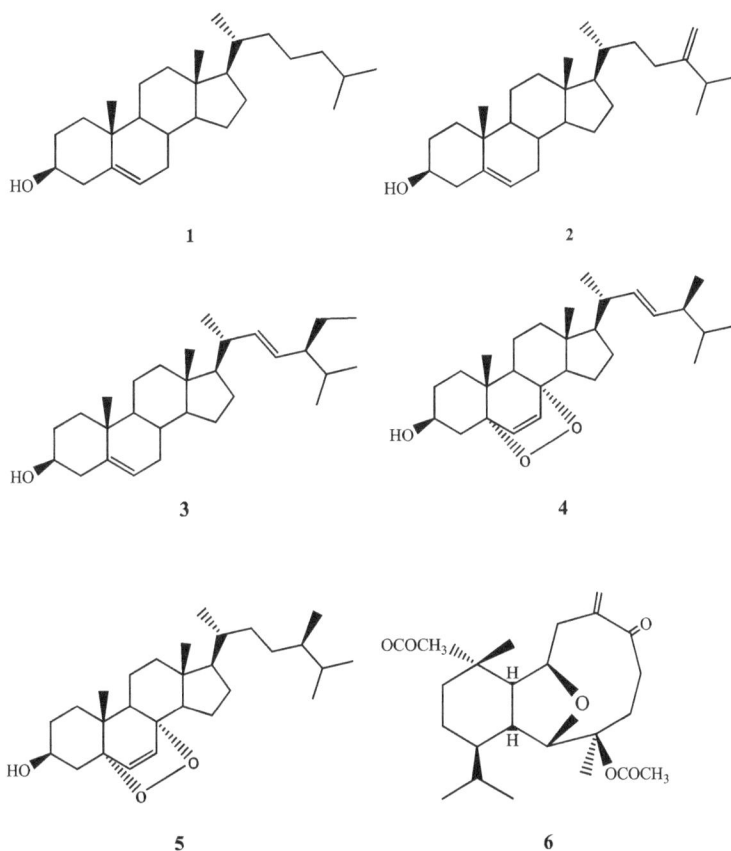

Figure 2 Chemical structures of six compounds isolated from the white gorgonian *E. singularis*. Five sterols (**1-5**): 5α-cholest-5-en-3β-ol (**1**); ergosta-5,22-dien-3β-ol (**2**); 24- ethylcholesta-5,22-dien-3b-ol (**3**); 5α,8α-epidioxyergosta 6,22-dien-3β-ol (**4**) and 3β-hydroxy- 5α,8α-epidioxyergosta-6-ene (**5**); and one diterpenoid: palmonine D (**6**).

a potent inhibitor of cyclooxygenase-2. The percent inhibition of edema at dose levels of 50, 100 and 200 mg/kg were 42.61%, 56.47% and 64.31% (at 3 h), respectively (Table 1). The semi-purified fractions (F-Ac, F-EtOH, F-MeOH/CH$_2$Cl$_2$) were assessed for anti-inflammatory effect at 25 and 50 mg/kg. A dose-related anti-inflammatory property was observed for the three fractions with highly significant activity of F-EtOH at dose 50 mg/kg with a percentage of inhibition of 66.12% at 3 h. While F-Ac and F-MeOH/CH$_2$Cl$_2$ at a dose of 50 mg/kg reduced

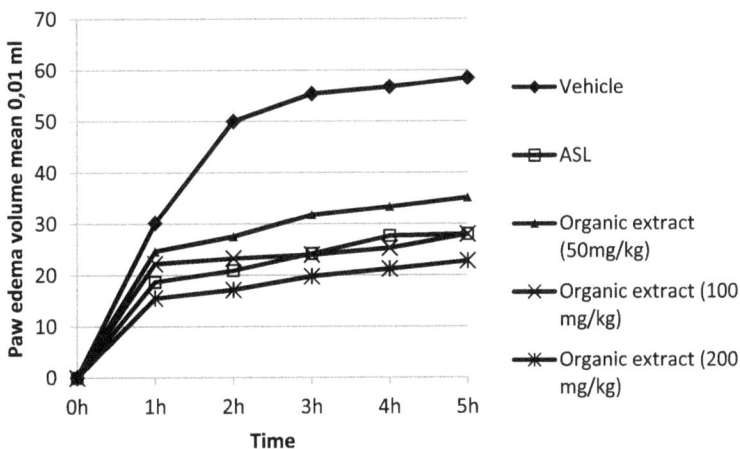

Figure 3 Effect of intraperitoneal administration of the organic extract from *E. singularis* on the carrageenan-induced rat paw edema. Values are mean ± SEM.

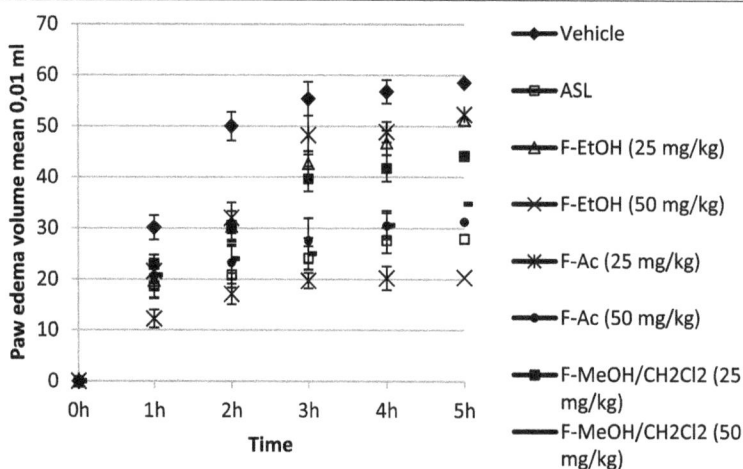

Figure 4 Effect of intraperitoneal administration of semi-purified fractions (F-Ac, F-EtOH and F-MeOH/CH2Cl2 from *E. singularis* on the carrageenan-induced rat paw edema. Values are mean ± SEM.

edema with a percentage of 50.22 and 54.78% (at 3 h), respectively. ASL as a reference standard drug inhibited the edema formation due to carrageenan to an extent of 56.32% (at 3 h) at the dose of 300 mg/kg. The development of edema induced by carrageenan corresponds to the events in the acute phase of inflammation mediated by histamine, bradykinin and prostaglandins produced under an effect of cyclooxygenase-2 (COX-2) [25]. This enzyme is an inducible cyclooxygenase which boosts the inflammatory response by COX-2 mediated prostaglandin E_2 (PGE_2) [26]. Hence, it is probably that the organic extract and its semi-purified fractions from the gorgonian *E. singularis* reduced inflammation by blocking the cyclooxygenase2 (COX-2). Morever, several studies reported that steroids isolated from other species of the genus

Eunicella have anti-inflammatory activity such as secosteroids [11]. The high anti-inflammatory activity of the fraction F-EtOH can be related with the presence of its main steroid constituents. The chemical analysis of this fraction (F-EtOH) revealed the presence of five sterols: 5α-cholest-5-en-3β-ol (cholesterol) (**1**); ergosta-5,22-dien-3β-ol (ergosterol) (**2**); 24-ethylcholesta-5,22-dien-3b-ol (stigmasterol) (**3**); 5α,8α-epidioxyergosta 6,22-dien-3β-ol (**4**) and 3β-hydroxy-5α,8α-epidioxyergosta-6-ene (**5**).

The gastroprotective effect of *E. singularis* organic extract and its semi-purified fractions against HCl/EtOH induced gastric damage in rats is shown in (Table 2) and the results are comparable to that of the reference drugs ranitidine, histamine H_2 receptor antagonist, and omeprazole, a proton pump inhibitor [27]. Oral administration of

Table 1 Anti-inflammatory effect of the intraperitoneal administration of *E. singularis* organic extract and its semi-purified fractions (F-EtOH, F-Ac and F-MeOH/CH$_2$Cl$_2$) and of reference drug (Acetylsalicylate of Lysine; ASL) in carrageenan-induced rat paw edema test

Treatment	Dose (mg/kg)	Edema (10^{-2}ml) (mean±s. e. m)			Edema inhibition (%)		
		1 h	3 h	5 h	1 h	3 h	5 h
Vehicle	-	30.12±2.38	55.35±3.3	58.5±4.69	-	-	-
Organic extract	50	24.62±2.8	31.76±3.6**	35.14±4.1*	18.26	42.61	39.92
	100	22.22±2.9	23.94±4.1**	27.95±1.5**	32.84	56.47	52.21
	200	15.5±3.2*	19.75±2.4**	22.75±3.6**	48.53	64.31	61.11
F-EtOH	25	19.73±1.6	42.74±2.7	51.26±2.6	34.49	22.78	12.36
	50	12.25±1.5**	18.75±2**	20.37±2.4**	59.32	66.12	65.17
F-Ac	25	21.55±2.6	48.24±2.4	52.33±3.5	28.42	12.84	10.53
	50	20.63±2.4	27.55±3.2**	31.27±2.7*	31.48	50.22	46.54
F-MeOH/CH$_2$Cl$_2$	25	22.85±3.2	39.67±2.6	44.2±4.8	24.12	28.32	24.43
	50	20.82±2.4	25.02±2.9**	34.79±3.4*	30.86	54.78	40.52
ASL	300	19.66±3.4	24.17±2.7**	27.95±3.1**	34.71	56.32	52.22

Values are expressed as mean±SEM; n=6 animals. *P<0.01, **P<0.001.

Table 2 Effect of *E. singularis* organic extract and its semi-purified fractions (F-EtOH, F-Ac, F-MeOH/CH$_2$Cl$_2$), and of reference drugs (ranitidine and omeprazol) on gastric ulcer induced by HCl/ethanol in rats

Treatment	Dose (mg/kg)	Ulcer index (mm)	Inhibition (%)
Vehicle	-	78.5±3,49	-
Organic extract	50	31.52±2,42**	59.84
	100	24.46±2,48**	68.84
	200	19.49±3,48**	75.16
F-EtOH	5	43.36±1,52*	44.76
	10	37.20±3,05**	52.61
	25	23.33±1**	70.27
F-Ac	25	61.97±0,7	21.05
F-MeOH/CH$_2$Cl$_2$	5	66.59±2,33	15.17
	10	58.78±2,82	25.11
	25	29.17±4,04**	62.84
Ranitidine	60	27.47±2.3**	65
Omeprazol	30	9.78±0,81*	87.53

Values are expressed as mean±SEM; n=6 animals. *P<0.01, **P<0.001.

HCl/EtOH produced gastric mucosal damage with severe hemorrhage with lesion index of 78.5 mm in the untreated group. Treatment of rats by organic extract of *E. singularis* produced a significant decrease in gastric hemorrhage and the lesion index was inhibited by 60, 68 and 75% at doses of 50, 100 and 200 mg/kg, respectively. The semi-purified fractions were assessed for gastroprotective activity at 5, 10 and 25 mg/kg. A dose-related gastroprotective effect was observed for the fractions F-EtOH and F-MeOH/CH$_2$Cl$_2$ with highly significant activity for the ethanolic fraction (F-EtOH) at 25 mg/kg. The lesion index was inhibited by 44, 52 and 70% at doses of 5, 10 and 25 mg/kg, respectively; while in the ranitidine treated animals (60 mg/kg) the inhibition was 65%. F-Ac failed to protect stomach tissues from mucosal damage. The two classical ulcer drugs ranitidine and omeprazole showed a significant activity with a percentage of inhibition of gastric lesions of 65 and 87%, respectively. Some reports on the gastroprotective effect of diterpenes belonging to different structural skeletons are published [28]. In addition, another studies demonstrated that several terpenes or their derivatives posses gastroprotective activity in different models of induced gastric lesions in animals [29]. This gastroprotective effect seems to be related with an increase of the defensive mechanisms of the stomach, such as prostaglandin synthesis and mucus production [30]. Therefore, the involvement of diterpenoids palmonine D **6** isolated from the active fraction F-EtOH is hypothesized and can be responsible for its high activity.

Furthermore, various phenolic compounds (alkaloids, glycosides, and saponins) detected in *E. singularis* organic extract and fractions [6] may be responsible for its activity.

Several studies reported that alkaloids have anti-inflammatory and gastroprotective effects [31]. Also, Glycosides, terpenoids and steroids detected in our samples are known to have anti-inflammatory and gastroprotective properties [10,32] The synergic effect of different compounds of *E. singularis* ethanolic fraction may be responsible for its higher anti-inflammatory and gastroprotective activities. Furthermore, the high free radical scavenging activity of F-EtOH in the DPPH test [6] suggests that the antioxidant activity may be one of the mechanisms of its gastroprotective and anti-inflammatory properties, because both ulcerous and inflammatory processes are related to an increase of free radicals [33].

Conclusion

In conclusion, the obtained results demonstrated that the ethanolic fraction of *E. singularis* had the highest activity in the two tests (anti-inflammatory and gastroprotective). The structure elucidation of compounds isolated from this fraction revealed the presence of five sterols and a eunicellan-based diterpenoid which may be responsible for its activity.

Competing interests

The authors declare that they have no competing interests.

Authors' contributions

AB and HBJ were the supervisors and designed the study. MD carried out pharmacological activities. CF and LG contribute to the chemical study. SDM and MVDA carried out the structure elucidation. RBS made contribution to preparation of organic extract and fractions from *E. singularis*. All authors read and approved the final manuscript.

Author details

[1]Laboratoire de développement chimique, galénique et pharmacologique des médicaments (LR12ES09). Equipe de Pharmacologie marine, Faculté de pharmacie de Monastir, Université de Monastir, Monastir, Tunisie. [2]Department of Pharmacy, University of Naples "Federico II", via D. Montesano 49, I- 80131 Napoli, Italy. [3]Laboratoire de chimie hétérocyclique, produits naturels et réactivité. Equipe de chimie médicinale et produits naturels (LR11ES39), Faculté des sciences de Monastir, Université de Monastir, Monastir, Tunisie. [4]Institut National des Sciences et Technologie de la Mer (INSTM), Salambo, Tunis, Tunisie.

References

1. Gori A, Bramanti L, Lopez-Gonzalez P, Thoma JN, Gili GM, Grinyo J, Uceira V, Rossi S: Characterization of the zooxanthellate and azooxanthellate morphotypes of the Mediterranean gorgonian *Eunicella singularis*. *Mar Biol* 2012, **159**:1485-1496.
2. McEnroe FJ, Fenical W: Structures and synthesis of some new antibacterial sesquiterpenoids from the gorgonian coral *Pseudopterogorgia rigida*. *Tetrahedron* 1978, **34**:1661-1664.

3.   Groweiss A, Look S, Fenical W: Solenolides, new antiinflammatory and antiviral diterpenoids from a marine octocoral of the genus *Solenopodium*. *J Org Chem* 1988, **53**:2401-2406.

4.   Wei X, Rodriguez AD, Baran P, Raptis RG, Sanchez JA, Ortega-Barria E, Gonzalez J: **Antiplasmodial cembradiene diterpenoids from a Southwestern Caribbean gorgonian octocoral of the genus *Eunicea*.** *Tetrahedron* 2004, **60**:11813-11819.

5.   Qi SH, Zhang S, Qian PY, Xiao ZH, Li MY: **Ten new antifouling briarane diterpenoids from the South China Sea gorgonian *Junceella juncea*.** *Tetrahedron* 2006, **62**:9123-9130.

6.   Deghrigue M, Dellai A, Bouraoui A: **In vitro antiproliferative and antioxidant activities of the organic extract and its semi-purified fractions from the Mediterranean gorgonian *Eunicella singularis*.** *Int J Pharm Pharm Sci* 2013, **5**:432-439.

7.   Sheu JH, Sung PJ, Cheng MC, Liu HY, Fang LS, Duh CY, Chiang MY: **Novel Cytotoxic Diterpenes, Excavatolides A-E, Isolated from the Formosan Gorgonian *Briareum excavatum*.** *J Nat Prod* 1998, **61**:602-608.

8.   Grode SH, James TR, Cardellina JH, Onan KD: **Molecular structures of the briantheins, new insecticidal diterpenes from *Briareum polyanthes*.** *J Org Chem* 1983, **48**:5203-5207.

9.   Berrue F, Kerr RG: **Diterpenes from gorgonian corals.** *Nat Prod Rep* 2009, **26**:681-710.

10. Ioannou E, Abdel-Razik AF, Alexi X, Vagias C, Alexis MN, Roussis V: **Pregnanes with antiproliferative activity from the gorgonian *Eunicella cavolini*.** *Tetrahedron* 2008, **64**:11797-11801.

11. Ioannou E, Abdel-Razik AF, Alexi X, Vagias C, Alexis MN, Roussis V: **9,11-Secosterols with antiproliferative activity from the gorgonian *Eunicella cavolini*.** *Bioorg Med Chem* 2009, **17**:4537-4541.

12. Hossain H, Al-Mansur A, Akter S, Sara U, Ahmed MR, Jahangir AA: **Evaluation of anti-inflammatory activity and total tannin content from the leaves of *Bacopa monnieri* (Linn.).** *IJPSR* 2014, **5**(4):1246-1252.

13. Kupchan SM, Britton RW, Ziegler MF, Sigel CW: **Bruceantin, a new potent antileukemic simaroubolide from *Brucea antidysenterica*.** *J Org Chem* 1973, **38**:178-179.

14. Winter CA, Risley EA, Nuss GW: **Carrageenan induced edema hind paw of the rat as an easy for anti-inflammatory drugs.** *Proc Soc Exp Biol Med* 1962, **3**:544-547.

15. Mizui T, Doteuchi M: **Effect of polyamines on acidified ethanol-induced gastric lesions in rats.** *Japanese J Pharmacology* 1983, **33**:939-945.

16. Acimovic J, Rozman D: **Steroidal triterpenes of cholesterol synthesis.** *Molecules* 2013, **18**:4002-4017.

17. Lages BG, Fleury BG, Hovell AMC, Rezende CM, Pinto AC, Creed JC: **Proximity to competitors changes secondary metabolites of non-indigenous cup corals, *Tubastraea* spp., in the southwest Atlantic.** *Mar Biol* 2012, **159**:1551-1559.

18. Wang X, Zhang M, Zhao Y, Wang H, Liu T, Xin Z: **Pentadecyl ferulate, a potent antioxidant and antiproliferative agent from the halophyte *Salicornia herbacea*.** *Food Chem* 2013, **141**:2066-2074.

19. Harneti D, Supriadin A, Ulfah M, Safari A, Supratman U, Awang K, Hayashi H: **Cytotoxic constituents from the bark of *Aglaia eximia* (Meliaceae).** *Phytochem Lett* 2014, **8**:28-31.

20. Sgarbi DBG, da Silva AJR, Carlos IZ, Silva CL, Angluster J, Alviano CS: **Isolation of ergosterol peroxide and its reversion to ergosterol in the pathogenic fungus *Sporothrix schenckii*.** *Mycopathologia* 1997, **139**:9-14.

21. Wei-Guang M, Xing-Cong L, De-Zu W, Chong-Ren Y: **Ergosterol peroxides from *Cryptoporus volvatus*.** *Acta Bot Yunnanica* 1994, **16**(2):196-200.

22. Ortega MJ, Zubia E, Salva J: **A new cladiellane diterpenoid from *Eunicella labiata*.** *J Nat Prod* 1997, **60**:485-487.

23. Roussis V, Fenical W, Vagias C, Kornprobst JM, Miralles J: **Labiatamides A, B, and other eunicellan diterpenoids from the Senegalese gorgonian *Eunicella labiata*.** *Tetrahedron* 1996, **52**:2735-2742.

24. Hanson JR: **Diterpenoids.** *Nat Prod Rep* 2001, **18**:88-94.

25. Borgi W, Ghedira K, Chouchane N: **Antiinflammatory and analgesic activities of Zizyphus lotus root barks.** *Fitoterapia* 2007, **78**:16-19.

26. Inoue H, Ohshima H, Kono H, Yamanaka M, Kubota T, Aihara M, Hiroi T, Yago N, Ishida H: **Supressive effects of tranilast on the expression of inducible cyclooxygenase (COX-2) in interleukin-1-β-stimulated fibroblasts.** *Biochem Pharmacol* 1997, **53**:1941-1944.

27. Ishihara M, Ito M: **Influence of aging on gastric ulcer healing activities of cimetidine and omeprazole.** *Eur J Pharmacol* 2002, **444**:209-215.

28. Schmeda-Hirschmann G, Astudillo L, Rodriguez J, Theoduloz C, Yanez T: **Gastroprotective effect of the Mapuche crude drug Araucaria araucana resin and its main constituents.** *J Ethnopharmacol* 2005, **101**:271-276.

29. Farina C, Pinza M, Pifferi G: **Synthesis and anti-ulcer activity of new derivatives of glycyrrhetic, oleanolic and ursolic acids.** *Il Farmaco* 1998, **53**:22-32.

30. Hiruma-Lima CA, Gracioso JS, Toma W, Paula ACB, Almeida ABA, Brasil DD, Muller AH, Souza-Brito AR: **Evaluation of the gastroprotective activity of cordatin, a diterpene isolated from Aparisthmium cordatum (Euphorbiaceae).** *Biol Pharm Bull* 2000, **23**:1465-1469.

31. Moulin M, Coquerel A: *Pharmacologie, connaissance et pratique*. 2èmeth edition. Paris: Masson; 2002:845.

32. Radjasa OK, Vaske YM, Navarro G, Vervoort HC, Tenney K, Linington RG, Crews P: **Highlights of marine invertebrate-derived biosynthetic products: their biomedical potential and possible production by microbial associants.** *Bioorg Med Chem* 2011, **19**:6658-6674.

33. Pedernera AM, Guardia T, Guardia Calderon C, Rotelli AE, de la Rocha NE, Di Genaro S, Pelzer LE: **Anti-ulcerogenic and anti-inflammatory activity of the methanolic extract of *Larrea divaricata* Cav. In rats.** *J Ethnopharmacol* 2006, **105**:415-420.

7

Aspirin use and bleeding volume in skin cancer patients undergoing surgery

Arman Engheta[1], Shahryar Hadadi Abianeh[2*], Ali Atri[1] and Mehdi Sanatkarfar[3]

Abstract

We investigated the occurrence of bleeding complications in patients who underwent skin tumor surgery and compared it between Aspirin users and a placebo control group. In this double blind randomized controlled trial, 32 patients who continued taking aspirin (intervention group) and 38 patients who stopped taking Aspirin (placebo group) before surgery were compared in terms of intraoprative and postoperative bleeding problems, hematoma and local signs of coagulopathy. There was no statistically significant difference in intraoprative bleeding between the study groups ($P = 0.107$). We concluded that continuation of Aspirin therapy had no significant effect on bleeding complications in patients who underwent skin tumor surgery.

Trial registration: IRCT201602049768N5

Keywords: Acetyl salicylic acid, Skin cancer, Surgery, Bleeding, Complication, Aspirin

Abbreviations: BT, Bleeding time; BUN, Blood urea nitrogen; CT, Clotting time; FBS, Fasting blood sugar; INR, International normalized ratio; PT, Prothrombin time; PTT, Partial thromboplastin time; SPSS, Statistical Package for the Social Sciences

Discontinuation of anticoagulant or anti platelet agents before skin surgery is still a challenge due to the lack of proper recommendations in the current guidelines [1]. For the decision making, the surgeon should consider several patient-related factors, such as indication of the treatment, patient's condition and the underlying disease, in order to decide about the continuation or interruption of the drug [2, 3]. Skin surgeries are considered as one of the safest and simplest surgeries. However, rapid increase in the use and new indications of anticoagulant drugs, particularly aspirin, requires specific attention toward their use in skin surgeries [4, 5].

However, the evidence regarding the continuation or discontinuation of Aspirin before skin surgery is inconsistent. In the present study, we aimed to monitor the bleeding complications in patients who underwent skin tumor surgery and compared it between Aspirin users and a placebo control group.

In this double-blind randomized controlled trial, we enrolled patients with non-bleeding skin tumors who were under treatment with aspirin due to any indication. The inclusion criteria were use of Aspirin for at least 3 months before surgery with a daily dose of 80 mg, age between 40 and 75 years, giving an informed consent for taking part in the study, and international normalized ratio (INR) of 1–1.5. Our exclusion criteria included as follows; Having dementia, movement disorder, simultaneous participation in another trial, patients with life-threatening cardiovascular diseases (i.e. New York Heart Association class III or more, history of previous myocardial infarction, severe heart valve disease), bleeding disorders, use of antiplatelets other than Aspirin or anticoagulants and positive history of gastrointestinal bleeding. Moreover, patients who did not follow the prescription rules, those who had a disease that required Aspirin discontinuation or Aspirin intolerance were also excluded. In order to make sure about the

* Correspondence: H_abianeh@yahoo.com
[2]Department of Plastic Surgery, Razi Hospital, Tehran University of Medical Sciences, Vahdat Eslami st, Tehran, Iran
Full list of author information is available at the end of the article

drug compliance of the patients, they were asked to bring the blister pack of the consumed tablets.

Using block randomization, patients were randomized into intervention and control groups, matched for age and sex. Both groups were asked to discontinue their Aspirin 7 days before the surgery and they received packed drugs of the trial including Aspirin (80 mg) for the intervention group and placebo for the control group.

Before operation, demographic and baseline clinical characteristics were collected from the patients. The clinical data included the presence of bleeding risk factors, type of skin tumor, number and size of the tumor(s), location of the lesion, drug history and blood test. For every patient, standard resection for the tumor was performed regarding its size and other clinical characteristics. Type of operation and data regarding anesthesia, cautery, need for osteotomy and other surgical characteristics were recorded for the patient. We measured the bleeding by weighing the dressing gases during and after operation up to 24 h. The nurse who was in charge of weighing the gases was blinded to the study protocol. Primary endpoint of the study was the amount of bleeding within and early after surgery. Secondary endpoints were need for early changing of the dressing, development of hematoma or local anticoagulation disorders such as petechia or ecchymosis.

Categorical variables were analyzed by the chi-square test. Continuous variables are presented as means ± standard deviation, or as median and interquartile ranges, as appropriate. Differences between groups in normally and non-normal continuous variables were assessed using the unpaired Student's t test and the Mann–Whitney U test,

Table 1 Comparison of the baseline characteristics between the study groups

Characteristic[a]	Intervention (n = 32)	Placebo (n = 38)	P-value[†]
Age, year	65.8 ± 2.3	64.1 ± 1.7	0.218
Male gender, n (%)	24 (75)	29 (76.3)	0.683
Diabetes, n (%)	13 (40.6)	5 (13.2)	0.009
Hypertension, n (%)	23 (71.9)	19 (50)	0.063
Cardiovascular diseases, n (%)	21 (65.6)	11 (28.9)	0.002
Smoking, n (%)	4 (12.5)	5 (13.2)	0.999
Opium abuse, n (%)	3 (9.4)	4 (10.5)	0.999
FBS, mg/dl	123.9 ± 58.0	121.7 ± 44.9	0.696
BUN, mg/dl	37.3 ± 8.9	33.7 ± 8.7	0.064
Creatinine, mg/dl	0.94 ± 0.24	0.95 ± 0.25	0.723
Hemoglobin, g/dl	13.7 ± 1.3	14.9 ± 4.4	0.054
Platelet, 1/mm^3	208.4 ± 81.9	200.3 ± 45.1	0.925
INR	2.1 ± 4.7	1 ± 0.01	0.096
PT, sec	13.3 ± 3.2	12.9 ± 2.3	0.001
PTT, sec	28.1 ± 4.1	28.9 ± 3.2	0.114
CT, sec	327.3 ± 72.2	321.7 ± 62.9	0.669
BT, sec	152.7 ± 59.7	148.7 ± 44.6	0.791

BT Bleeding time, BUN Blood urea nitrogen, CT clotting time, FBS Fasting blood sugar, INR International normalized ratio, PT Prothrombin time, PTT Partial thromboplastin time

[a]Variables are shown as mean ± standard deviation or frequency (percentage) where appropriate

[†]P < 0.05 was considered as statistically significant

Table 2 Comparison of the tumoral and operative characteristics between the study groups

Characteristic[a]	Intervention (n = 32)	Placebo (n = 38)	P-value[†]
Location			0.908
Face	10 (29.4)	13 (30.9)	
Nose	6 (17.6)	4 (9.5)	
Ear	4 (11.7)	5 (11.9)	
Neck	0 (0)	1 92.3)	
Scalp	9 (26.4)	14 (33.3)	
Other	5 (14.7)	5 (11.9)	
Type			0.675
Basal cell carcinoma	24 (75)	32 (84.2)	
Squamous cell carcinoma	5 (15.6)	5 (13.2)	
Melanoma	1 (3.1)	0 (0)	
Not reported	2 (6.2)	1 (2.6)	
Size of lesion			0.17
< 3 cm	15 (46.9)	14 (35)	
3–6 cm	15 (46.9)	24 (60)	
> 6 cm	1 (3.1)	2 (5)	
Not reported	1 (3.1)	0 (0)	
Number of lesions			0.478
1 lesion	22 (68.8)	29 (76.3)	
2 lesions	3 (9.4)	6 (15.8)	
3 lesions	2 (6.2)	1 (2.6)	
4 lesions and more	3 (9.4)	1 (2.6)	
Not reported	2 (6.2)	1 (2.6)	
Type of surgery			0.72
Flap	24 (70.6)	28 (68.3)	
Graft	9 (56.4)	13 (31.7)	
Other	1 (2.9)	0 (0)	
Type of anesthesia			0.999
Sedative	31 (96.9)	38 (100)	
Not reported	1 (3.1)	0 (0)	
Cautery			0.999
Monopolar	31 (96.9)	37 (97.4)	
Bipolar	1 (3.1)	1 (2.6)	
Need for osteotomy	0 (0)	1 (2.6)	
Volume of bleeding, ml	30 [20, 80]	30 [17, 40]	0.107

[a]Variables are shown as frequency (percentage) or median [interquartile range] where appropriate

[†]P < 0.05 was considered as statistically significant

respectively. All probability values were two-tailed and a P-value < 0.05 was considered significant. Data were analyzed with Statistical Package for the Social Sciences (SPSS) for Windows, version 15.0 (SPSS Inc., Chicago, Ilinois, United States of America).

In the present study, 38 patients were randomized to the intervention group and 38 patients were included in the control group. However, after randomization it was revealed that three patients had used antiplatelet or anticoagulant drugs and three other patients refused to continue the study; so, they were excluded from the final analysis ($n = 32$ for the intervention group). The frequency of diabetes and cardiovascular disease was significantly higher in the intervention group ($P = 0.009$ and $P = 0.002$, respectively). Details of the demographic and baseline clinical characteristics of the study groups are shown in Table 1.

Based on the pathology report, characteristics of the tumors and operation were comparable between the two groups as shown in Table 2.

Bleeding in all participants was restricted to the operation time and none of the participants had postoperative bleeding. Median volume of bleeding was 30 gram in both groups ($P = 0.107$) (Table 2). None of the patients required early change of wound dressing and we observed no case of hematoma or local coagulation disorder.

We found no significant difference between patients who used Aspirin perioperatively and those who discontinued it beforehand. This finding is in line with similar previous studies [6–8], while the strength of our study is its randomized controlled trial design and its uniform population that consisted of skin cancer patients. We also observed no complication within the study period.

Based on our findings, perioperative Aspirin therapy had no significant effect on bleeding complications in patients who underwent skin tumor surgery. Currently, surgical bleedings can be controlled easily by electrocauterization and are not potentially life-threatening. It seems that dermasurgeons should be more informed about the safety of Aspirin use in skin surgeries based on the current body of knowledge. Larger studies can also contribute to the elucidation of the use of multiple antiplatelet and anticoagulant agents during skin surgeries.

Acknowledgements
This study was supported by Razi Hospital and Tehran University of Medical Sciences, Tehran, Iran.

Authors' contribution
Study design: SHA, AA. Randomization, Data collection: AE. Statistical Analysis and drafting: AE, MS. Manuscript revision and final approval: All authors.

Competing interests
The authors declare that they have no competing interests.

Declarations
All participants signed a written informed consent. The protocol of this study was approved by the institutional ethical committee and board of research and is in accordance with the Declaration of Helsinki.

All the authors have read the article and gave consent for its publication as a letter to editor.
Data and material of this study is available via the corresponding author.

This work was funded by Tehran University of Medical Sciences.

Author details
[1]Department of Plastic Surgery, Imam Khomeini Hospital, Tehran University of Medical Sciences, Tehran, Iran. [2]Department of Plastic Surgery, Razi Hospital, Tehran University of Medical Sciences, Vahdat Eslami st, Tehran, Iran. [3]Department of Anesthesiology, Razi Hospital, Tehran University of Medical Sciences, Tehran, Iran.

References
1. Alam M, Goldberg LH. Serious adverse vascular events associated with perioperative interruption of antiplatelet and anticoagulant therapy. Dermatol Surg. 2002;28(11):992–8.
2. Alcalay J, Alkalay R. Controversies in perioperative management of blood thinners in dermatologic surgery: continue or discontinue? Dermatol Surg. 2004;30(8):1091–4.
3. Burger W, Chemnitius JM, Kneissl GD, et al. Low-dose aspirin for secondary cardiovascular prevention - cardiovascular risks after its perioperative withdrawal versus bleeding risks with its continuation - review and meta-analysis. J Intern Med. 2005;257(5):399–414.
4. Bordeaux JS, Martires KJ, Goldberg D, et al. Prospective evaluation of dermatologic surgery complications including patients on multiple antiplatelet and anticoagulant medications. J Am Acad Dermatol. 2011;65(3):576–83.
5. Gerstein NS, Schulman PM, Gerstein WH, et al. Should more patients continue aspirin therapy perioperatively?: clinical impact of aspirin withdrawal syndrome. Ann Surg. 2012;255(5):811–9.
6. Eichhorn W, Kluwe L, Heiland M, et al. Lack of evidence for increased risk of postoperative bleeding after cutaneous surgery in the head and neck in patients taking aspirin. Br J Oral Maxillofac Surg. 2014;52(6):527–9.
7. Dixon AJ, Dixon MP, Dixon JB. Bleeding complications in skin cancer surgery are associated with warfarin but not aspirin therapy. Br J Surg. 2007;94(11):1356–60.
8. Dhiwakar M, Khan NA, McClymont LG. Surgical resection of cutaneous head and neck lesions: does aspirin use increase hemorrhagic risk? Arch Otolaryngol Head Neck Surg. 2006;132(11):1237–41.

8

Ionic liquid phase microextraction combined with fluorescence spectrometry for preconcentration and quantitation of carvedilol in pharmaceutical preparations and biological media

Mohsen Zeeb[*] and Behrooz Mirza

Abstract

Background: Carvedilol belongs to a group of medicines termed non-selective beta-adrenergic blocking agents. In the presented approach, a practical and environmentally friendly microextraction method based on the application of ionic liquids (ILs) was followed by fluorescence spectrometry for trace determination of carvedilol in pharmaceutical and biological media.

Methods: A rapid and simple ionic liquid phase microextraction was utilized for preconcentration and extraction of carvedilol. A hydrophobic ionic liquid (IL) was applied as a microextraction solvent. In order to disperse the IL through the aqueous media and extract the analyte of interest, IL was injected into the sample solution and a proper temperature was applied and then for aggregating the IL-phase, the sample was cooled in an ice water-bath. The aqueous media was centrifuged and IL-phase collected at the bottom of the test tube was introduced to the micro-cell of spectrofluorimeter, in order to determine the concentration of the enriched analyte.

Results: Main parameters affecting the accuracy and precision of the proposed approach were investigated and optimized values were obtained. A linear response range of 10–250 $\mu g\ l^{-1}$ and a limit of detection (LOD) of 1.7 $\mu g\ l^{-1}$ were obtained.

Conclusion: Finally, the presented method was utilized for trace determination of carvedilol in commercial pharmaceutical preparations and biological media.

Keywords: Carvedilol, Hydrophobic ionic liquid, Spectrofluorimetry, Real samples

Background

Carvedilol belongs to a group of medicines termed non-selective beta-adrenergic blocking agents (Figure 1). This drug is useful in treatment of congestive heart failure. In addition, carvedilol is applied to treat high blood pressure (hypertension) and for prevention of heart attacks [1,2].

In order to assay the presence of carvedilol in pharmaceutical and biological samples, some analytical approaches including chromatography [3-6], spectrophotometery [7], electrochemistry [8,9] and fluorimetry [10] have been developed. These methods suffer form some limitations including poor sensitivity, high cost of analysis, unsuitable selectivity and high time of analysis. One of the best choices for overcoming the mentioned problems is the combination of a practical sample enrichment method with analytical instruments.

In recent years, analytical chemists have developed some practical liquid phase microextraction methods and among these sample pretreatment methods, dispersive liquid-liquid microextraction (DLLME) has received much attention [11,12]. Unfortunately, one of the most important disadvantages of these microextraction methods is the usage of toxic solvents as the extraction solvent such as $CHCl_3$, CCl_4 and etc. In order to remove these toxic materials from microextraction procedures, ionic liquids (ILs) are the best choice. ILs offer many

* Correspondence: Zeeb.mohsen@gmail.com
Department of Applied Chemistry, Faculty of science, Islamic Azad University, South Tehran Branch, Tehran, Iran

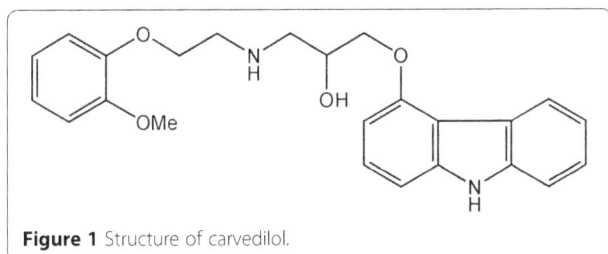

Figure 1 Structure of carvedilol.

advantages such as low vapor pressure, tunable solubility, desire thermal stability and etc. [13].

In recent years, some microextraction methods based on the application of ILs such as ionic liquid-based dispersive liquid-liquid microextraction (IL-DLLME) [14-16], ionic liquid cold-induced aggregation dispersive liquid-liquid microextraction (IL-CIA-DLLME) [17-19], ionic Liquid-based ultrasound-assisted in situ solvent formation microextraction [20], temperature-controlled ionic liquid dispersive liquid phase microextraction (TCIL-DLPME) [21], etc. have been introduced.

Solubility of ILs depends on the aqueous media temperature; hence it is possible to control the solubility of ILs by changing the temperature. In the presented ionic liquid phase microextraction, in order to disperse the IL-phase into the sample solution and increase the extraction recovery, a high temperature was applied. For collecting the IL-phase, sample solution was cooled and centrifuged.

Our previous studies revealed that the solubility of ILs depends on ionic strength of aqueous media, which has a negative influence on reproducibility and accuracy [18,19]. For solving this problem, a common ion of IL was introduced to the aqueous media. As a result, the solubility of IL phase was not affected by variations of ionic strength, and reproducible volume of enriched phase was obtained.

Some analytical instrument such as spectrofluorimetry offer many advantages such as proper sensitivity, selectivity, cost of analysis, speed of quantitative measurements and etc. In addition, by coupling a microextraction method with fluorescence spectrometry and due to the proper selectivity of this analytical technique, it is avoided the need of employing a high performance separation instrumental for pretreatment of biological samples prior to measurement.

As a part of our continuing efforts for quantitation of drugs using combination of new and benign sample enrichment methods with inexpensive, selective and sensitive analytical instrument [18,21], herein, for the first time a practical and environmentally friendly microextraction method based on the application of ILs was followed with spectrofluorimetry for trace determination of carvedilol in real samples. All variable were evaluated in details and optimized values were obtained.

Material and methods

Instrumentation

Detection of fluorescence signals were performed using a Perkin-Elmer LS 50 spectrofluorimeter. This instrument was equipped with xenon discharge lamp, and quartz micro-cell with a volume of 100 µl. Excitation and emission slits were fixed at 15 nm. In order to perform microextraction and optimization steps, a centrifuge from Hettich (Tuttlingen, Germany), a pH-meter, an adjustable sampler (10–100 µL) and a 1 ml syringe was prepared.

Reagents and materials

Analytical-reagent grade of 1-Hexyl-3-methylimidazolium hexafluorophosphate [Hmim][PF_6], acetone, acetonitrile, methanol, ethanol, HCl, NaOH and sodium hexafluorophosphate ($NaPF_6$) were obtained from Merck (Darmstadt, Germany). A working solution of $NaPF_6$ (250 mg ml^{-1}) was prepared. For preparing stock solution of carvedilol (1000 mg l^{-1}) (Fluka, Switzerland), proper amount of this drug was dissolved in methanol and diluted with ultra pure water. Standard solutions were prepared by dilution of the stock solution with ultra pure water. Tablets containing 12.5 mg and 25 mg carvedilol were purchased from a local pharmacy.

Sample pretreatment procedure

In this sample pretreatment method, ten milliliters of sample solution (10–250 µg l^{-1} of carvedilol) was transferred to a centrifuge tube. The pH of the solution was adjusted at 9. Afterwards, 60 mg of 1-Hexyl-3-methylimidazolium hexafluorophosphate [Hmim][PF_6] ionic liquid and 0.7 ml of hexafluorophosphate ($NaPF_6$) (250 mg ml^{-1}) was injected into the aqueous sample solution. After mixing the extractor with sample solution, the resultant solution was transferred into a hot water batch equipped with a thermostat. The temperature of the water batch was fixed at 50°C for 4 min. Under driving the temperature, IL-phase was dissolved and dispersed through the aqueous media. In order to aggregate the IL-phase, the sample was cooled at 0°C for 7 min. In order to collect the enriched phase, sample solution was centrifuged (6 min, 4000 r.p.m). After removing the aqueous media, the enriched phase was diluted with ethanol to 200 µl and transferred into the micro-cell of the spectrofluorimeter. Finally, quantitation of carvedilol was performed. Schematic diagram of the designed method is shown in Figure 2.

Preparation of pharmaceutical preparations, human urine and human plasma

To obtain pharmaceutical solutions for quantification, eight carvedilol tablets containing 12.5 or 25 mg drug were powdered, mixed and weighted. Required amount of the resultant material containing 10 mg carvedilol

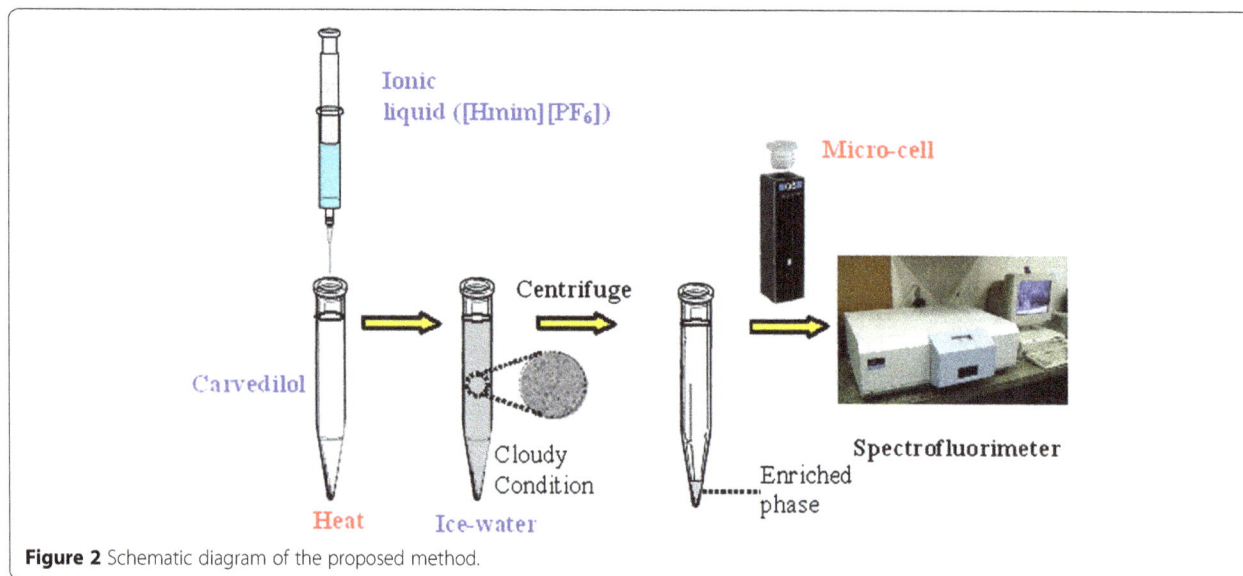

Figure 2 Schematic diagram of the proposed method.

was dissolved in methanol with signification. After filtration, the solution was transferred into a 100 ml volumetric vessel and diluted with ultra pure water. In order to set the concentration of carvedilol within the linear response range, further dilution was performed.

For preparing human plasma samples, different concentrations of carvedilol were added to one milliliter of human plasma. After this step, the real sample was deproteinized using 5 ml of acetonitrile. After centrifugation (12 min, 4000 r.p.m), 2.0 ml of the upper phase (clear condition) was diluted with ultra pure water and 10.0 ml of the obtained sample was utilized for quantitation.

In order to prepare human urine samples, ten milliliters of urine were centrifuged (5 min, 4000 r.p.m). Then, 2.0 ml of the upper clear phase was placed in centrifuge test tube and different amount of carvedilol was added to

this and diluted to 10.0 ml. Finally, the defined quantitation procedure was performed.

Results and discussion

In recent work, a simple and benign sample pretreatment method based on the application of ILs was combined with fluorescence spectrometry for enrichment and determination carvedilol in real samples. Main parameters affecting the accuracy and precision of the proposed approach were investigated and optimized values were obtained.

Fluorescence spectra properties and linear dynamic range

Native Fluorescence intensities of molecules with π-electron and cyclic structure are relatively high. As a result, measurement of fluorescence intensity provides a

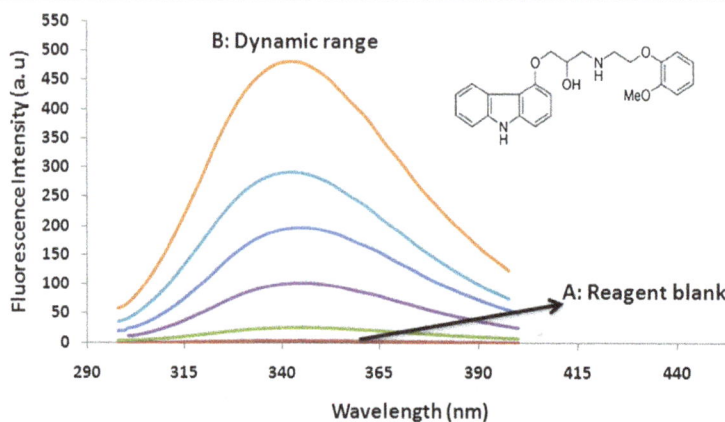

Figure 3 Fluorescence spectra of reagent blank and carvedilol. (A) Fluorescence spectrum of reagent blank after applying microextraction procedure. (B) Fluorescence spectra of carvedilol within linear dynamic range (10, 50, 100, 150, 250 µg l^{-1}) after applying microextraction procedure. Applied parameters: sample volume 10 ml; IL 60 mg; NaPF$_6$ 175 mg; pH 9; temperature 50°C; λ_{ex} 285 ± 5 nm; λ_{em} 345 ± 5 nm.

practical tool for sensitive quantitative analysis. After applying the designed microextraction procedure, fluorescence spectra of carvedilol (100 μg l^{-1}) was recorded (Figure 3). In this study, emission peaks were recorded at 345 ± 5 nm (excitation wave length was fixed at 285 ± 5 nm).

In order to evaluate the spectra properties of reagent blank, sample pretreatment method was performed without analyte of interest and the fluorescence spectra were recorded at 345 ± 5 nm. No main measurable influence of reagent blank on the quantitative analysis of carvedilol was observed. As a result, these excitation and emission wavelengths were selected for further quantitation of carvedilol.

Kind of ionic liquid
Based on the results obtained in our previous studies [18,19], three factors must be considered, in order to select a proper IL: (a) the density of IL as the extraction solvent must be higher than aqueous media, (b) IL must illustrate a desire hydrophobicity, (c) IL must be liquid and (d) these ionic material must be inexpensive. ILs with imidazolium scaffold which contain Cl$^-$, BF$_4^-$ and CF$_3$SO$_3^-$ show hydrophilic properties and those contain PF$_6^-$ and (CF$_3$SO$_2$)$_2$N$^-$ show hydrophobic properties.

According to these factors, [Hmim][PF$_6$] was used as an optimum microextraction solvent in all tests.

Optimization of diluting solvent
The viscosity of ionic liquids is relatively high; hence their direct transfer into the micro-cell of spectrofluorimeter for analyzing carvedilol is difficult. As a result, enriched-phase was conditioned and diluted. For this goal, some conditioner solvents such as methanol, ethanol, acetonitrile and acetone were evaluated as the diluting solvent. The obtained data showed that reproducible and sensitive

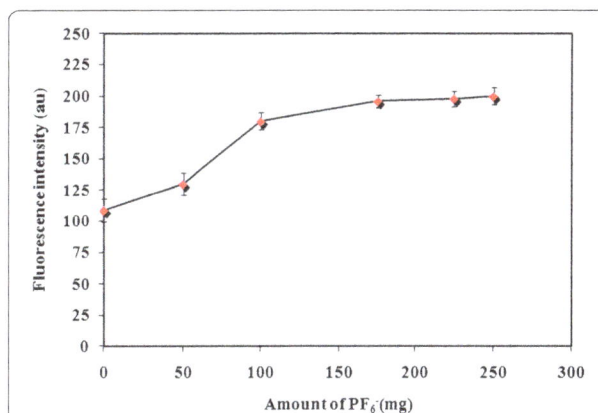

Figure 5 Effect of PF$_6^-$ Applied parameters: Carvedilol concentration 100 μg l^{-1}; Sample volume 10 ml; IL 60 mg; pH 9; temperature 50°C; λ_{ex} 285 ± 5 nm; λ_{em} 345 ± 5 nm. Indicated analytical signals are the average of three independent measurements and error bars correspond to their standard deviations.

signals were obtained in using ethanol as a conditioner agent. Due to the better data stability and ethanol environmental safety (less toxicity), this organic solvent was preferred and used in all experiments.

Optimization of IL amount
As it was mentioned, in this microextraction procedure, IL was applied as the microextraction phase. In this kind of sample pretreatment method, one of the major parameters affecting the performance is the amount of IL. This parameter has a significant effect on the reproducibility and sensitivity. In order to optimize the amount of extraction solvent, this parameter was tested within the range of 10–100 mg (Figure 4). Stable and sensitive fluorescence signals were obtained at 60 mg and this value was used for the rest of the work.

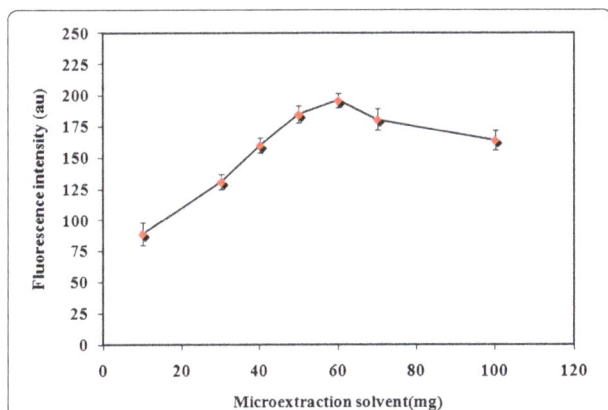

Figure 4 Effect of IL as the microextraction phase. Applied parameters: Carvedilol concentration 100 μg l^{-1}; sample volume 10 ml; NaPF$_6$ 175 mg; pH 9; temperature 50°C; λ_{ex} 285 ± 5 nm; λ_{em} 345 ± 5 nm. Indicated analytical signals are the average of three independent measurements and error bars correspond to their standard deviations.

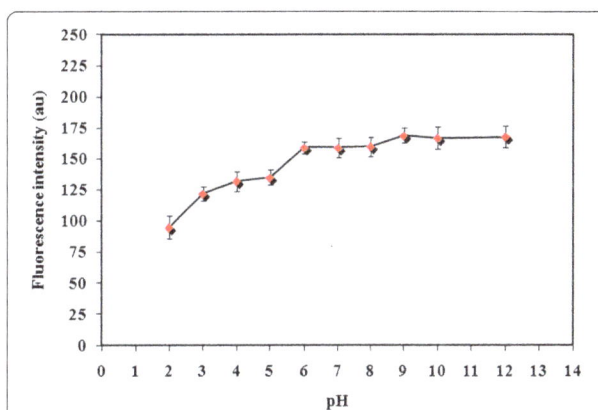

Figure 6 Effect of pH. Applied parameters: Carvedilol concentration 100 μg l^{-1}; sample volume 10 ml; IL 60 mg; NaPF$_6$ 175 mg; temperature 50°C; λ_{ex} 285 ± 5 nm; λ_{em} 345 ± 5 nm. Indicated analytical signals are the average of three independent measurements and error bars correspond to their standard deviations.

Table 1 Analytical characteristics of the presented work

Analytical factor	Values
Linear analytical response range (μg l^{-1})	10-250
Correlation coefficient (R^2)	0.9980
LOD[a] (μg l^{-1})	1.7
RSD[b] (%) (n = 4) (C$_{carvedilol}$ = 100 μg l^{-1})	3.8
PF[c]	50
Sample volume (mL)	10

[a]Limit of detection.
[b]Relative standard deviation.
[c]The ratio of diluted settled phase volume to aqueous volume gives the preconcentration factor (PF).

Optimization of PF$_6^-$ amount and ionic strength

As it was demonstrated in our previous works [18,19], dissolving a common ion of IL like PF$_6^-$, significantly reduce the solubility of IL. This act improves the extraction performance of carvedilol and provides better analytical sensitivity. Effect of this parameter was examined in the range of 0–250 mg (see Figure 5). A value of 175 mg was selected as an optimum value, in order to obtain proper signal stability and reproducibility.

One of the most important parameters which affects on the extraction performance is ionic strength of the aqueous media. An increase in ionic strength causes a considerable increase in solubility of IL. As a result, the volume of the settled phase depends on the salt content of the sample solution. This phenomenon has a negative influence on the stability of analytical data. Fortunately, presence of PF$_6^-$ (as a common ion) solves this problem and fixes the volume of the enrich phase. The effect of ionic strength was studied within the range of 0–40% (w/v) using NaNO$_3$ as an electrolyte. In the studied range, no significant influence on fluorescence signal was observed.

Table 2 Comparison of the proposed methodology with reported methods

Method	Sample	LOD (μg l^{-1})	LR (μg l^{-1})	Reference
DLLME-HPLC[a]	Human Urine, Human Plasma	4, 14	50-750, 20-1000	[6]
SPE-CE[b]	Human Urine	50	50-500	[23]
Synchronous fluorimetry	Pharmaceutical preparations	1	5-100	[24]
LLE-HPLC[c]	Human serum	2.5	5-500	[25]
Ionic liquid phase microextraction-spectrofluorimetry	Human Urine, Human Plasma, Pharmaceutical preparations	1.7	10-250	This work

[a]Dispersive liquid-liquid microextraction.
[b]Solid phase extraction-capillary electrophoresis.
[c]Liquid-liquid extraction.

Table 3 Results of recoveries of spiked biological samples

Sample	Carvedilol added (μg l^{-1})	Carvedilol found (μg l^{-1})[a]	RSD (%)	Recovery (%)
Urine	50	53.2	6.1	106.4
	100	98.3	5.9	98.3
	150	146.1	3.8	97.4
Plasma	50	44.6	5.6	89.2
	100	107.3	7.1	107.3
	150	154.8	4.2	103.2

[a]Average of four independent measurements.

Optimization of pH

In the case of microextraction of molecules like carvedilol, which have ionizable property, pH of the aqueous media reveals a significant role. In order to obtain the highest extraction efficiency, the uncharged condition of carvedilol must be prevalent (pK$_a$ value of carvedilol is 7.97) [22]. The effect of sample pH on the analytical sensitivity and reproducibility was tested within the range of 2–12 (Figure 6). In the recent experiments, HCl and NaOH were used for adjusting the pH. Based on the results obtained in this study, in order to obtain a compromise between sensitivity and reproducibility, pH 9 was selected for further experiments.

Influence of temperature

In this microextraction procedure, IL-phase is dispersed into the aqueous media under increasing the temperature. The effect of this parameter was evaluated in the range of 25–80°C. Finally, a temperature of 50°C was used as an optimum value. In order to collect the IL-phase after extraction, the sample solution must be cooled. For the recent goal, the aqueous media was placed in ice-water bath and kept at 0°C for 7 min.

Interference study

For studying the possible interferences coming form other compounds, which exist in real samples, some ions and compounds were subjected to the recent combined methodology. In this investigation, the effect of 100-fold of K$^+$, Na$^+$, Mg$^+$, F$^-$, Cl$^-$, NO$_3^-$, SO$_4^{2-}$, glucose, urea, lactic acid, sucrose, ascorbic acid and fructose as the interfering or quenching agents on the determination of

Table 4 Analysis of carvedilol tablets by the present work and the reported method (5)

Claimed (mg/tablet)	Proposed method (mg)[a]	Reported method (mg)[a]	Error (%)[b]	Error (%)[c]
12.5	12.3 (±0.5)	12.6 (±0.4)	−1.6	−2.9
25	25.5 (±1.0)	25.7 (±1.1)	+2.0	−0.7

[a]Values in parenthesis give the standard deviation based on four determinations.
[b]Error against the tablet value.
[c]Error against the reported method.

carvedilol (100 µg L^{-1}) was evaluated. No change in signals over than 4.5% was observed.

Analytical figures of merits

Linear analytical response range was defined by analyzing standard solutions of carvedilol. The obtained results revealed that analytical responses are linear from 10 to 250 µg l^{-1}. Other analytical figures of merits obtained by the ionic liquid phase microextraction-spectrofluorimetry are shown in Table 1. Limit of detection (LOD) was determined using a conventional equation, LOD = ks_{bl}/m. This equation is resulted from the equation showed below:

$$S_m = S_{bl} + ks_{bl}$$
$$S_m = mc_m + S_{bl}$$
$$c_m = \frac{S_m - S_{bl}}{m} = \frac{ks_{bl}}{m}$$

S_m, S_{bl}, s_{bl}, K, m and C_m show the minimum distinguishable analytical signal, average of blank analytical signal, blank standard deviation, constant value equal with 3 (confidence level of 95%), calibration graph slope and detection limit, respectively. Using this way, a value of 1.7 µg l^{-1} carvedilol was achieved. In order to determine the relative standard deviation (RSD), four 100 µg l^{-1} of carvedilol was subjected to the designed methodology and finally a value of 3.8% was obtained.

Comparison with reported methods

In order to show the analytical advantages of the proposed method for the quantitation of carvedilol, some details were compared with reported methods in literature, and these results are shown in Table 2. As it can be seen, considerable LOD and relatively wide dynamic range were obtained. In addition, in most of the reported methods, tedious sample pretreatment procedures, toxic solvents and expensive analytical instrument have been used for quantification. In contrast, in the proposed method, a rapid, benign and simple ionic liquid phase microextraction was utilized for preconcentration and extraction of carvedilol. No hazardous material was used in this sample pre-treatment method. In addition, an inexpensive and sensitive analytical instrument was applied for quantitation.

Analysis of carvedilol in real samples

In order to demonstrate the analytical application of the presented technique, real samples including human urine and human plasma were spiked with different amounts of carvedilol and analyzed. Results of this investigation are shown in Table 3. At it can be seen, the averages of recoveries are placed in the range of 97.4-106.2% (urine) and 89.2-107.3% (plasma). It can be concluded that in the case of accuracy and reproducibility,

satisfactory results were obtained. In the next step, some commercial pharmaceutical formulations involving carvedilol capsules and tablets were subjected to the designed method, in order to determine concentration of carvedilol (Table 4). The results obtained with the present work were compared with a reported method [5]. These data reveal the practical analytical application of the proposed method for analyzing the analyte of interest in pharmaceutical preparations.

Conclusion

A rapid, benign and simple ionic liquid phase microextraction was utilized for preconcentration and extraction of carvedilol. The enriched-phase was introduced to spectrofluorimeter for quantitation of carvedilol. No toxic and hazardous material was used in this sample pre-treatment method. In addition, an inexpensive and sensitive analytical instrument was applied for quantitative measurements. Finally, the combined methodology was successfully applied for quantitation of carvedilol in real samples.

Competing interests
The authors declare that they have no competing interests.

Authors' contributions
All authors contributed equally. Both authors read and approved the final manuscript.

Acknowledgment
Support of this investigation by the Islamic Azad University Tehran south branch through grant is gratefully acknowledged.

References
1. Packer M, Colicci WS, Sacker-Bernstein JD. Placebo-controlled study of the effects of carvedilol in patients with moderate to severe heart failure, the PRECISE trial. Circulation. 1996;94:2793–9.
2. Bristow MR, Gilbert EM, Abraham WT, Adams KF, Fowler MB, Hershberger RE, et al. Carvedilol produces dose related improvements in left ventricular function and survival in subjects with chronic heart failure. Circulation. 1996;94:2807–16.
3. Hokama N, Hobara N, Kameya H, Ohshiro S, Sakanashi M. Rapid and simple micro-determination of carvedilol in rat plasma by high performance liquid chromatography. J Chromatogr, B. 1999;732:233–8.
4. Machida M, Watanabe M, Takechi S, Kakinoki S, Nomura A. Measurement of carvedilol in plasma by high-performance liquid chromatography with electrochemical detection. J Chromatogr, B. 2003;798:187–91.
5. Zarghi A, Foroutan SM, Shafaati A, Khoddam A. Quantification of carvedilol in human plasma by liquid chromatography using fluorescence detection: application in pharmacokinetic studies. J Pharm Biomed Anal. 2007;44:250–3.
6. Zamani-Kalajahi M, Fazeli-Bakhtiyari R, Amiri M, Golmohammadi A, Afrasiabi A, Khoubnasabjafari M, et al. Analysis of losartan and carvedilol in urine and plasma samples using a dispersive liquid–liquid microextraction isocratic HPLC–UV method. Bioanalysis. 2012;4:2805–21.
7. Cardoso SG, Ieqqli CV, Pomblum SC. Spectrophotometric determination of carvedilol in pharmaceutical formulations through charge-transfer and ion-pair complexation reactions. Pharmazie. 2007;62:34–7.
8. Radi A, Elmogy T. Differential pulse voltammetric determination of carvedilol in tablets dosage form using glassy carbon electrode. Il Farmaco. 2005;60:43–6.

9. Soleymanpour A, Ghasemian M. Chemically modified carbon paste sensor for the potentiometric determination of carvedilol in pharmaceutical and biological media. Measurement. 2015;59:14–20.

10. Silva RA, Wang CC, Fernandez LP, Masi AN. Flow injection spectrofluorimetric determination of carvedilol mediated by micelles. Talanta. 2008;76:166–71.

11. Zeeb M, Ganjali MR, Norouzi P. Dispersive liquid-liquid microextraction followed by spectrofluorimetry as a simple and accurate technique for determination of thiamine (vitamin B$_1$). Michrochim Acta. 2010;168:317–24.

12. Bidari A, Jahromi EZ, Assadi Y, Hosseini MRM. Monitoring of selenium in water samples using dispersive liquid-liquid microextraction followed by iridium-modified tube graphite furnace atomic absorption spectrometry. Microchem J. 2007;87:6–12.

13. Zeeb M, Ganjali MR, Norouzi P, Kalaei MR. Separation and preconcentration system based on microextraction with ionic liquid for determination of copper in water and food samples by stopped-flow injection spectrofluorimetry. Food Chem Toxicol. 2011;49:1086–91.

14. Yao C, Anderson JL. Dispersive liquid-liquid microextraction using an in situ metathesis reaction to form an ionic liquid extraction phase for the preconcentration of aromatic compounds from water. Anal Bioanal Chem. 2009;395:1491–502.

15. Yao C, Li T, Wu P, Pitner WR, Anderson JL. Selective extraction of emerging contaminants from water samples by dispersive liquid-liquid microextraction using functionalized ionic liquids. J Chromatogr A. 2011;1218:1556–66.

16. Gharehbaghi M, Shemirani F, Baghdadi M. Dispersive liquid-liquid microextraction based on ionic liquid and spectrophotometric determination of mercury in water samples. Int J Environ Anal Chem. 2009;89:21–33.

17. Zeeb M, Sadeghi M. Modified ionic liquid cold-induced aggregation dispersive liquid-liquid microextraction followed by atomic absorption spectrometry for trace determination of zinc in water and food samples. Microchim Acta. 2011;175:159–65.

18. Zeeb M, Ganjali MR, Norouzi P. Modified ionic liquid cold-induced aggregation dispersive liquid-liquid microextraction combined with spectrofluorimetry for trace determination of ofloxacin in pharmaceutical and biological samples. Daru. 2011;19:446–54.

19. Zeeb M, Ganjali MR, Norouzi P. Preconcentration and Trace Determination of Chromium Using Modified Ionic Liquid Cold-Induced Aggregation Dispersive Liquid-Liquid Microextraction: Application to Different Water and Food Samples. Food Anal Method. 2013;6:1398–406.

20. Zeeb M, Mirza B, Zare-Dorabei R, Farahani H. Ionic Liquid-based Ultrasound-Assisted In Situ Solvent Formation Microextraction Combined with Electrothermal Atomic Absorption Spectrometry as a Practical Method for Preconcentration and Trace Determination of Vanadium in Water and Food Samples. Food Anal Method. 2014;7:1783–90.

21. Zeeb M, Tayebi-Jamil P, Berenjian A, Ganjali MR, Talei BOMR. Quantitative analysis of piroxicam using temperature controlled ionic liquid dispersive liquid phase microextraction followed by stopped-flow injection spectrofluorimetry. Daru. 2013;6:1398–406.

22. Stojanovic J, Vladimirov S, Marinkovic V, Velickovic D, Sibinovic P. Monitoring of the photochemical stability of carvedilol and its degradation products by the RP-HPLC method. J Serb Chem Soc. 2007;72:37–44.

23. Mazzarino M, De La Torre X, Mazzei F, Botre F. Rapid screening of beta-adrenergic agents and related compounds in human urine for anti-doping purpose using capillary electrophoresis with dynamic coating. J Sep Sci. 2009;32:3562–70.

24. Xiao Y, Wang HU, Han J. Simultaneous determination of carvedilol and ampicillin sodium by synchronous fluorimetry. Spectrochim Acta, Part A. 2005;61:567–73.

25. Gannu R, Yamsani VV, Rao YM. New RP-HPLC method with UV-detection for the determination of carvedilol in human serum. J Liq Chromatogr Rel Technol. 2007;30:1677–85.

9

Pharmacokinetics of calycopterin and xanthmicrol, two polymethoxylated hydroxyflavones with anti-angiogenic activities from *Dracocephalum kotschyi Bioss*

Seyedeh-Somayeh Zamani[1], Mohsen Hossieni[2], Mahmoud Etebari[1], Pirooz Salehian[3] and Soltan Ahmad Ebrahimi[4*]

Abstract

Background: Recently flavonoids have attracted the attention of researchers in the fight against cancer. Calycopterin and xanthomicrol, are two polymethoxylated flavonoids found in the aerial parts of *Dracocephalum kotschyi* Bioss.. We have recently shown that these compounds possess antiangiogenic activity and may be of value as potential anticancer agents. In order to demonstrate putative in vivo antitumor effect of these compounds we needed preliminary information on both pharmacokinetics and toxicological properties of these two agents.

Method: A new online SPE HPLC method for measurement of calycopterin and xanthomicrol in rat plasma was developed. Pharmacokinetic parameters of calycopterin and xanthomicrol, after i.v. administration in rats, were determined.

Results: The plasma half-life for both agents was around 4 h, however, the volume of distribution of calycopterin appeared to be about 8 times greater than xanthomicrol. This was probably due the greater hydrophobicity of the former which had other consequences such as much smaller maximum plasma concentration of calycopterin compared to its less methoxylated congener. Preliminary toxicological study of xanthomicrol failed to show any behavioral, histological and biochemical adverse effects after repeated administrations of high doses.

Keywords: Calycopterin, Xanthomicrol, Flavonoids, *Dracocephalum kotschyi*, Pharmacokinetics

Background

The demonstration of antiproliferative effects of a number of flavonoids against cancer cell lines, has attracted the interest of researchers in these chemicals as potential therapeutic agents for the prevention and/or treatment of different forms of neoplasms [1]. The in vitro effects of flavonoids range from being generally cytotoxic [2] to showing selective effects against some cell lines and not others [3]. The molecular mechanisms involved in the cellular effects of flavonoids reflect a similar diversity: from a change in inner mitochondrial membrane permeability leading to cell death by many flavonoids [4] to selective regulation of the miR-101/MKP-1/MAPK pathway to decrease the inflammatory response [5] by genkwanin. Structure activity relationship (SAR) studies have been able to delineate the link between molecular structure and selectibity of cytotoxic effects for some of these compounds [6]. For example, data obtained by Moghadam et al. [6] suggests that polymethoxylated hydroxyflavones like xanthomicrol and calycopterin (Fig. 1) appear to have more selective activities against cancer cell lines compared to hydroxyflavones with no methoxy groups such as luteolin or apigenin. It can be reasoned that a xenobiotic with across the board cytoxicity does not get us any nearer to finding new therapeutic agents with less side-effects than the currently used drugs and thus the more selective agents should be better candidates for further research. However, as

* Correspondence: ebrahimi.sa@iums.ac.ir
[4]Department of Pharmacology, Iran University for Medical Sciences, Tehran, Iran
Full list of author information is available at the end of the article

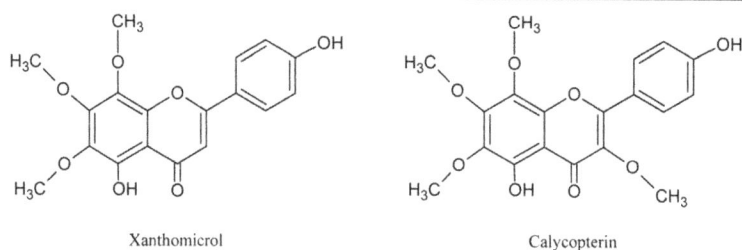

Fig. 1 Structures of calycopterin and xanthomicrol

our knowledge about the in vitro mode of action of these agents increases, we obtain a better understanding why those flavonoids which are not globally cytotoxic against a multitude of malignant cell lines, may help decrease tumor size in vivo and therefore have potential anticancer activity with little or no direct cytotoxic effects on neoplastic cells making up the bulk of the tumor. Recent work in our laboratory on calycopterin and xanthomicrol has shown these compounds to possess, in addition to their selective cytotoxic effects, potent antiangiogenic activities which appear to be due to inhibition of endothelial cell proliferation via decreased VEGF activity [7]. The importance of angiogenesis in tumor growth and metastasis was first suggested by Folkman [8] and later demonstrated by many other workers [9–11] and may provide an explanation for the antineoplastic effect of many flavanoids e.g., genistein [12]. It is also worth remembering that currently there are a number of agents under clinical trial as antitumor drugs with this mechanism of action [13].

The demonstration of in vitro antiangiogenic activities for these two polymethoxylated flavones has to be followed by investigations into the in vivo antitumor effects of xanthomicrol and calycopterin. However, these efforts are hampered by a lack of pharmacokinetic and toxicological data about these agents. In other words, we not only have to obtain data which links administered dose to plasma flavonoid concentrations but also have to provide preliminary evidence on the lack of overt toxicity. This study was undertaken to achieve these goals.

Methods
Plant material
Aerial parts of *Dracocephalum kotschyi* Bioss. were obtained from a herbalist in the city of Isfahan and the identity of the specimen was confirmed by Dr Gh Amin, Faculty of Pharmacy, Tehran University of Medical Sciences (voucher specimen number at the faculty of pharmacy herbarium: PMP-304).

Isolation and purification of xanthomicrol and calycopterin, identity confirmation, recovery calculations
Xanthomicrol and calycopterin were isolated and purified as previously reported [6] with some modifications to the HPLC step. Briefly, 10 kg of dried aerial parts of Dracocephalum kotschyi Bioss. were manually powdered and extracted in 50 g batches by overnight extraction with 400 mL ethyl acetate using a Soxhelt apparatus. The extract aliquots from 10 kg plant material were dried in vacuo, combined and finally dissolved in 8 L chloroform and filtered through Whatman No. 1 filter paper to remove particulate matter. The flavonoid content was extracted in 1 L batches into 1 L 1 M ammonia solution. The intensely yellow ammonia solution was acidified to pH 1 using concentrated HCl and the flavonoid content was back extracted into 200 mL ethylacetate. The non-methoxylated hydroxyflavones were removed by treatment with alumina. The organic solvent was evaporated in vacuo. The material obtained in this step was subjected to semipreparative HPLC purification as follows. A 10 μm Nucleosil ODS column from Macherey Nagel (21x250mm) was equilibrated with a mobile phase containing 37 % ACN, 24 % MeOH, 38.5 % Water and 0.5 % triethylamine, adjusted to pH 6 with acetic acid. A saturated solution of the extract in mobile phase was centrifuged at 10000 g for 5 min and 1.7 mL of the supernatant was injected onto the column. The column eluent (5 mL/min) was monitored at 226 nm using a LKB Uvicord UV detector connected to a Younglin (Younglin, South Korea) data acquisition module. Fractions containing xanthomicrol, calycopterin and circimaritin were collected and dried by lyophilization. Peak identities were confirmed by infrared spectroscopic analysis [6]. The flavones content (μg per gram of dried aerial parts of the plant material) was calculated. Purity of isolated compounds was examined using analytical HPLC on a 4.6x150mm, ODS-2, 5 μm, Tracer Excell column (Technochroma, Spain) using the same mobile phase as described above, pumped isocratically while detecting at 263 nm.

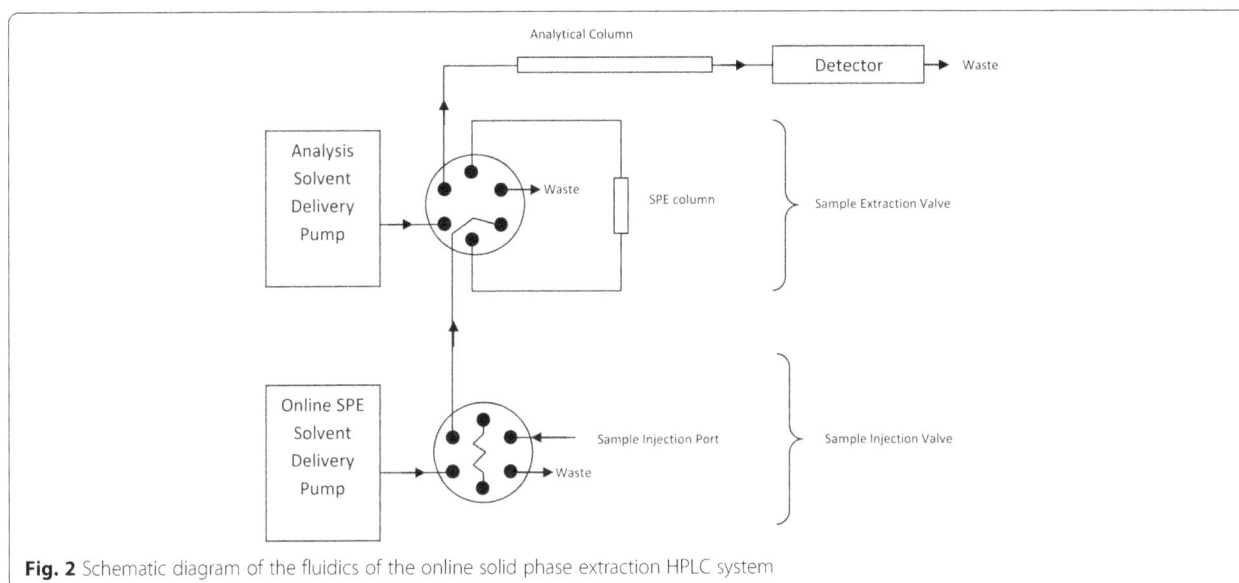

Fig. 2 Schematic diagram of the fluidics of the online solid phase extraction HPLC system

Analytical HPLC method for measurement of xanthomicol and calycopterin

Confirmation of calycopterin, xanthomicrol and circimaritin identity was carried out using HPLC analysis of purified compound compared to the material obtained from previous work [6] and also IR spectroscopy. A HPLC method with online solid phase extraction was developed for the analysis of xanthomicrol and calycopterin in biological fluids (Fig. 1) using circimaritin as internal standard (IS). 100 μL of plasma and 10 μL of 500 μg/mL IS were mixed in a 2 mL microcentrifuge tube. 40 μL of 10 mg/mL $ZnSO_4$ was added to the tube and the content was mixed. After addition of 200 μL acetonitrile, the tube was placed in an orbital shaker for 10 min. The samples were subsequently centrifuged at 14000 g for 10 min the supernatant was subjected to online extraction/HPLC analysis as follows:

At the start of every run, the sample injection valve and the sample extraction valve were switched to load position (Fig. 1). 250 μL of sample was injected into the sample loop of the sample injection valve. The valve was switched to the inject position which diverted the flow from the online SPE (solid phase extraction) solvent delivery pump (500 μL/min) through the sample loop which in turned carried the sample onto the online SPE column (3×15mm, ODS-2, 5 μm). After 2 min, the sample extraction valve was switched to inject position. This allowed the mobile phase from the analysis solvent delivery pump (1 mL/min) to wash any material retained by the online SPE system, onto the analytical column (4.6×150mm, ODS-2, 5 μm, Tracer Excell, Technochroma, Spain) for separation and measurement. The mobile phase pumped by online SPE solvent delivery pump consisted of acetonitrile:water (35:65) and the mobile phase pumped by the analysis

solvent delivery pump was composed of acetonitrile:-methanol:water:triethylamine (37:24:38.5:0.5). 16 min after the start of analysis, the mobile phase pumped by the analysis solvent delivery pump was switched to methanol:te-trahydrofurane:dichloromethane (80:10:10) for 3 min. This allowed for highly non-polar compounds retained by the SPE and analytical column to be flushed. Detection was at 263 nm.

The assay system was calibrated for both xanthomicrol and calycopterin over the concentration range of 125 to 1500 ng/mL. In order to estimate the recovery of the assay, the calibration curve with online SPE was compared to a standard curve injected directly into the analytical column, without the SPE step. Inter-day and intra-day variation and S/N ratio were calculated for this analytical system.

Rat femoral vein cannulation

All procedures involving animals were carried out after the approval and under the supervision of the Ethics Committee for Animal Expreiments of Iran University for Medical Sciences. In order to be able to withdraw blood samples at predefined time points during pharmacokinetic studies, femoral vein of male Wistar rats, in the weight range of 280 to 300 g, were catheterized,

Table 1 Flavone content of *Dracocephalum kotschyi Bioss.* dried aerial parts

Flavone	Specific amount (μg flavone / g plant material)
Xanthomicrol	95.2
Calycopterin	38
Circimaritin	15

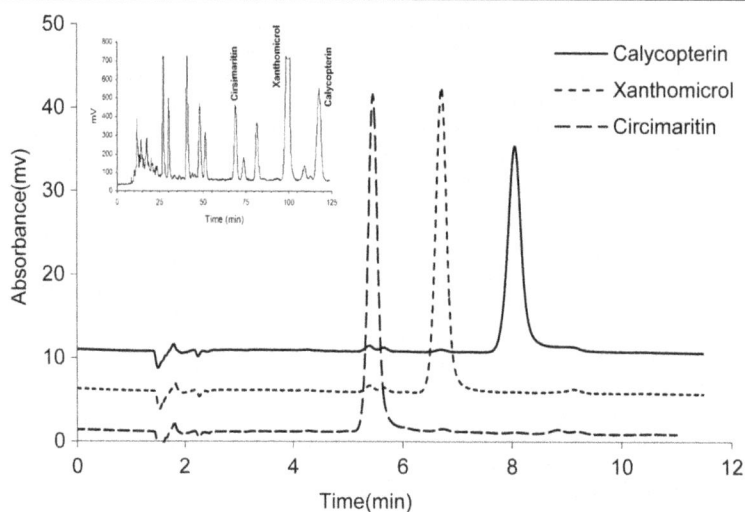

Fig. 3 Purity of isolated flavonoids as determined by analytical HPLC. The inset shows a preparative chromatogram of *Dracocephalum kotschyi Biossy* flavonoid fraction

under anaesthesia, using the method described by Jespersen et al. [14]. After the placement of the catheter, the animals were allowed to recover for 24 h, during which time, the rats were checked for signs of bleeding and the catheters were checked for patency.

Pharmacokinetic study

Xanthomicrol or calycopterin was dissolved in 200 µL of dimethylsulfoxide (DMSO) and injected into the dorsal tail vein of rats. Just before drug injection (time zero) and at 1, 5, 10, 20, 60, 120 and 240 min after drug injection, 300 µL of blood were withdrawn via the femoral vein which had been catheterized previously. In order to prevent phlebotomy induced hypovolemia, 200 µL normal saline was injected via the femoral catheter after each blood sample withdrawal. Blood samples were centrifuged at 4 °C for 10 min at 4000 g. Plasma was collected and stored frozen at -80 °C until needed.

Toxicological studies in mice

Toxicity studies were carried out using Balb/C mice in the 25-30 g weight range. Drug administration was via the I.P. methoud. Animals were assigned to

five groups of three: one-Control groups which received no treatment, two-Vehicle control which received 60 µL of DMSO (dimethyl sulfoxide) for 6 days, 3- Test group one which received 30 mg/kg body weight xanthomicrol in 60 µL of DMSO per day, 4- Test group two which received 40 mg/kg body weight xanthomicrol on 60 µL of DMSO per day and 5- Test group three which received 50 mg/kg body weight xanthomicrol on 60 µL of DMSO per day. The animals were weighed and examined for changes in skin tone, signs of fur loss and changes in bowl function [15]. On the seventh day, the animals were anaesthetized under an atmosphere of chloroform. Once fully anaesthetized, blood samples were collected from the heart and the animals were killed by cervical dislocation. Serum samples were analyzed for hepatic enzymes AST and ALT [16] and also for creatinin levels [17]. Kidneys, liver, lung, intestines and stomach were removed from animals and placed in 10 % formalin solution for subsequent paraffin embedding, sectioning, staining and histological studies. Tissue sections were examined for fibrotic, inflammatory and vascular changes by a qualified pathologist [18].

Table 2 Validation parameters for the HPLC assay of calycopterin and xanthomicrol

Compound	Calibration Equation $Y = mX + C$, R^2	Interday at 500 ng/mL	Intraday at 500 ng/mL	LOD (ng/mL) (S/N) = 3	LOQ (ng/mL) (S/N) = 10
Calycopterin	$Y = 0.0002X + 0.0014$ $R^2 = 0.998$	4.3 %	2.5 %	10	34
Xanthomircol	$Y = 0.0001X + 0.0023$ $R^2 = 0.999$	3.9 %	2.2 %	8	32

S/N, signal to noise ratio

Results

Isolation and purification of xanthomicrol, calycopterin and circimaritin, identity confirmation

Processing of 10 kg of dried aerial parts of *Dracocephalum kotschyi Bioss.* yielded 476 mg of xanthomicrol, 190 mg of calycopterin and 60 mg of circimaritin. The compounds obtained appeared to be pure as demonstrated by the existence of single peak in HPLC analysis (Fig. 2). The identities of isolated flavones were confirmed HPLC analysis and IR spectroscopy in comparison with standard material previously obtained [6]. The flavones contents were determined (Table 1).

Analytical HPLC method for measurement of xanthomicol and calycopterin

Plasma samples spiked with calycopterin (125 to 1500 ng/mL) or xanthomicrol (125 to 2000 ng/mL) were extracted as described above and subsequently analyzed by analytical HPLC using online extraction (Fig. 3). Both calibration curves were linear over the concentration ranges described (Table 2). Recovery of the extraction method was investigated by comparing the peak areas of 500 ng/mL of calycopterin and xanthomicrol and 1430 ng/mL circimaritin (as IS) obtained from injection of mixtures using the on-line SPE method with the same flavone mixtures injected directly onto the analytical column, without the online solid phase extraction step. Recoveries of calycopterin and xanthomicrol were 94 % and 92 % respectively.

Pharmacokinetic study

Figure 4 shows the plots of plasma flavones concentration against time for both xanthomicrol and calycopterin. For both xanthomicrol and calycopterin, two-compartment models were found to adequately describe the changes in concentration with time (Fig. 5). Pharmacokinetic parameters obtained from constructing the residual concentration verses time curve for these two-compartmental models are presented in Table 3. Rate constants for transfer between the central and peripheral compartments (K_{21} and K_{12}) and also the elimination process (K_{el}) were also calculated.

Toxicological studies in mice

There were no significant differences in serum creatinin content, alanine transaminase (ALT) and aspartic acid transaminase (AST) activities between control, vehicle and test groups of mice which had received xanthomicrol at 30, 40 or 50 mg/kg body weight (Table 4). The weight of animals in control group (27.1 g ± 1.2), on different days, were not significantly different compared to the animals in xanthomicrol groups (27.7 ± 1.7 g), on corresponding days.

Histological examination of tissue samples from kidney, small and large intestines, lung and heart of test animals showed absence of significant pathological

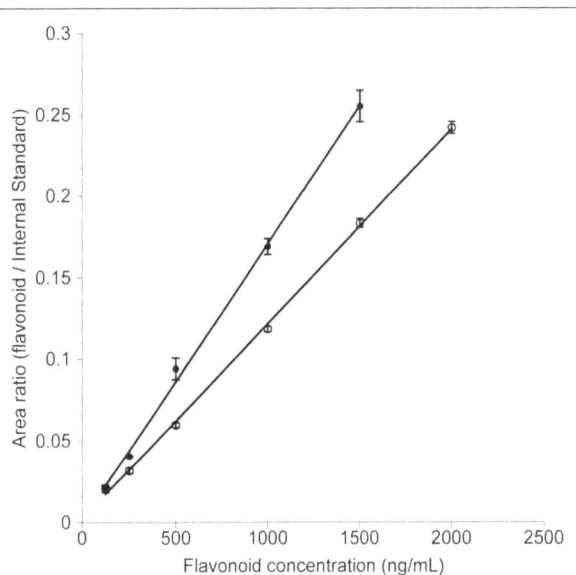

Fig. 4 Calibration curve for xanthomicrol (o) and calycopterin (●) spiked in plasma. The values are mean ± SEM for three independent analyses

change in animals receiving xanthomicrol compared to the control group (Fig. 6) (Table 5).

Discussion

The research into the proposed antineoplastic properties of Spinal-Z, an Iranian herbal remedy, composed of peganum harmala seeds extracted and *Dracocephalum kotschyi Bioss.* leaves extract has been going on in our laboratory for more than 15 years. The inhibitory effects of β-carbolines found in peganum harmala seeds on topoisomerase activity [19] was demonstrated first, however, further work suggested a more prominent role for selective

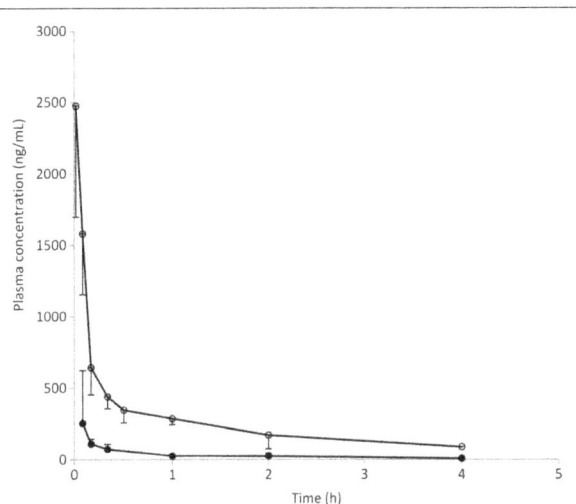

Fig. 5 Plasma concentration-time profile of calycopterin (●) and xanthomicrol (o) in rats after IV administration of 20 mg/kg of the flavnoid. Values are mean ± SEM, n = 4

Table 3 Pharmacokinetic parameters for xanthomicrol and calycopterin after i.v. bolus administration to rats

	C_0 (µg/L)	V_c (L)	$t_{1/2}$ (h)	K_{21} (h^{-1})	K_{12} (h^{-1})	K_{el} (h^{-1})	Cl_a (L/h)
Calycopterin (20 mg/kg)	312	63.9	3.8	0.52	1.39	0.26	16.8
Xanthomicrol (20 mg/kg)	2345	8.5	4.2	0.46	1.88	0.21	1.8

C_0: Initial plasma concentration; V_c: Volume of distribution of the central compartment; t_{half}: Biological half-life; K_{21}: Rate constant of transfer from the central compartment into the peripheral compartment; K_{12}: Rate constant of transfer from the peripheral compartment into the central compartment; K_{el}: Rate constant of elimination from the central compartment, Cl_a: Clearance rate of the central compartment

cytotoxic activity of flavonoids found in *Dracocephalum kotschyi Bioss.* leaves extract [20]. Recently we were able to show calycopterin and xanthomicrol to have anti-angiogenic activity in ex vivo and in vitro models of angiogenesis [7]. Although there is some data suggesting antineoplastic effects for xanthomicrol in mice (data not published), in order to proceed to investigate the in vivo antineoplastic effects of calycopterin and xanthomicrol, one has to have information about pharmacokinetic parameters of these two flavonoids, particularly the maximum attainable plasma concentration after a particular dose and drug half-life. Also any toxic effects they may possess in whole animals will be of great interest. The current work was carried out to furnish such data.

In order to speed up the purification process and increase the productivity of the semi-preparative HPLC purification, the procedure for extraction, isolation and purification of xanthomicrol and calycopterin reported previously [6] was modified. Inclusion of an alumia treatment step after alternate alkali/acid extraction of the flavanoid fraction, helped remove the unmethoxylated hydroxyflavones. This treatment, decreased the complexity of the extract to the extent that a new mobile phase containing triethylamine could be used for the semi-preparative HPLC phase. The solubility of the crude extract in the new mobile phase was about 10 times greater than the previously reported simple mobile phase, which meant that during each semi-preparative HPLC step, 10 times greater quantities of calycopterin and xanthomicrol were obtained. Also, the change in mobile phase helped shorten the run time to 70 min compared to the previously reported 125 min. Taken

together, the efficiency of the new purification process was increased by about 20 fold. However, the total recovery of xanthomicrol, calycopterin and circimaritin, were similar to what had been reported previously (Table 1) [6].

During the pharmacokinetic study, one has to withdraw multiple blood samples from the test animal over a few hours. In order to ensure relatively constant physiological homeostasis during the pharmacokinetic study, it is best to withdraw as little a blood sample as possible. This in turn means a small amount of plasma harvested for analytical purposes, typically about 100 µL for the rat, increasing the sensitivity and repeatability constrains of the assay method. Therefore, in order to measure calycopterin and xanthomicrol in rat plasma, a HPLC method was developed and validated that utilized online solid phase extraction, offering enhanced sensitivity and improved low-concentration precision. The method was simple in that plasma deprotination was acheived by addition of zinc sulphate and acetonitrile. The total volume of deproteinated sample was 350 µL, of which, after centrifugation, 250 µL was injected onto the column. In other words, the content of greater that 70 % of the plasma sample was loaded onto the analytical HPLC column, maximizing the total material loaded. Also, the on-line SPE, concentrated the sample's flavonoid content, helping tominimize band broadening through the analytical column, again enhancing the detection and quantification limits of the assay (Table 2). Although the quantitation of xanthomicrol or calycopterin in plasma has not been reported before, workers have measured other flavanoids in human or animal serum: Busby et al. [21] used 1000 µL of human serum to measure isoflavones genistein and daidzein. They achieved a LOQ of 1.7 and 3 µg/mL for genistein and daidzein respectively. These values are approximately 30 times higher than those obtained for xanthomicrol and calycopterin in the current work. Biasutto [22] measured quercetin in rat plasma. Using 200 µL samples and a sample deproteination step involving solvent extraction, they achieved a LOQ of 50 ng/mL for this flavonoid [22]. This is similar to the value obtained in the present work, however, their method was more elaborate and time consuming.

The assay thus developed in this study was applied to the pharmacokinetic study of xanthomicrol and calycopterin in rats. The I.V. route for drug administration was

Table 4 Effects of different doses of xanthomicrol on kidney and liver functions

Group	Serum Creatinin (mg/mL)	Serum ALT (IU/L)	Serum AST (IU/L)
Control	0.36 ± 0.019	43 ± 15	180 ± 48
Vehicle	0.35 ± 0.015	49 ± 29	228 ± 94
30 mg/kg Xanthomicrol	0.36 ± 045	38 ± 8.8	138 ± 37
40 mg/kg Xanthomicrol	0.35 ± 0.036	22 ± 19	130 ± 49
50 mg/ kg Xanthomicrol	0.39 ± 0.02	30 ± 3.0	316 ± 163

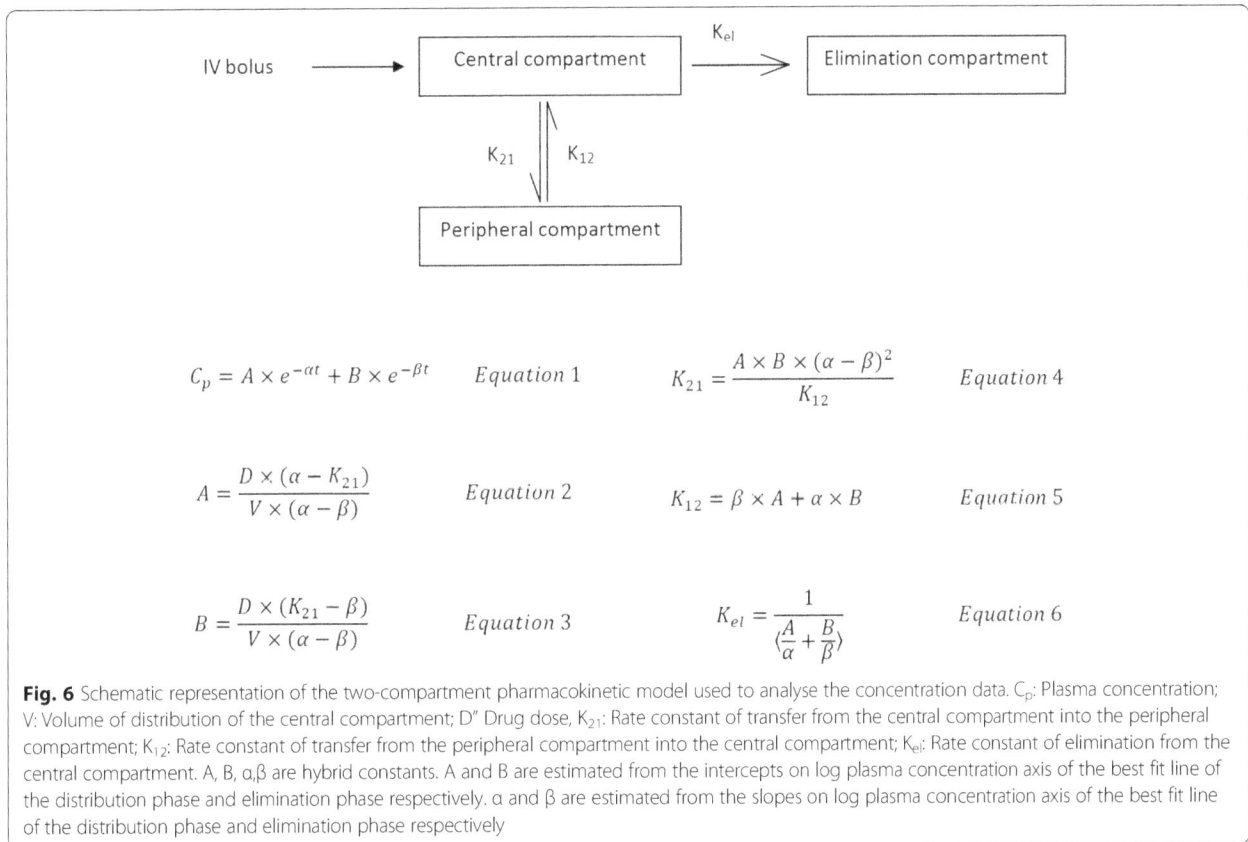

$$C_p = A \times e^{-\alpha t} + B \times e^{-\beta t} \qquad Equation\ 1$$

$$A = \frac{D \times (\alpha - K_{21})}{V \times (\alpha - \beta)} \qquad Equation\ 2$$

$$B = \frac{D \times (K_{21} - \beta)}{V \times (\alpha - \beta)} \qquad Equation\ 3$$

$$K_{21} = \frac{A \times B \times (\alpha - \beta)^2}{K_{12}} \qquad Equation\ 4$$

$$K_{12} = \beta \times A + \alpha \times B \qquad Equation\ 5$$

$$K_{el} = \frac{1}{\left(\frac{A}{\alpha} + \frac{B}{\beta}\right)} \qquad Equation\ 6$$

Fig. 6 Schematic representation of the two-compartment pharmacokinetic model used to analyse the concentration data. C_p: Plasma concentration; V: Volume of distribution of the central compartment; D" Drug dose, K_{21}: Rate constant of transfer from the central compartment into the peripheral compartment; K_{12}: Rate constant of transfer from the peripheral compartment into the central compartment; K_{el}: Rate constant of elimination from the central compartment. A, B, α, β are hybrid constants. A and B are estimated from the intercepts on log plasma concentration axis of the best fit line of the distribution phase and elimination phase respectively. α and β are estimated from the slopes on log plasma concentration axis of the best fit line of the distribution phase and elimination phase respectively

chosen because this ensured all administered dose would reach the systemic circulation, without the need to take into account loss during oral absorption and less than complete bioavailability. Therefore the data obtained from I.V. administration of the flavonoids, would give more direct estimates of pharmacokinetic parameters of interest in this study which would enable us to design more valid in vivo antitumor assays for these two agents.

Both agents are relatively hydrophobic and thus do not dissolve in water based solvent systems. A number of solvents which were able to dissolve xanthomicrol and calycopterin were investigated as vehicles for the delivery of these compounds into the blood stream. DMSO was chosen as it is relatively benign in terms of toxicological effects (a number of drug formulations or medical devices containing DMSO are marketed e.g., RIMSO-50 from Bioniche Pharma, USA and Dolicur from Schering, Germany). Also, the volume required as vehicle (200 μL) was small compared to total blood volume in rat (about 20 mL) and would be unlikely to have an appreciable effect on pharmacokinetics of flavonoids being studied.

In order to keep to a predefined sample withdrawal schedule, a cannula was inserted into the rat's vein at least 24 h before pharmacokinetic study. Cannulation procedure for the femoral artery [14] proved to be easier

than that of the carotid artery with faster recovery of the animal after the procedure. Blood sampling schedule was designed to ensure there were enough samples in the initial period after drug administration, during which time changes in drug concentration were likely to be rapid. Plots of the logarithm of both calycopterin and xanthomicrol plasma concentrations verses time were not linear which suggested that the one compartment model would be unsuitable for analysis of concentration data. Two compartment analyses were successfully applied.

Calycopterin has one methoxy group more than xanthomicrol and is thus expected to be more hydrophobic. This is confirmed by the longer retention time of the former during reverse phase chromatography (Fig. 3). However, the extent of the effect of this increased hydrophobicity on disposition of calycopterin in rat, was unexpected. When administered at 20 mg/kg, xanthomicrol had a calculated initial plasma concentration of 2345 μg/L while the corresponding value for calycopterin was 312 μg/L (Table 3). This is probably because, compared to xanthomicrol, calycopterin distributes more rapidly into various organs thus leaving blood or the "central compartment" in our model, more quickly. This, which is also reflected in the difference in the V_c

Table 5 Effects of different doses of xanthimcrol on tissue histology

Animal	Tissue	Inflammation structural change	Fibrosin	Vascular change	Notes
Vehicle 1	Lung/Liver/Heart/ Kidney	Absent	Absent	None	Normal
Vehicle 2	Small intestine/ Large intestine/ Gastric wall	Focal inflammation in gastric wall	Absent	None	Normal
Vehicle 3	Lung/Liver/Heart/ Kidney	Absent	Absent	Hypermic	Increased type II pneumocytes
Test group 1,1	Small intestine/ Large intestine/ Gastric wall	Absent	Absent	None	Normal
Test group 1, 2	Lung/Liver/Heart/ Kidney	Absent	Absent	None	Normal
Test group 1, 3	Small intestine/ Large intestine/ Gastric wall	Absent	Absent	None	Normal
Test group 2, 1	Lung/Liver/Heart/ Kidney	Focal inflammation in lung tissue	Absent	Increased vascularization in lung sample	Increased type II pneumocytes
Test group 2, 2	Small intestine/ Large intestine/ Gastric wall	Absent	Absent	None	Normal
Test group 2,3	Lung/Liver/Heart/ Kidney	Lymphocyte infilteration in lung sample, Subcapsular inflammation in liver sample	Absent	Hypermic	Normal
Test group 3,1	Small intestine/ Large intestine/ Gastric wall	Absent	Absent	None	Increased type II pneumocytes
Test group 3,2	Lung/Liver/Heart/ Kidney	Focal inflammation in lung sample	Absent	None	Increased type II pneumocytes
Test group 3,3	Lung/Liver/Heart/ Kidney	Absent	Absent	None	Normal

values for these flavonoids (Table 3), is also confirmed by the difference in the K_{12} rate constants. The rate constant for transfer of calycopterin into the central compartment is smaller than that of xanthomicrol which suggests a tendency for calycopterin to distribute more easily into tissues. The elimination rate constants are not very different, which may explain similar $t_{1/2}$ of elimination for these two flavonoids (Table 3).

Our previous research had shown that at 500 ng/mL, both calycopterin and xanthomicrol inhibited capillary-like tube formation by HUVEC cell [7]. Our aim in this work was to find doses of these flavonoids which could produce such plasma levels over extended periods. This would let us investigate the in vivo effects of these compounds on experimentally induced tumors at therapeutically relevant plasma concentrations. The models generated, were used to predict the plasma concentration-time profiles for different doses of calycopterin and xanthomicrol (Fig. 7). After a single I.V. dose of 30 mg/kg, xanthomicrol plasma concentration would be greater than 500 ng/

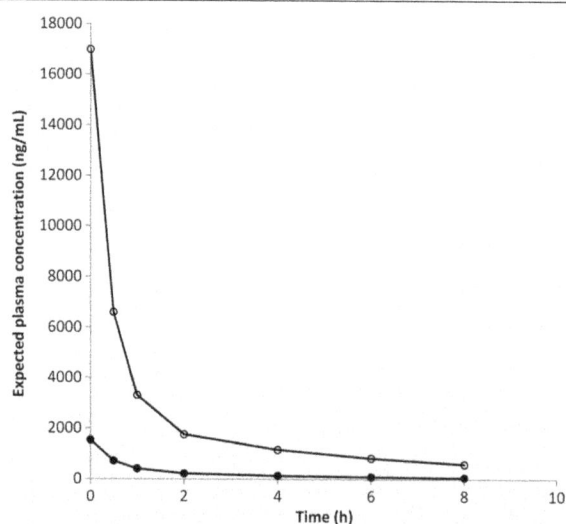

Fig. 7 Predicted plasma calycopterin (●) and xanthomicrol (○) concentration-time profiles after a single IV bolus dose of 30 mg/kg or either compound in the rat. The values were calculated based upon the two compartment models developed in this work

mL for more than 6 h while calycopterin's plasma concentration would dip below 500 ng/mL 30 min after administration.

The pharmacokinetic superiority, in terms of maximum attainable concentration and the time it took to leave the central compartment, meant that xanthomicrol had the greater potential as an anti-angiogenic agent. Thus, the potential toxic effects of xanthomicrol at 30, 40 and 50 mg/kg/day for six days, were studied. As none of the animals displayed xanthomicrol induced toxic effects with in the first 24 h after the highest dose, this flavonoid appears not to have acute toxic effects. None of the animal died in any of the administered dose groups. After six days of drug treatment, none of the animals AST levels, which are indicative of liver damage, were not significantly different amongst control, vehicle and test groups. Histological examination (Fig. 8) was unable to find xenobiotic induced damage to vital organs. There was no change in animal weights compared to control group and no animal showed any signs of motor or behavioral abnormalities. Xanthomicrol, at administered doses, did not appear to have toxic effects in mice. However, it is important to remember that this study did not attempt to determine LD_{50} value for xanthomicrol or show long term safety. Future toxicological studies must determine LD_{50} and also examine sub-acute and chronic toxic effects.

Conclusion

Both calycopterin and xanthomicrol have anti-angiogenic properties however, our data suggests that from a pharmacokinetic point of view, xanthomicrol has greater potential as an antitumor agent.

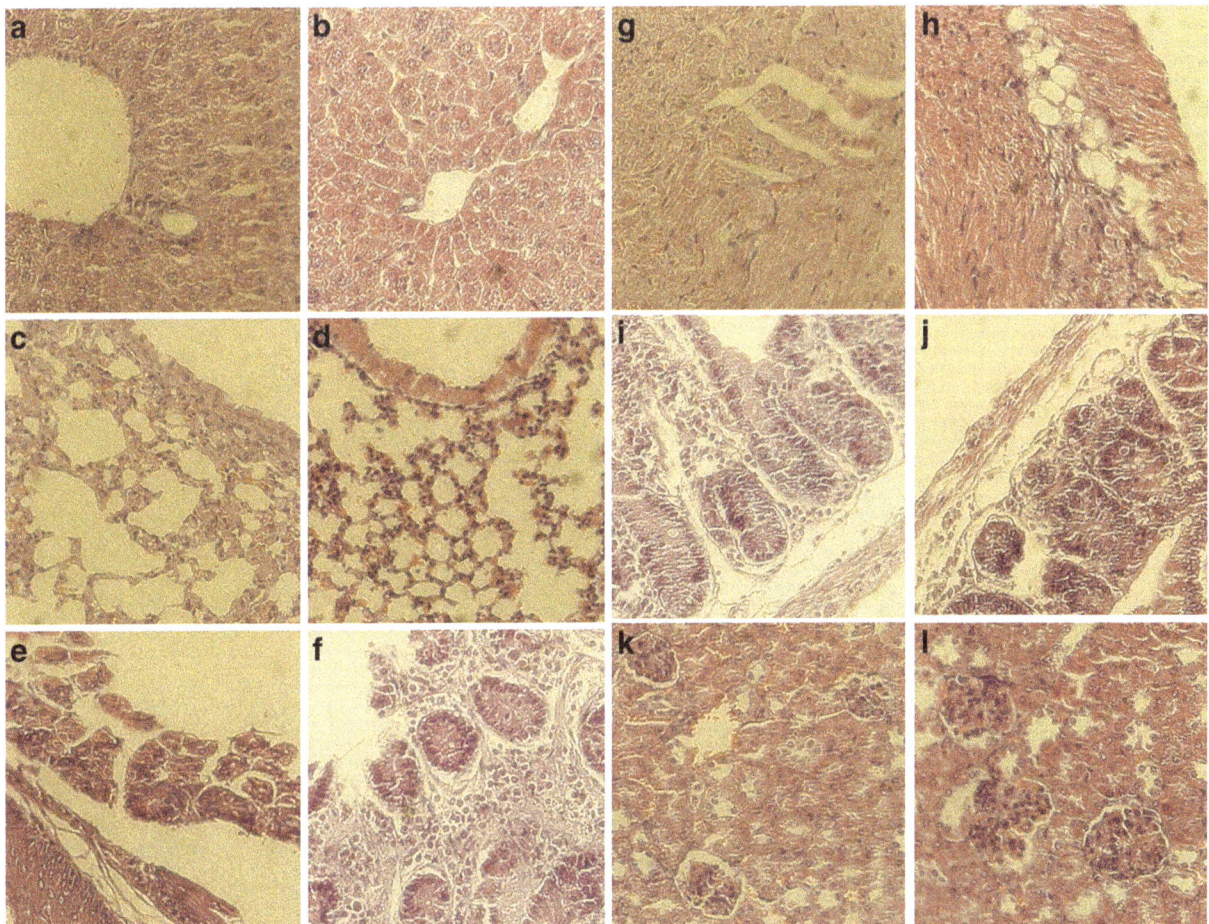

Fig. 8 Effect of xanthomicrol treatment on vital organ histology in mice. Images on the left have been selected from animals treated with 50 mg/kg xanthomicrol and images on the right are from control animals. **a** and **b** Liver, **c** and **d** Lung, **e** and **f** Stomach wall, **g** and **h** Heart muscle, **i** and **j** Small intestine, **k** and **l** Kidney

Abbreviations

AST: Aspartate transaminase; ALT: Alanine transaminase; DMSO: Dimethyl sulfoxide; SPE: Solid phase extraction; VEGF: Vascular endothelial growth factor

Acknowledgements

The authors would like to acknowledge that Iran University for Medical Sciences furnished the funding for this research (grant number 20919).

Authors' contributions

Separation, purification and kinetics of xanthomicrol was carried out by M Hosseini. Separation, purification and kinetics of calycopterin was carried out by S Zamani. Toxicological study of xanthomicrol was carried out by M Etebari. P Salehian was responsible for the histological work. S A Ebrahimi conceived the study and developed the HPLC assay for analysis of serum hydroxyflavones, analyzed serum concentration data, prepared the manuscript. All authors read and approved the final manuscript.

Competing interests

The authors declare that they have no competing interests.

Author details

[1]Department of Pharmacology and Toxicology, Isfahan Pharmaceutical Sciences Research Center, School of Pharmacy and Pharmaceutical Sciences, Isfahan University of Medical Sciences, Isfahan, Iran. [2]Department of Pharmaology, School of Medicine, Tehran University for Medical Sciences, Tehran, Iran. [3]Sarem Fertility and Infertility Research Centre, Sarem Hospital, P.O. Box 1396956111Shahrak-e-Ekbatan, Tehran, Iran. [4]Department of Pharmacology, Iran University for Medical Sciences, Tehran, Iran.

References

1. Kuete V, Sandjo LP, Djeussi DE, Zeino M, Kwamou GM, Ngadjui B, Efferth T. Invest New Drugs. 2014;32:1053–62.
2. Lam IK, Alex D, Wang YH, Liu P, Liu AL, Du GH, Lee SM. Mol Nutr Food Res. 2012;56:945–56.
3. Walle T. Semin Cancer Biol. 2007;17(5):354–62.
4. Yadegarynia S, Pham A, Ng A, Nguyen D, Lialiutska T, Bortolazzo A, Siv ryuk V, Bremer M, White JB. Nat Prod Commun. 2014;9:597–606.
5. Gao Y, Liu F, Fang L, Cai R, Zong C, Qi Y. PLos One. 2014;9:e96741.
6. Moghaddam GH, Ebrahimi SA, Rahbar-Roshandel N, Foroumadi A. Phytother Res. 2012;26:1023–28.
7. Abbaszadeh H, Ebrahimi SA, Akhavan MM. Phytother Res. 2014;28:1661–70.
8. Folkman J. Ann Intern Med. 1975;82:96–100.
9. Folkman J. Annu Rev Med. 2006;57:1–18.
10. Tanaka S, Sugimachi K, Yamashita Y, Shirabe K, Shimada M, Wands JR, Sugimachi K. J Gastroenterol. 2003;15:93–7.
11. Mojzis J, Varinska L, Mojzisova G, Kostova I, Mirossay L. Pharmacol Res. 2008; 57:259–65.
12. Luo Y, Wang SX, Zhou ZQ, Wang Z, Zhang YG, Zhang Y, Zhao P. Tumour Biol. 2014;35:11483–8.
13. Zhao Y, Adjei AA. Oncologist. 2015;20:660–73.
14. Jespersen B, Knupp L, Northcott CA. J Vis Exp. 2012;24:1–8.
15. Li X, Wang L, Li Y, Bai L, Xue M. Regul Toxicol Pharmacol. 2011;60:106–11.
16. Fernández I, Peña A, Del Teso N, Pérez V, Rodríguez-Cuesta J. J Am Assoc Lab Anim Sci. 2010;49:202–6.
17. Keppler A, Gretz N, Schmidt R, Kloetzer H-M, Groene H-J, Lelongt B, Meyer M, Sadick M, Pill J. Kidney Int. 2007;71:74–8.
18. Singh P, Mishra SK, Noel S, Sharma S, Rath SK. PLoS One. 2012;7.
19. Sobhani AM, Ebrahimi SA, Mahmoudian M. J Pharm Pharm Sci. 2002;5:19–23.
20. Jahaniani F, Ebrahimi SA, Rahbar-Roshandel N, Mahmoudian M. Phytochemistry. 2005;66:1581–92.
21. Busby MG, Jeffcoat AR, Bloedon LT, Koch MA, Black T, Dix KJ, Heizer WD, Thomas BF, Hill JM, Crowell JA, Zeisel SH. Am J Clin Nutr. 2002;75:126–36.
22. Biasutto L, Marotta E, Garbisa S, Zoratti M, Paradisi C. Molecules. 2010; 20(15):6570–9.

10

Hydroxylation index of omeprazole in relation to CYP2C19 polymorphism and sex in a healthy Iranian population

Maryam Payan[1], Mohammad Reza Rouini[1*], Nader Tajik[2], Mohammad Hossein Ghahremani[3] and Reza Tahvilian[4]

Abstract

Background: Polymorphism of *CYP2C19* gene is one of the important factors in pharmacokinetics of CYP2C19 substrates. Omeprazole is a proton pump inhibitor which is mainly metabolized by cytochrome P450 2C19 (*CYP2C19*). The aim of present study was to assess omeprazole hydroxylation index as a measure of CYP2C19 activity considering new variant allele (*CYP2C19*17*) in Iranian population and also to see if this activity is sex dependent.

Methods: One hundred and eighty healthy unrelated Iranian individuals attended in this study. Blood samples for genotyping and phenotyping were collected 3 hours after administration of 20 mg omeprazole orally. Genotyping of *2C19* variant alleles **2, *3* and **17* was performed by using polymerase chain reaction-restriction fragment length polymorphism (PCR-RFLP) and semi-nested PCR methods. Plasma concentrations of omeprazole and hydroxyomeprazole were determined by high performance liquid chromatography (HPLC) technique and hydxroxylation index (HI) (omeprazole/ hydroxyomeprazole) was calculated.

Results: The *CYP2C19*17* was the most common variant allele in the studied population (21.6%). Genotype frequencies of *CYP2C19*17*17, *1*17,* and **2*17* were 5.5%, 28.8% and 3.3% respectively. The lowest and the highest median omeprazole HI was observed in **17*17* and **2*2* genotypes respectively (0.36 vs. 13.09). The median HI of omeprazole in subjects homozygous for *CYP2C19*1* was 2.16-fold higher than individuals homozygous for *CYP2C19*17* (P < 0.001) and the median HI of *CYP2C19*1*17* genotype was 1.98-fold higher than *CYP2C19 *17*17* subjects (P < 0.001). However, subjects with *CYP2C19*2*17* (median HI: 1.74) and *CYP2C19*1*2* (median HI: 1.98) genotypes and also *CYP2C19*1*17* (median HI: 0.71) and *CYP2C19*1*1* (mean HI: 0.78) did not show any significantly different enzyme activity. In addition, no statistically significant difference was found between women and men in distribution of *CYP2C19* genotypes. Furthermore, the hydroxylation index of Omeprazole was not different between women and men in the studied population.

Conclusion: Our data point out the importance of *CYP2C19*2* and *CYP2C19*17* variant alleles in metabolism of omeprazole and therefore CYP2C19 activity. Regarding the high frequency of *CYP2C19*17* in Iranian population, the importance of this new variant allele in metabolism of CYP2C19 substrates shall be considered.

Keywords: CYP2C19, Enzyme activity, Genotype, Omeprazole, Phenotype

* Correspondence: rouini@tums.ac.ir
[1]Biopharmaceutics and Pharmacokinetics Division, Department of Pharmaceutics, School of Pharmacy, Tehran University of Medical sciences, Tehran, Iran
Full list of author information is available at the end of the article

Introduction

Cytochrome P450 includes a wide variety of phase I metabolizing enzymes which are involved in metabolism of drugs and endogenic substances [1,2]. CYP2C19 is one of the members of cytochrome iso enzyme superfamily which contributes in metabolism of important drugs such as proton pump inhibitors (PPI) [3] psychotic drugs like venlafaxine [4] and citalopram [5,6], voriconazol [7], and clopidogrel [8,9].

CYP2C19 is represented by a gene located on chromosome 10 [10]. Genetic polymorphism of CYP2C19 is one of the major reasons of inter-individual variability in response to CYP2C19 substrate [11-13]. The main CYP2C19 polymorphisms that are associated with difference in therapeutic response are attributed to CYP2C19*2, CYP2C19*3 and CYP2C19*17 [14,15].

A point mutation in exon 5 (681 G > A, designated *2) causes a cryptic splice defect (CYP2C19*2) and a single nucleotide polymorphism (SNP) in exon 4 (636 G > A designated *3) creates a stop codon. Both mutations predominantly result in decreased CYP2C19 activity [9,16]. A recently discovered SNP in 5′ −flanking region (−806 C > T and −3402 C > T) leads to increased CYP2C19 activity and therefore produces ultra rapid metabolizer phenotype [17,18].

The CYP2C19*2*2 and *3*3 genotypes are more prevalent in oriental and Asian populations than in Caucasian (12-23% vs 3-5%). In contrast the CYP2C19*17*17 is more frequent in Caucasian than in Asian populations (18-26% vs 0.4-1.4%) [19,20].

Omeprazole is a proton pump inhibitor that is administered in treatment of gastric acid related disease [21]. Polymorphism of CYP2C19 can affect pharmacokinetic and therefore efficacy of proton pump inhibitors [21,22]. Additionally non genetic factors like age, liver disease and combination therapy can result in resistance to *Helicobacter Pylori* eradication treatment [23,24].

Several studies have used hydroxylation index of omeprazole as an indicator of CYP2C19 activity however this enzyme activity, was mainly measured in relation to *2 and *3 variant alleles and not the new variant allele (*17) [16,25-28]. Although Sim et al. studied the effect of CYP2C19*17 variant allele on enzyme activity, they only reported this activity in extensive metabolizers (*17*17, *1*17 and *1*1) and they did not determine CYP2C19 activity in CYP2C19*2*17 carriers [17]. CYP2C19*2 leads to decreased enzyme activity and CYP2C19*17 causes increased enzyme activity [16,17] but the impact of combined alleles (CYP2C19*2*17) on CYP2C19 activity has not been reported comprehensively and it is unknown that the effect of which allele is more predominant in CYP2C19*2*17 carriers.

Furthermore there are some controversies in publications about impact of sex on CYP2C19 activity [29,30].

To our best knowledge, currently there is no published data regarding CYP2C19 activity in relation to new variant allele in Iranian population. Thus, the objects of this study were to assess effect of CYP2C19*17 on enzyme activity and also to see if there is any sex-dependent difference in CYP2C19 activity and finally to investigate genotype-phenotype relationship of CYP2C19 considering new variant allele (CYP2C19*17) in Iranian population.

Material and methods
Study subjects

The study protocol was approved by ethics committee of Tehran University of Medical Sciences (ethical no. 11208). Generally one hundred and eighty (60 women and 120 men) unrelated healthy Iranian volunteers with the mean age of between 20–55 years and average body weight of 45–89 kg took part in this study. All participants signed written informed consent of this project. The study was completed by contribution of faculties of pharmacy of Tehran, Yazd, Kermanshah and Kerman University of Medical Sciences. The participants were students or stuffs of pharmacy schools, with no history of any illness or medicine consumption. No smoking and consumption of medicine that would affect CYP2C19 activity was permitted for one week before and during the study.

CYP2C19 phenotyping

After an overnight fast for at least 8 hours, volunteers took 20 mg omeprazole capsule (Abidi pharmaceuticals) with 250 milliliter tap water. Ten ml venous blood sample was collected from each subject 3 hours after administration of omeprazole and transferred into tubes containing 10 µl of 10% EDTA. Five ml of blood samples were centrifuged for 5 min at 4000 rpm and the plasma was separated and transferred to Eppendorf tube and stored at −80°C up to the day of analysis. The other 5 ml blood samples were stored directly in −80°C for genotyping analysis.

Analytical procedure

Omeprazole powder was purchased from TMAD (Iran). 5-hydroxyomeprazole was a kind donation by AstraZeneca (Sweden). The concentration of omeprazole and 5-hydroxyomeprazole was analyzed by HPLC method as described by Rezk et al. with a few modifications [31]. Briefly 500 µl plasma was extracted by liquid-liquid extraction using 1500 µl ethyl acetate. After orbital mixing for 10 min and centrifuging at 4000 × g for 10 min, the upper organic layer was separated and transferred to glass tube and then evaporated to dryness under gentle stream of air. Finally the residue was dissolved in 250 µl mobile phase and 100 µl of this sample was injected to HPLC system. The mobile phase was a combination of dibasic sodium phosphate buffer (0.025 mol/lit, pH 6): acetonitrile: methanol (73: 18: 8 V/V/V). The HPLC apparatus consisted of a low pressure HPLC pump, UV detector (λ = 302 nm) all from Knauer (Berlin, Germany). The chromatographic separation was performed by using Chromolit™ Performance RP-18e 100 mm × 4.6 mm, 5 µm particle size. Flow rate was adjusted to 1 ml/min. The limits of quantification were about 15 µg/ml for both compounds. Intraday and between day precisions were < 5% for both omerpazole and 5-hydroxyomeprazole.

CYP2C19 genotyping

The DNA was extracted from blood leucocytes by standard salting out method as explained by Miller et al. [32]. The extracted DNA was dissolved in sterile distilled water and stored at 4 °C until the day of analysis. Amplification of CYP2C19*2 and *3 allele was implemented using polymerase chain reaction-restriction fragment length polymorphism (PCR-RFLP) as described by De Morias [33]. The PCR product of each reaction was digested by specific endonuclease (all from New England Biolabs GmbH, Frankfurt, Germany); the 169 bp CYP2C19*2 product was digested by SmaI to 40 and 129 bp fragments. The 329 bp PCR product of CYP2C19*3 was digested by BamHI to 233 and 96 bp pieces. Genotyping of CYP2C19*17 -3402 C > T and −806 C > T polymorphisms was done by PCR-RFLP and nested-PCR assays as defined by Sim et al. [17]. For CYP2C19*17 -3402 C > T the PCR product (504 bp) was digested by MnlI and resulted in 224 and 280 bp fragments. But the PCR product of CYP2C19*17 -806 C > T (200 bp) was separated directly on 2.5% agarose gel without any digestion. In all PCR-RFLP assays mutation caused abolishment of restriction site and thus PCR product was not digested.

Statistical analysis

The allele frequencies differences between population were estimated using two-tailed Fisher's exact test. The 95% confidence intervals (CI) were calculated using Confidence Interval Analysis software. The relation of sex and genotype was assessed by two tailed Fisher's exact test. The observed and expected frequencies were calculated by using Hardy-Weinberg equation. The two-tailed Fisher's exact test was used to evaluate deviation of genotype frequencies in the studied population from Hardy-Weinberg equilibrium. The enzyme activity was compared by using omeprazole hydroxylation index. The hydroxylation index (HI) of omeprazole 3 hours after administration of omeprazole was calculated by dividing omeprazole to 5-hydroxyomeprazol plasma concentration. The mean HI in different genotypes were compared by Mann–Whitney two tailed test. The impact of sex on HI of omeprazole was also evaluated using Mann–Whitney two tailed test. The inter-individual variability in metabolism of

omeprazole was represented by probit plot. For drawing probit plot, the log of HI was calculated, the antimode value was determined using Microsoft office excel 2010. The normality of HI distribution was analyzed by frequency distribution histogram and also by Kolmogorov-Smirnov test. All statistical analyses were performed by Sigma Plot version 12.0 and Graph Pad Prism version 5 softwares and P < 0.05 was considered as statistically significant difference.

Results

The genotype and allele frequencies of CYP2C19 are reported in Table 1. According to the data presented in Table 1, CYP2C19 *17*17, *1*17 and *1*1 were detected in 10 (5.5%), 52 (28.9%) and 75 (41.7%) subjects respectively. The CYP2C19 *2*17 and *1*2 were identified in 6 (3.3%) and 33 (18.3%) individuals and finally the CYP2C19*2*2 was recognized in 4 (2.2%) of volunteers. CYP2C19*17 was the most common variant allele in Iranian population.

The hydroxylation index of omeprazole as mean ± SD, median and 95% confidence interval is reported in Table 2. Subjects with CYP2C19 *17*17 genotype had a very high metabolic capacity with median hydroxylation index of 0.36 and were classified as Ultra-Rapid Metabolizers (URM). The median hydroxylation index of omeprazole in subjects homozygous for CYP2C19*1 was 2.17 fold higher than individual homozygous for CYP2C19*17 (P < 0.001) and the median hydroxylation index of CYP2C19*1*17 genotype was 1.97 fold higher than CYP2C19*17*17 subjects (P < 0.001). There was not a significant difference between HI of omeprazole in CYP2C19*1*17 and *1*1 carriers (P > 0.05) and these two groups were stratified as extensive metabolizers (EM).

The median HI of omeprazole was 1.74 in CYP2C19*2*17 and 1.98 in CYP2C19*1*2 carriers respectively. The difference in HI of omeprazole in CYP2C19*1*2 carriers were statistically significant with other CYP2C19 genotypes (P < 0.05) except for CYP2C19*2*17 genotype (p > 0.05). Individuals in these two groups had intermediate metabolic capacity and were designated as Intermediate-Metabolizers (IM). Homozygous carrier of CYP2C19*2 had a very low metabolic capacity with the median hydroxylation index of 13.03 and they were classified as poor metabolizers (PM). There was a significant difference between HI index of homozygous carriers of CYP2C19*2 with the other five genotypes (p < 0.001).

The plasma concentration of omeprazole and hydroxyomeprazole is illustrated in Figure 1. According to this figure there is a significant difference between omeprazole plasma concentration in individuals with CYP2C19*17*17 genotype with all other groups (P < 0.01), but the omeprazole plasma concentration was neither different between 1*17 and 1*1(EM) (P > 0.5) nor between 2*17 and 1*2 (IM)

Table 1 Genotype and allele frequencies of CYP2C19 in 180 healthy Iranian volunteers

CYP2C19 Genotype	Number of subjects		Frequency (%)	95% CI
	Men (120)	Women (60)		
*17*17	5	5	5.5	2.7 - 10.0
*1*17	37	15	28.8	22.4 - 36.1
*1*1	53	22	41.7	34.4 - 49.2
*1*2	20	13	18.3	13.0 - 24.7
*2*17	4	2	3.3	1.23 - 7.1
*2*2	1	3	2.2	0.6 - 5.5
CYP2C19 Alleles	**No. of alleles**		**Frequency (%)**	**95% CI**
CYP2C19*17	78		21.6	17.5 - 26.3
CYP2C19*1	235		65.3	60.1 - 70.2
CYP2C19*2	47		13.1	9.7 - 16.9
CYP2C19*3	0		0	0

*CI: Confidence Interval. (The 95% confidence intervals (CI) were calculated using Confidence Interval Analysis software).

genotypes. However, omeprazole plasma concentration was significantly different between EM (*1*17* and *1*1*) and IM (*2*17* and *1*2*). The plasma concentration of hydroxyomeprazole was significantly different between *2*2* and all other 5 genotypes while the plasma concentration of hydroxyomeprazole was not significantly different between other 5 genotypes (*17*17, 1*17, *1*1, 2*17, 1*2*).

Figure 2 indicates the hydroxylation index of omeprazole in 6 genotypes and also in predicted phenotype groups. As it is observed there is no significant difference between hydroxylation index of omeprazole in *1*17* and *1*1* groups or between *2*17* and *1*2* groups. While the difference between *17*17* or *2*2* with all other genotype groups were statistically significant.

The summary of omeprazole, hydroxyomeprazole plasma concentration and omeprazole HI in the total population, women and men is reported in Table 3. Omeprazole plasma concentration was significantly higher in *2*2* genotype than other genotype groups. Additionally there was a significant difference in omeprazole plasma concentration between different groups (P < 0.001) except for *CYP2C19*1*17* and *1*1* (P > 0.05), *CYP2C19*1*2* and *CYP2C19*2*17* (P > 0.05). Mean omeprazole plasma concentration was 19.0 fold higher in *CYP2C19*2*2* than *CYP2C19*17*17* and 11 fold higher than *CYP2C19*1*1* (P < 0.001), however hydroxyomeprazole concentration

was not statistically different among genotype groups (P > 0.05) except for *CYP2C19*2*2*. Moreover, omeprazole and hydroxyomeprazole plasma concentrations as well as omeprazole HI were not statistically different among women and men in the studied population (P > 0.05).

The effect of sex on hydroxylation index of omeprazole is illustrated in Figure 3. According to this figure there is not any significant difference between median hydroxylation index in women (0.84) and men (0.86) (p > 0.05).

The frequency distribution histogram of omeprazole hydroxylation index in 180 healthy Iranian volunteers is indicated in Figure 4. The graph shows a bimodal distribution with the antimode of around 0.8. Kolmogorov-Smirnov test showed that the omeprazole hydroxylation index was not normally distributed in the studied population (K-S Dist. = 0.296 p < 0.001). The bimodal distribution was also confirmed by probit plot.

The correlation of CYP2C19 genotype and phenotype was tested using Spearman rank correlation, and the results showed a well correlation between CYP2C19 genotype and phenotype (r_s = 0.64, P < 0.0001).

Discussion

Inter-individual variability in drug response always has been one of the main concerns in drug discovery and development. The important factors resulting in such

Table 2 Hydroxylation index of omeprazole (omeprazole/hydroxyomeprazole) in relation to CYP2C19 genotype in 180 healthy Iranian subjects

	*17*17	*1*17	*1*1	*2*17	*1*2	*2*2
Mean (SD)	0.35(0.06)	0.75(0.28)	0.85(0.30)	2.02(0.84)	2.27(1.04)	13.59(3.13)
Median	0.36[a]	0.71	0.78	1.74[b]	1.98[b]	13.03[a]
95% CI	0.31 - 0.39	0.68 -0.83	0.79 – 0.92	1.33 – 2.72	1.92 – 2.63	10.51– 16.67

[a]Represent statistically significant difference with other 5 genotypes.
[b]Represent statistically significant difference with *17*17, *1*17, *1*1 and *2*2.
CI: Confidence Interval.

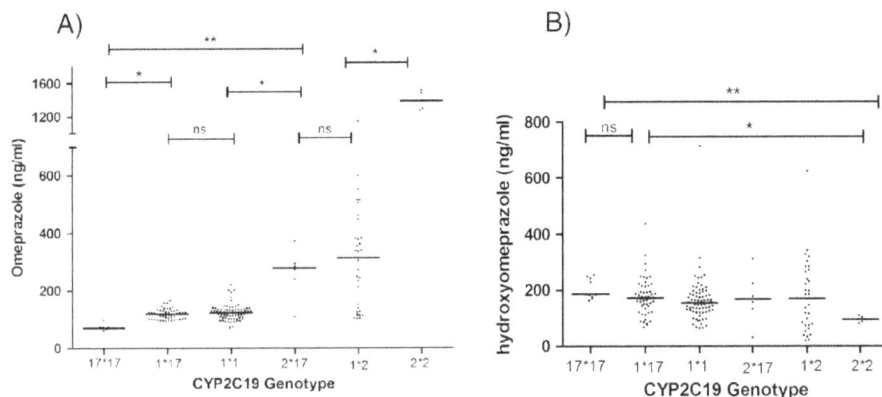

Figure 1 Plasma concentrations of Omeprazole (A) and hydroxyomerpazole (B) in different genotypes 3 hours after administration of **Omeprazole orally.** ns: not significant, * p < 0.05, ** p < 0.001.

variation include genetic, nongenetic and physiologic agents like change in protein structure, combination therapy, alcohol, smoking, sex, age and disease condition [34].

*CYP2C19*17* is a new variant allele which is associated with increased gene transcription and therefore higher enzyme activity [17]; which may lead to several clinical consequences including the lower susceptibility to breast cancer risk [35], higher risk of peptic ulcer disease [36], greater response to clopidogrel treatment and more risk of bleeding [37] in addition to a better treatment with tamoxifen [38].

In this study, omeprazole HI after 3 hours administration of omeprazole was used as indicator of CYP2C19 activity. The HI in *CYP2C19*17*17* was significantly different with *CYP2C19*1*17* and *CYP2C19*1*1* genotypes and people in this group had very high metabolic activity, which is in agreement with what was reported by Sim *et al.* They found that median HI of omeprazole in homozygous carriers of *CYP2C19*1* is 2 fold higher than homozygous carriers of *CYP2C19*17* and 1.2 fold higher

than *CYP2C19*1*17* [17]. Ramsjö *et al.* has also reported that mean HI of omeprazole in *CYP2C19*1*1* was 3.2 fold higher than *CYP2C19*17*17* and 1.1 fold higher than *CYP2C19*1*17* [27].

*CYP2C19*2* allele is associated with decreased enzyme activity and *CYP2C19*17* variant allele is connected with increased enzyme activity. In Most of the genotype phenotype studies of *CYP2C19*17* variant allele, only HI of omeprazole in *CYP2C19*17*17*, *CYP2C19*1*17* and *CYP2C19*1*1* genotypes has been reported [17,27]. However, the capacity of CYP2C19 enzyme activity in people carrying both defective mutant alleles of *2 and *17 (*CYP2C19*2*17*) was still unclear. Although Ragia *et al.* in the study for evaluation of distribution of *CYP2C19*17* genetic polymorphism in Greece people defined CYP2C19*2*17 carriers as EM and people with *CYP2C19*1*2* as IM, they only predicted phenotype based on genotype and CYP2C19 activity was not determined by using a probe drug [39]. Sugimito *et al.* did not see any difference between metabolic capacities of *CYP2C19*1*1, *1*17, 2*17 and 1*2* for metabolism of

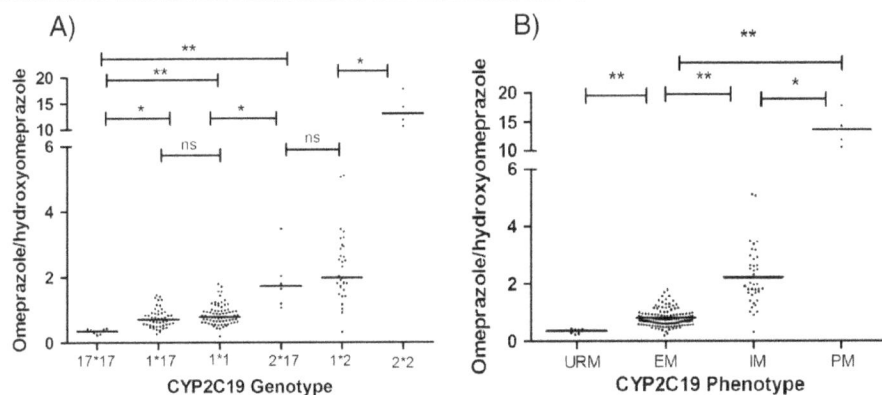

Figure 2 The hydroxylation index of Omeprazole in different genotypes (A) and in predicted phenotype groups (B) 3 hours after administration of Omeprazole orally. ns: not significant, * p < 0.05, ** p < 0.001.

Table 3 Plasma concentration of omeprazole (OMP) and hydroxyomeprazole (OH-OMP) and hydroxylation index (HI) of omeprazole in relation to genotype in 60 women and 120 men 3 hour after administration of single oral dose of 20 mg omeprazole

Genotype	No of subjects	Mean OMP concentration (ng/ml) ± SD	Mean OH-OMP concentration (ng/ml) ± SD	Mean HI ± SD
17*17	Total (10)	71.01 ± 10.28	203.31 ± 34.93	0.35 ± 0.06
	Women (5)	68.32 ± 5.73	204.92 ± 41.35	0.34 ± 0.08
	Men (5)	73.71 ± 13.67	201.69 ± 32.08	0.36 ± 0.04
1*17	Total (52)	118.28 ± 10.19	177.05 ± 37.53	0.75 ± 0.28
	Women (15)	120.22 ± 20.12	174.51 ± 28.01	0.72 ± 0.18
	Men (37)	117.49 ± 16.10	178.07 ± 44.57	0.77 ± 0.32
1*1	Total (75)	124.75 ± 27.18	163.74 ± 32.25	0.85 ± 0.30
	Women (22)	128.06 ± 39.90	194.40 ± 60.84	0.78 ± 0.27
	Men (53)	123.38 ± 20.83	151.01 ± 26.38	0.89 ± 0.30
2*17	Total (6)	289.01 ± 97.45	172.79 ± 63.58	2.02 ± 0.54
	Women (4)	324.25 ± 39.90	178.72 ± 33.59	1.97 ± 0.62
	Men (2)	271.39 ± 118.56	169.82 ± 84.95	2.05 ± 0.67
1*2	Total (33)	319.45 ± 150.34	177.79 ± 38.39	2.27 ± 1.04
	Women (13)	364.92 ± 265.16	194.66 ± 52.56	2.24 ± 0.79
	Men (20)	289.89 ± 167.55	165.53 ± 23.55	2.29 ± 1.19
2*2	Total (4)	1388.99 ± 123.41	104.67 ± 10.55	13.59 ± 3.13
	Women (3)	1359.84 ± 133.23	105.03 ± 13.80	13.37 ± 3.80
	Men (1)	1476.4	103.58	14.25

HI = (omerprazole concentration/hydroxyomeprazole concentration).

omeprazole and stratified these individuals as EM [20]. The omeprazole HI in subjects with CYP2C19*2*17 genotype in this study was not significantly different from CYP2C19*1*2 genotype (P = 0.33) so we designated them as IM. It seems that in heterozygous carriers of CYP2C19*2 and *17 allele, the effect of *2 allele is more predominant than *17 allele and it can suppress induced enzyme activity by *17 allele. This observation is in agreement with classification of CYP2C19*2*17 as IM by Gurbel et al. based on the study for genotype phenotype analysis of 2C19 in stented patient [40]. In contrast to these findings, in a study for evaluation of

CYP2C19 enzyme activity in Turkish children using lansoprazole as a probe drug, individuals with CYP2C19*2*17 had similar enzyme activity to CYP2C19*1*17 and CYP2C19*1*1; and this activity was significantly different from CYP2C19*1*2 [41]. Involvement of individual with different age groups could possibly explain such different observations. Our study was conducted in adult individuals with the average age of 32 years but Gumus implemented the study in children with mean age of 10.2 years. The lower frequency of CYP2C19*2*17 in our studied subjects in comparison to Turkish individuals (6 vs 16) can be considered as another justification.

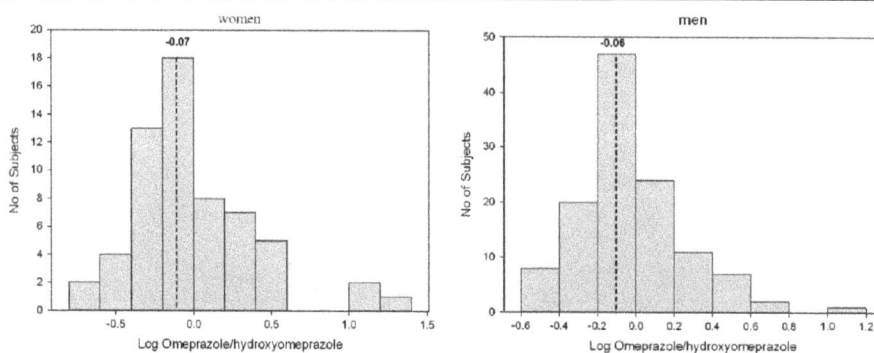

Figure 3 The effect of sex on hydroxylation index of omeprazole in 60 women and 120 men. The median hydroxylation index is indicated by dashed line.

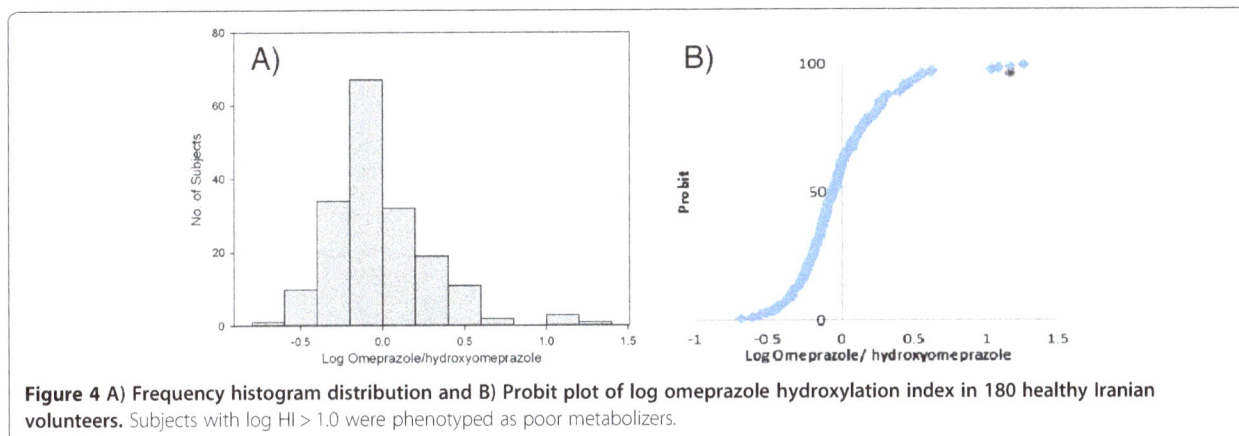

Figure 4 A) Frequency histogram distribution and B) Probit plot of log omeprazole hydroxylation index in 180 healthy Iranian volunteers. Subjects with log HI > 1.0 were phenotyped as poor metabolizers.

In the present study effect of CYP2C19 genetic polymorphism and sex on metabolic activity of CYP2C19 was also assessed. Sex is an important factor in activity of some cytochrome P450 enzymes. CYP3A4 is an example of cytochrome enzymes which has higher activity in women than men [2]. There were some controversies in the previous published reports for impact of sex on CYP2C19 activity. Ramsjö et al. indicated a sex difference in CYP2C19 activity between Korean subjects and not in Swedish volunteers using Omeprazole as a probe drug [27]. Tamminga et al. observed a sex related decreased CYP2C19 activity in women when used mephenytoin as a probe for evaluation of CYP2C19 activity, however the author declared this reduction was more obvious in those who used oral contraceptive [42]. In contrast, Hägg et al. did not see any sex differences in CYP2C19 activity after administration of mephenytoin in Norwegian population [43]. By considering these reports one may conclude that sex dependency of CYP2C19 activity is influenced by environmental and epigenetic factors like diet and ethnic differences. The other possibility can be attributed to some new genetic mutation in some populations which has not been studied well. The result of this study represents no effect of sex on CYP2C19 activity which is in line with what is reported in Swedish and Norwegian population.

The frequency of PM and URM in Iranian population in this study was about 2.2% and 5.5% which is close to the study by Zand et al. [44] and other Caucasian population. In previous report by Akhlaghi et al. in Iranian patients with coronary artery disease the genotype frequency of CYP2C19*2*2 was reported 4.7% which is quite different from our results [45]. This can be due to difference in studied population (healthy volunteer's vs specific patients). The genotype frequency of CYP2C19*17*17 (URM) was 4% in Swedish and 3% in Ethiopian [17], 5.1% in Danish [19], 3.18% in Greece [39], 7% in Saudi Arabian [46] 1.2% in Indian [16] and 0% in Japanese, Korean and Thai population [20,27,47]. Accordingly the genotype frequency of

CYP2C19*2*2 (PM) is 2.2% in Danish [19], 2.1% in Greece [39], 0.4% in Saudi Arabian [46], 18.4% in Indian [16] and 18% in Japanese people [20].

To the best of authors' knowledge, this is the first study evaluating CYP2C19 genotype and phenotype in Iranian population in relation to new variant allele (CYP2C19*17). In the previous report, Zendehdel et al. investigated impact of CYP2C19 on therapeutic efficacy of omeprazole in Iranian patients with erosive reflux esophagitis; patients were genotyped only for CYP2C19*2 and CYP2C19*3, Individuals with HetEM genotype had better response to treatment with omeprazole than EM (95% vs 43% successful treatment response respectively) [48]. The high frequency of CYP2C19*17 allele (21.6%) detected in this study maybe one justification for 50% resistance rate in the EM group in Iranian patients in previous report. However impact of this variant allele (CYP2C19*17) on the efficacy of PPIs like omeprazole shall be evaluated in controlled clinical trials.

In this study the antimode of 0.8 was calculated for Iranian population. Different antimodes for HI of omeprazole have been reported in different ethnics groups: 14.4 in Indian [16], 7.0 in Koreans [25] and Thai population [47], 0.63 in Colombians [26], and 3.98 in West Mexicans [49]. The calculated antimode for Iranian population is similar to Colombian population, indicating comparable CYP2C19 activity in Iranians and Colombians and faster enzyme activity than Asian people.

A complete genotype phenotype correlation was observed in this study. However it should be noted that enzyme activity and therefore metabolic ratio may vary during some disease condition which may result in discrepancy in genotype-phenotype relationship of specific enzyme. Kimura et al. [50] indicated discordance of genotype-phenotype relationship of omeprazole in 14.5% of EM patients who had peptic ulcer disease. However this discrepancy was not observed in healthy individuals. Reduced hepatic enzyme activity as a result of old age or liver disease was reported as an explanation for such finding. Long term treatment with omeprazole which has auto inhibition effect was the other possibility. Williams *et al.* [51] also did not see genotype-phenotype relationship of 2C19 using omeprazole in patients with advanced cancer. The authors concluded that increased level of some signaling molecules like interleukin (IL) and tumor necrosis factors (TNFα) may result in down-regulation of metabolizing enzymes [51,52]. So it should be considered that factors like age, disease state, and concomitant medication may have pronounced effect on enzyme activity. Although omeprazole hydroxylation index has been used as an indicator of CYP2C19 activity, it should be considered that hydroxyomeprazole which is formed by CYP2C19 is further metabolized by CYP3A4 to hydroxyomeprazole sulfone [53] which in turn may indirectly affect the hydroxylation index of omeprazole. Therefore the high concentration of CYP3A4 in liver microsomes of some human can explain the deviation from CYP2C19 genotype and also the sex dependent enzyme activity observed in some ethnic groups [54].

The prevalence of *CYP2C19*2*17* in this study was only 6% which is a limitation of this study. Future studies to investigate impact of *CYP2C19*2*17* genotype on CYP2C19 enzyme activity in larger groups specially by using drugs with narrow therapeutic window is suggested.

In conclusion, the result of this study shows that *CYP2C19*2*17* has an intermediate metabolic activity which maybe important for drug dose adjustment regimens for treatment, specially in those having narrow therapeutic indices like clopidogrel. Additionally no effect of sex on CYP2C19 activity was observed in this study. Regarding the high frequency of *CYP2C19*17* in Iranian population, the importance of this new variant allele in metabolism of CYP2C19 substrates shall be considered.

Abbreviations
CYP2C19: Cytochrome P450 2C19; PCR-RFLP: Polymerase chain reaction-restriction fragment length polymorphism; HPLC: High performance liquid chromatography; HI: Hydxroxylation index; SNP: Single nucleotide polymorphism; URM: Ultra-rapid metabolizers; EM: Extensive metabolizers; IM: Intermediate metabolizers; PM: Poor metabolizers; OMP: Omeprazole; OH-OMP: Hydroxyomepazole.

Competing interests
The authors declare that they have no competing interests.

Authors' contributions
M-RR, MP, NT, M-H GH and RT conceived the study. MP performed the experimental work. All authors were involved in data analysis and interpretation. MP prepared the manuscript. All authors read and approved the final version.

Acknowledgement
This project was supported by a grant from Tehran University of Medical Sciences. We thank Dr. Kjell Andersson, AstraZeneca, Sweden, for kind donation of pure powder of 5 -hydroxyomeprazole. We are grateful to Dr. Mehdi Ansari Dogaheh, Department of Pharmaceutics, Faculty of Pharmacy, Kerman Medical Sciences and Dr. Mohsen Nabimeybodi, Department of pharmaceutics, Faculty of Pharmacy, Yazd University of Medical Sciences, for kind assistance in collection of blood samples.

Author details
[1]Biopharmaceutics and Pharmacokinetics Division, Department of Pharmaceutics, School of Pharmacy, Tehran University of Medical sciences, Tehran, Iran. [2]Cellular and Molecular Research Center (CMRC), Iran University of Medical Sciences, Tehran, Iran. [3]Department of Pharmacology and Toxicology, School of Pharmacy, Tehran University of Medical sciences, Tehran, Iran. [4]Department of pharmaceutics, School of Pharmacy, Kermanshah University of Medical Sciences, Kermanshah, Iran.

References
1. Sim SC, Nordin L, Andersson TM-L, Virding S, Olsson M, Pedersen NL, Ingelman- Sundberg M: Association Between CYP2C19 Polymorphism and Depressive Symptoms. *Am J Med Genet* 2010, **153**(B):1160–1166.
2. Zanger UM, Schwab M: Cytochrome P450 enzymes in drug metabolism: Regulation of gene expression, enzyme activities, and impact of genetic variation. *J Pharmacol Ther* 2013, **138**:103–141.
3. Qiao H-L, Hu Y-R, Tian X, Jia L-J, Gao N, Zhang L-R, Guo Y-z: Pharmacokinetics of three proton pump inhibitors in Chinese subjects in relation to the CYP2C19 genotype. *Eur J Clin Pharmacol* 2006, **62**:107–112.
4. Weide JVD, Baalen-Benedek EHV, Kootstra-Ros JE: Metabolic ratios of psychotropics as indication of cytochrome P450 2D6/2C19 genotype. *Ther Drug Monit* 2005, **27**:478–483.
5. Yu B-N, Chen G-L, He N, Ouyang D-S, Chen X-P, Liu Z-Q, Zhou HH: Pharmacokinetic of citalopram in relation to genetic polymorphism of CYP2C19. *Drug Metabol Dispos* 2003, **31**(10):1255–1259.
6. Mrazek DA, Biernacka JM, O'Kane DJ, Black JL, Cunningham JM, Drews MS, Snyder KA, Stevens SR, Rush AJ, Weinshilboum RM: CYP2C19 variation and citalopram response. *Pharmacogenet Genomics* 2011, **21**:1–9.
7. Wang G, Lei HP, Li Z, Tan Z-R, Guo D, Fan L, Chen Y, Hu D-L, Wang D, Zhou H-H: The CYP2C19 ultra rapid metabolizer genotype influences the pharmacokinetics of voriconazol in healthy male volunteers. *Eur J Clin Pharmacol* 2009, **65**:281–285.
8. Sibbing S, Koch W, Gebhard D, Schuster T, Braun S, Stegherr J, Morath T, Scho¨mig A, Beckerath NV, Kastrati A: Cytochrome 2C19*17 allelic variant, platelet aggregation, bleeding events, and stent thrombosis in clopidogrel-treated patients with coronary stent placement. *Circulation* 2010, **121**:512–518.
9. Hulot JS, Collet JP, Silvain J, Pena A, Bellemain-Appaix A, Barthélémy O, Cayla G, Beygui F, Montalescot G: Cardiovascular risk in clopidogrel-treated patients according to cytochrome P450 2C19*2 loss-of-function allele or proton pump inhibitor coadministration: a systematic meta-analysis. *J Am Coll Cardiol* 2010, **56**(2):134–143.
10. Mathijssen RHJ, Schaik RHN: Genotyping and phenotyping cytochrome P450: Perspectives for cancer treatment. *Eur J Cancer* 2006, **42**:141–148.
11. Gabriella Scordo M, Caputi AP, D'Arrigo C, Fava G, Spina E: Allele and genotype frequencies of CYP2C9, CYP2C19 and CYP2D6 in an Italian population. *Pharmacol Res* 2004, **50**:195–200.
12. Ingelman-Sundberg M, Sim SC, Ingelman-Sundberg A, Rodriguez-Antona C: Influence of cytochrome P450 polymorphism on drug therapies: Pharmacogenetic and clinical aspects. *Pharmacol Ther* 2007, **116**:496–526.
13. Chaudhry AS, Kochrar R, Kohli KK: Genetic polymorphism of CYP2C19 & therapeutic response to proton pump inhibitors. *Indian J Med Res* 2008, **127**(6):521–530.
14. Lee S-J, Kim W-Y, Kim H, Shon J-H, Lee SS, Shin J-G: Identification of new CYP2C19 variants exhibiting decreased enzyme activity in the metabolism of S-Mephenytoin and Omeprazole. *Drug Metab Dispos* 2009, **37**(11):2262–2269.
15. Li-Wan-Po A, Girard T, Farndon P, Cooley C, Lithgow J: Pharmacogenetics of CYP2C19: functional and clinical implications of a new variant CYP2C19*17. *Br J Clin Pharmacol* 2010, **69**(3):222–230.
16. Rosemary J, Adithan C, Padmaja N, Shashindran CH, Gerard N, Krishnamoorthy R: The effect of the CYP2C19 genotype on the hydroxylation index of Omeprazole in south Indians. *Eur J Clin Pharmacol* 2005, **61**:19–23.
17. Sim SC, Risinger C, Dahl ML, Aklillu E, Christensen M, Bertilsson L, Ingelman-Sundberg M: A common novel CYP2C19 gene variant causes ultrarapid drug metabolism relevant for the drug response to proton pump inhibitors and antidepressants. *Clin Pharmacol Ther* 2006, **79**:103–113.

18. Anichavezhi D, Roa C, Shewade DG, Krishnamoorthy R, Adithan C: Distribution of *CYP2C19*17* allele and genotype in an Indian population. *J Clin Pharmacy Ther* 2012, 37:313–318.

19. Pedersen RS, Brasch-Andersen C, Sim SC, Bergmann TK, Halling J, Petersen MS, Weihe P, Edvardsen H, Kristensen VN, Brøsen K, Ingelman-Sundberg M: Linkage disequilibrium between the *CYP2C19*17* allele and wide type CYP2C8 and CYP2C9 alleles: identification of CYP2C haplotypes in healthy Nordic population. *Eur J Clin Pharmacol* 2010, 66:1199–1205.

20. Sugimito K, Uno T, Yamazaki H, Tateishi T: Limited frequency of the *CYP2C19*17* allele and its minor role in a Japanese population. *Br J Clin Pharmacol* 2008, 65(3):437–439.

21. Sakai T, Aoyama N, Kita T, Sakaeda T, Nishiguchi K, Nishitora Y, Hohda T, Sirasaka D, Tamura T, Tanigawara Y, Kasuga M, Okumura K: CYP2C19 genotype and pharmacokinetics of three proton pump inhibitors in healthy subjects. *Pharm Res* 2001, 18(6):72–77.

22. Cho H, Choi MK, Cho DY, Yeo CW, Jeong HE, Shon JH, Lee JY: Effect of CYP2C19 genetic polymorphism on pharmacokinetics and pharmacodynamics of a new proton pump inhibitor, ilaprazole. *J Clin Pharmacol* 2012, 52(7):976–984.

23. Ammon S, Treiber G, Kees F, Klotz U: Influence of age on the steady state disposition of drugs commonly used for the eradication of *Helicobacter pylori*. *Aliment Pharmacol Ther* 2000, 14(6):759–766.

24. Ishizawa Y, Yasui-Furukori N, Takahata T, Sasaki M, Tateishi T: The effect of aging on the relationship between the cytochrome P450 2C19 genotype and Omeprazole pharmacokinetics. *Clin pharmacokinetics* 2005, 44:1179–1189.

25. Chong E, Ensom M: Pharmacogenetics of the Proton Pump Inhibitors: A Systematic Review. *Pharmacotherapy* 2003, 23(4):460–471.

26. Isaza C, Henao J: Isaza Martínez J H, Sepúlveda Arias J, Beltrán L: Phenotype-genotype analysis of CYP2C19 in Colombian mestizo individuals. *BMC Clin Pharmacol* 2007, 7(6):1–5.

27. Ramsjö M, Aklillu E, Bohman L, Ingelman-Sundberg M, Roh HK: CYP2C19 activity comparison between Swedish and Koreans: effect of genotype, sex, oral contraceptive use and smoking. *Eur J Clin Pharmacol* 2010, 66:871–877.

28. Niioka T, Uno T, Sugimoto K, Sugawara K, Hayakari M, Tateishi T: Estimation of CYP2C19 activity by the Omeprazole hydroxylation index at a single point in time after intravenous and oral administration. *Eur J Clin Pharmacol* 2007, 63(11):1031–1038.

29. Xie HG, Huang SL, Xu ZH, Xiao ZS, He N, Zhou HH: Evidence for the effect of gender on activity of (S)-mephenytoin 4′-hydroxylase (CYP2C19) in a Chinese population. *Pharmacogenetics* 1997, 7(2):115–119.

30. Laine K, Tybring G, Bertilsson L: No sex-related differences but significant inhibition by oral contraceptives of CYP2C19 activity as measured by the probe drugs mephenytoin and Omeprazole in healthy Swedish white subjects. *Clin Pharmacol Ther* 2000, 68(2):151–159.

31. Rezk NL, Brown KC, Kashuba ADM: A simple and sensitive bioanalytical assay for simultaneous determination of Omeprazole and its three major metabolites in human blood plasma using RP-HPLC after a simple liquid–liquid extraction procedure. *J Chromatogr B* 2006, 844:314–321.

32. Miller SA, Dykes DD, Polesky HF: A simple salting out procedure for extracting DNA from human nucleated cells. *Nucleic Acids Res* 1988, 16:1215.

33. De Morais SM, Wilkinson GR, Blaisdell J, Nakamura K, Meyer UA, Goldstein JA: The major genetic defect responsible for the polymorphism of S-mephenytoin metabolism in humans. *J Bio Chem* 1994, 269(22):15419–15422.

34. Qiang M, Anthony YHL: Pharmacogenetics, Pharmacogenomics, and Individualized Medicine. *Pharmacol Rev* 2011, 63:2437–2459.

35. Justenhoven C, Hamann U, Pierl CB, Baisch C, Harth V, Rabstein S, Spickenheuer A, Pesch B, Brüning T, Winter S, Ko YD, Brauch H: CYP2C19*17 is associated with decreased breast cancer risk. *Breast Cancer Res Treat* 2009, 115(2):391–396.

36. Musumba CO, Jorgensen A, Sutton L, Eker DV, Zhang E, Hara NO, Carr DF, Pritchard DM, Pirmohamed M, Eker DV, Zhang E, Hara NO, Carr DF, Pritchard DM, Pirmohamed M: CYP2C19*17 Gain-of-function polymorphism is associated with peptic ulcer disease. *Clin Pharmacol Ther* 2013, 93(2):195–203.

37. Li Y, Tang HL, Hu YF, Xie HG: The gain-of-function variant CYP2C19*17: a double-edged sword between thrombosis and bleeding in clopidogrel-treated patients. *J Thromb Haemost* 2012, 10(2):199–206.

38. Schroth W, Antoniadou L, Fritz P, Schwab M, Muerdter T, Zanger UM, Simon W, Eichelbaum M, Brauch H: Breast cancer treatment outcome with adjuvant tamoxifen relative to patient CYP2D6 and CYP2C19 genotypes. *J Clin Oncol* 2007, 25(33):5187–5193.

39. Ragia G, Arvanitidis KI, Tavridou A, Manolopoulos VG: Need for reassessment of reported CYP2C19 allele frequencies in various populations in view of *CYP2C19*17* discovery: the case of Greece. *Pharmacogenomics* 2009, 10(1):43–49.

40. Gurbel PA, Shuldiner AR, Bliden KP, Ryan K, Pakyz RE, Tantry US: The relation between CYP2C19 genotype and phenotype in stented patients on maintenance dual antiplatelet therapy. *Am Heart J* 2011, 161:598–604.

41. Gumus E, Karaca O, Babaoglu MO, Baysoy G, Balamtekin N, Demir H, Uslu N, Bozkurt A, Yuce A, Yasar U: Evaluation of lansoprazole as a probe for assessing cytochrome P450 2C19 activity and genotype-phenotype correlation in childhood. *Eur J Clin Pharmacol* 2012, 68(5):629–636.

42. Tamminga WJ, Wemer J, Oosterhuis B, Weiling J, Wilffert B, de Leij LF, de Zeeuw RA, Jonkman JH: CYP2D6 and CYP2C19 activity in a large population of Dutch healthy volunteers: indications for oral contraceptive-related gender differences. *Eur J Clin Pharmacol* 1999, 55(3):177–184.

43. Hägg S, Spigset O, Dahlqvist R: Influence of gender and oral contraceptives on CYP2D6 and CYP2C19 activity in healthy volunteers. *Br J Clin Pharmacol* 2001, 51(2):169–173.

44. Zand N, Tajik N, Moghaddam AS, Milanian I: Genetic polymorphisms of cytochrome P450 enzymes 2C9 and 2C19 in a healthy Iranian population. *Clin Exp Pharmacol Physiol* 2007, 34(1–2):102–105.

45. Akhlaghi A, Shirani S, Ziaie N, Pirhaji O, Yaran M, Shahverdi G, Sarrafzadegan N, Khosravi A, Khosravi E: Cytochrome P450 2C19 Polymorphism in Iranian Patients with Coronary Artery Disease. *ARYA Atheroscler* 2011, 7(3):106–110.

46. Saeed LH, Mayet AY: Genotype-Phenotype analysis of CYP2C19 in healthy Saudi individuals and its potential clinical implication in drug therapy. *Int J Med Sci* 2013, 10:1497–1502.

47. Tassaneeyakul W, Tawalee A, Tassaneeyakul W, Kukongaviriyapan V, Blaisdell J, Goldstein JA, Gaysornsiri D: Analysis of the CYP2C19 polymorphism in a North-eastern Thai population. *Pharmacogenetics* 2002, 12:221–225.

48. Zendedel N, Biramijamal F, Hossein-Nezad A, Zendedel N, Sarie H, Doughaiemoghaddam M, Pourshams A: Role of Cytochrome P450 2C19 genetic polymorphism in the therapeutic efficacy of omeprazole in Iranian patients with erosive reflux esophagitis. *Arch Iran Med* 2010, 13(5):406–412.

49. Gonzalez HM, Romero EM, Peregrina AA, de J Chavez T T, Escobar-Islas E, Lozano F, Hoyo-Vadillo C: CYP2C19- and CYP3A4-dependent Omeprazole metabolism in West Mexicans. *J Clin Pharmacol* 2003, 43:1211–1215.

50. Kimura M, Ieiri I, Wada Y, Mamiya K, Urae A, Iimori E, Sakai T, Otsubo K, Higuchi S: Reliability of the omeprazole hydroxylation index for CYP2C19 phenotyping: possible effect of age, liver disease and length of therapy. *Br J Clin Pharmacol* 1999, 47(1):115–119.

51. Williams ML, Bhargava P, Cherrouk I, Marshall JL, Flockhart DA, Wainer IW: A discordance of the cytochrome P450 2C19 genotype and phenotype in patients with advanced cancer. *Br J Clin Pharmacol* 2000, 49(5):485–488.

52. Helsby NA, Lo WY, Sharples K, Riley G, Murray M, Spells K, Dzhelai M, Simpson A, Findlay M: CYP2C19 pharmacogenetics in advanced cancer: compromised function independent of genotype. *Br J Cancer* 2008, 99(8):1251–1255.

53. Hagymási K, Müllner K, Herszényi L, Tulassay Z: Update on the pharmacogenomics of proton pump inhibitors. *Pharmacogenomics* 2011, 12(6):873–888.

54. Yamazaki H, Inoue K, Shaw PM, Checovich WJ, Guengerich FP, Shimada T: Different contributions of cytochrome P450 2C19 and 3A4 in the oxidation of omeprazole by human liver microsomes: effects of contents of these two forms in individual human samples. *J Pharmacol Exp Ther* 1997, 283(2):434–442.

11

Raloxifene adjunctive therapy for postmenopausal women suffering from chronic schizophrenia

Gilda Kianimehr[1], Farzad Fatehi[2], Sara Hashempoor[3], Mohammad-Reza Khodaei-Ardakani[3], Farzin Rezaei[4], Ali Nazari[4], Ladan Kashani[5] and Shahin Akhondzadeh[6*]

Abstract

Background: Cumulative evidence from epidemiological, preclinical and clinical studies suggests estrogens may have psychoprotective effects in schizophrenic patients. Selective Estrogen Receptor Modulators could have therapeutic benefits in schizophrenia for both sexes without being hazardous to gynecological tissues or having feminizing effects. Few studies have been conducted regarding the effects of raloxifene on postmenopausal women suffering from schizophrenia. We conducted this placebo-controlled trial to compare the add-on effect of raloxifene to risperidone versus risperidone with placebo.

Methods: This was an 8-week, parallel-group, placebo-controlled trial undertaken at two universities affiliated psychiatric Hospitals in Iran. Forty-six postmenopausal women with the definite diagnosis of schizophrenia were enrolled in the study. Patients received risperidone (6 mg/day in 3 divided doses) combined with either placebo (N = 23) or 120 mg/day of raloxifene (N = 23) for 8 weeks. Patients were assessed by a psychiatrist at baseline and at 2 and 8 weeks after the start of medical therapy. Efficacy was defined as the change from baseline to endpoint in score on Positive and Negative Syndrome Scale (PANSS).

Results: For PANSS scores, the main effect comparing two types of intervention was not significant [$F_{(1, 48)} = 1.77$, $p = 0.18$]. For positive subscale scores, there was marginal significant interaction between intervention type and time [$F_{(2, 47)} = 2.93$, $p = 0.06$] and there was substantial main effect for time [$F_{(2, 47)} = 24.39$, $p = 0.001$] within both groups showing reduction in positive subscale scores across the three time periods. In addition, the main effect comparing two types of intervention was significant [$F_{(1, 48)} = 3.78$, $p = 0.02$]. On the other hand, for negative subscale scores, the main effect comparing two types of intervention was not significant [$F_{(1, 48)} = 1.43$, $p = 0.23$]. For general subscale scores, the main effect comparing two types of intervention was not significant [$F_{(1, 48)} = 0.03$, $p = 0.86$].

Conclusions: According to our findings, raloxifene as an adjunctive treatment to risperidone was only superior in improvement of positive symptoms and it was not effective in treating negative and general psychopathology symptoms.

Trial registration: The trial was registered at the Iranian registry of clinical trials: IRCT201205131556N42

Keywords: Schizophrenia, Menopause, Raloxifene, Selective estrogen receptor modulators

* Correspondence: S.akhond@neda.net
[6]Psychiatric Research Center, Roozbeh Psychiatric Hospital, Tehran University of Medical Sciences, South Kargar Street 13337, Tehran, Iran
Full list of author information is available at the end of the article

Background

Cumulative evidence from epidemiological, preclinical and clinical studies suggests estrogens may provoke psychoprotective effects in schizophrenic patients [1]. In addition, Selective Estrogen Receptor Modulators (SERMs) could have therapeutic benefits on both sexes with schizophrenia without any hazard to gynecological tissues or feminizing effects [1]. There are several lines of evidence that support the estrogen hypothesis of schizophrenia [2]. Most antipsychotics cause prolactin-inducing effects, and ensuing negative feedback on estrogen levels [2]. Sex differences in the incidence, onset and course of schizophrenia have led to the hypothesis that estrogens play a protective role in the pathophysiology of this disorder [3]. Estrogen treatment may boost the recovery of schizophrenia in women. However, adverse effects on uterine and breast tissue and other physical side effects may limit the long-term therapeutic use of estrogen [4-6]. Raloxifene hydrochloride is a selective estrogen receptor modulator that acts as an estrogen antagonist in breast tissue and may have agonistic actions in the brain, potentially offering mental health benefits with few estrogenic side effects [4].

Prognosis and severity of schizophrenia is different between males and females and as a result, it is suggested that estrogen may play a role in the pathogenesis of schizophrenia [1,3]. sex differences is a fascinating aspect of schizophrenia, which have been described for nearly all features of the illness, including the peak age of onset, symptoms and treatment response [7]. Estradiol and some SERMs are neuroprotective in a variety of experimental models of neurodegeneration; they could lessen the inflammatory response of glial cells, decrease anxiety and depression, and endorse cognition. Moreover, they are able to modulate synaptic plasticity in the hippocampus of rodents [8]; however, long term estrogen application may cause significant complications especially in menopausal women. Therefore, administration of Selective Estrogen Receptor Modulators (SERMs) may reduce such side effects. Raloxifene is a SERM that has similar dopaminergic and serotonergic effects as estrogen. Few studies have been conducted regarding the effects of raloxifene on postmenopausal women suffering from schizophrenia [9,10]. However, the sample size of these studies was relatively small [9.10]. We conducted this placebo-controlled trial to compare the add-on effect of raloxifene to risperidone in comparison with risperidone and placebo.

Methods

Trial organization

This was an 8-week, parallel-group, placebo-controlled trial undertaken at two universities affiliated psychiatric Hospitals in Iran (Roozbeh and Razi Hospital) from June 2012 to December 2013. The trial protocol was approved by the Institutional Review Board (IRB) of Tehran University of Medical Science (Grant No: 17215) and was conducted in agreement with the Declaration of Helsinki and its subsequent revisions. The trial was registered at the Iranian registry of clinical trials (www.irct.ir; registration number: (IRCT201205131556N42). Written informed consent was obtained from all eligible patients and/or their legally authorized representatives. Patients were informed that they are free to withdraw from the study at any time without any influence on their relationship with their health care provider.

Study population

Forty-six postmenopausal women with the definite diagnosis of schizophrenia were enrolled in the study. The diagnosis of schizophrenia was made according to DSM-IV TR. Diagnosis was made based on a Structured Clinical Interview for DSM-IV-TR Axis I Disorders (SCID) and was confirmed with chart review and senior physician interview. Inclusion criteria were postmenopausal (be in postmenopause is defined as period of one year spontaneous amenorrhea, a serum FSH level of >20 and clinical symptoms such as hot flashes,...) women who met the diagnostic criteria for schizophrenia according to DSM IV-TR consisting of Positive and Negative Syndrome Scale (PANSS) [11] score above 60 and disease onset over 2 years. Exclusion criteria were the concurrent presence of neurologic or organic disorders; IQ lower than 70; illicit drug use in past 6 months, consumption of antipsychotic drugs in the previous week or a long-acting antipsychotic drug in previous 2 months, receiving any antidepressant and mood stabilizer drugs during the trial, former hormone replace therapy, electroconvulsive therapy in past 2 weeks; endocrine abnormality; hepatic or renal dysfunction; and history of thromboemboli, abnormal uterine bleeding or breast and uterine cancer, and stroke.

Study design

Forty-six postmenopausal women with DSM-IV-TR diagnosed chronic schizophrenia received risperidone (6 mg/day in 3 divided doses) (Janssen Pharmaceuticals, Toronto, Canada; 2 mg tablet) combined with either placebo (N = 23) or 120 mg/day of raloxifene (Eli Lilly) (N = 23) for 8 weeks. Patients were assessed by a psychiatrist at baseline and at 2 and 8 weeks after the start of medical therapy. Efficacy was defined as the change from baseline to endpoint in score on PANSS.

Outcome measurement

PANSS is one of the most important rating tools for computing symptom severity in patients with schizophrenia. It comprises 3 subscales (positive scale, negative scale, and general psychotherapy scale) with 30 items in total ranging in score between 1 and 7 which leads to a minimum total score of 30. PANSS has been used in a number of trials in Iran [12-15]. The mean decline in PANSS scale as well as subscales from baseline was regarded as the main outcome measure of response in schizophrenia to treatment. The scale was measured at baseline, week 2 and week 8. Efficacy will be defined as change from baseline to endpoint in score on PANSS. Adverse events were evaluated using a 25 –item checklist and Extra-pyramidal Symptoms Rating Scale (ESRS) [16].

Statistical analysis

SPSS software, version 20.0 for Windows, was used to analyze the data. Continuous data are presented as mean ± standard deviation (SD). We used Kolmogorov-Smirnov Z test to determine the normal distribution of all continuous variables and due to normal distribution of PNSS score and subscales (positive, negative, general), we used parametrical tests to analyze data. A mixed between-within subjects analysis of variance was conducted to assess the impact of two different interventions (Risperidone + Raloxifene, Risperidone + placebo) on patient scores on PANSS score, positive subscale, negative subscale, and general psychotherapy subscale, across three time periods (the start of study, week 2, and week 8).

Results

Figure 1 shows flow diagram of the patients. The mean age (±SD) of the raloxifene group was 61.96 ± 4.49 years versus 60.44 ± 5.28 years in the placebo group (non significant). Demographic data of the patients is presented in Table 1.

For PANSS scores, there was no significant interaction between intervention type and time [Wilks' Lambda = 0.89, F (2, 47) = 2.79, p = 0.07]. There was substantial main effect for time [Wilks' Lambda = 0.36, F (2, 47) = 42.56, p < 0.01] within both groups showing a reduction in PANSS scores across three time periods (Table 2, Figure 2). Furthermore, the main effect comparing two types of intervention was not significant [F (1, 48) = 1.77, p = 0.18].

For positive subscale scores, there was marginal significant interaction between intervention type and time [Wilks' Lambda = 0.89, F (2, 47) = 2.93, p = 0.06] and there was substantial main effect for time [Wilks' Lambda = 0.44, F (2, 47) = 24.39, p < 0.01] within both groups showing a reduction in positive subscale scores across the three time periods (Table 2, Figure 3). In addition, the main effect comparing two types of intervention was significant [F (1, 48) = 3.78, p = 0.02] suggesting superior effectiveness of Risperidone plus Raloxifene over Risperidone plus Placebo.

For negative subscale scores, there was no significant interaction between intervention type and time [Wilks' Lambda = 0.99, F (2, 47) = 0.12, p = 0.73]. There was

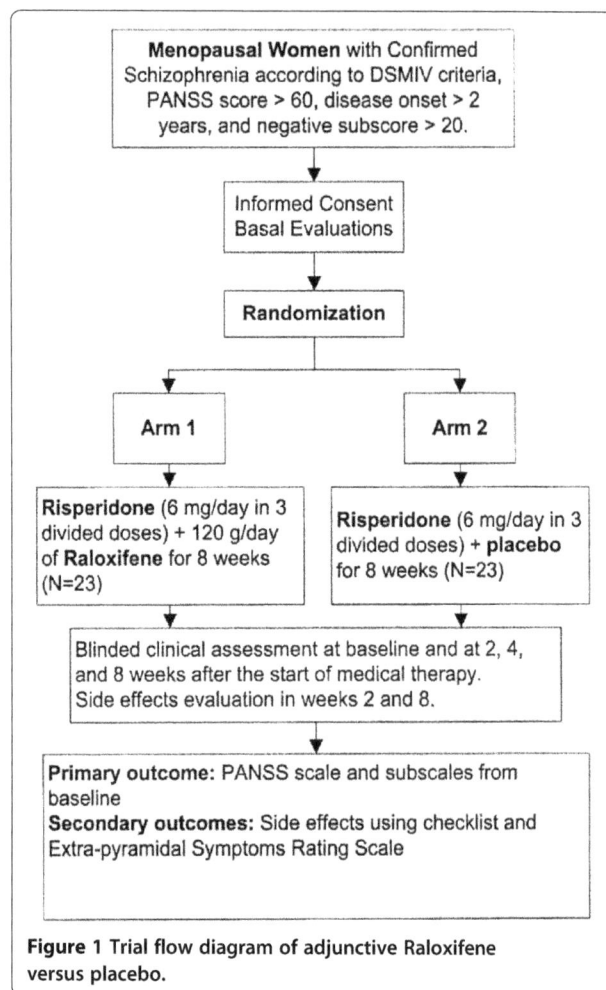

Figure 1 Trial flow diagram of adjunctive Raloxifene versus placebo.

substantial main effect for time [Wilks' Lambda = 0.46, F (2, 47) = 55.65, p < 0.01] within both groups showing a reduction in negative subscale scores across three time periods (Table 2, Figure 4). Additionally, the main effect comparing two types of intervention was not significant [F (1, 48) = 1.43, p = 0.23] suggesting no difference in effectiveness of the two therapies on negative subscale scores.

For general subscale scores, there was significant interaction between intervention type and time [Wilks' Lambda = 0.78, F (2, 47) = 6.78, p < 0.01]. There was substantial main effect for time [Wilks' Lambda = 0.34, F (2, 47) = 46.13, p < 0.01] within both groups showing a reduction in general subscale scores across the three time periods (Table 2, Figure 5). However, the main effect comparing two types of intervention was not significant [F (1, 48) = 0.03, p = 0.86] suggesting no difference in the effectiveness of the two therapies on general subscale scores.

Main adverse events included constipation (3 patients in Raloxifene group and 2 patients in placebo group), tremor (1 in each group), dry mouth (2 patients in raloxifene group), restless leg syndrome (1 patient in Raloxifene

Table 1 Demographic data of the raloxifene group versus the placebo group

		Risperidone + Raloxifene group (N = 25)	Risperidone + Placebo group (N = 25)	p-value
Age (±SD)		61.96 ± 4.49	60.44 ± 5.28	p > 0.05
Education	Illiterate	4 (36.36%)	7 (63.64%)	p > 0.05
	School	17 (51.52%)	16 (48.48%)	
	University	3 (50%)	3 (50%)	
Positive family history		13 (42%)	15 (60%)	p > 0.05
Age of onset		34.96 ± 11.69	29.40 ± 8.57	p > 0.05
Duration		17.24 ± 12.03	13.64 ± 12.41	p > 0.05
Previous treatment	Risperidone	7 (41.12%)	10 (58.88%)	p > 0.05
	Other atypical	3 (75.0%)	1 (25.0%)	
	Typical	11 (50.0%)	11 (50.0%)	
	Combination	4 (57.14%)	3 (42.86%)	
IQ	Normal	24 (52.17%)	22 (47.83%)	p > 0.05
	Borderline	1 (25.0%)	3 (75.0%)	

group), drowsiness (2 patients in placebo group), and loss of appetite (1 patient in placebo group). In addition, there was no ESRS difference between the two groups at weeks 2 and 8 [F (1, 48) = 1.04, p = 0.30].

Discussion

Adjunctive therapy and polypharmacy is used routinely for several chronic diseases. Medications with different mechanisms of action are used in polypharmacy. The use of adjunctive therapy in schizophrenia has been a major concern especially in recent years. The potential therapeutic efficacy of estrogens in schizophrenia is being identified and Selective Estrogen Receptor Modulators (SERMs) seem to be a better option in view of safety concerns. According to our findings, Raloxifene as an adjunctive treatment to risperidone was only superior

for positive symptoms and it was not effective in treating negative and general psychopathology symptoms.

Recently, some studies have pointed to the adjunctive efficacy of raloxifene in improving schizophrenic symptoms [17]. In a 12-week, double-blind, randomized, placebo-controlled study [10], 33 postmenopausal women with schizophrenia were randomized to receive either adjuvant raloxifene (16 women) or adjuvant placebo (17 women) for three months. The addition of raloxifene produced significant differences in some aspects of memory and executive function in patients treated with raloxifene. In another 12-week, double-blind, randomized, placebo-controlled study, 33 postmenopausal women with schizophrenia and prominent negative symptoms were randomized to either adjunctive raloxifene or adjunctive placebo for 12 weeks [9]. The addition of raloxifene

Table 2 PANSS and subscale scores for the intervention type across three time periods

	Time period	Risperidone + Raloxifene (n = 25) Mean ± SD	Risperidone + Placebo (n = 25) Mean ± SD
PANSS score	Week 0	105.52 ± 16.96	105.00 ± 11.68
	Week 2	89.08 ± 16.14	94.16 ± 19.78
	Week 8	68.32 ± 21.04	82.00 ± 26.14
Positive subscale	Week 0	25.76 ± 8.00	26.68 ± 7.04
	Week 2	20.92 ± 5.41	24.28 ± 6.33
	Week 8	14.32 ± 4.33	21.12 ± 7.07
Negative subscale	Week 0	28.04 ± 8.64	30.76 ± 9.09
	Week 2	24.88 ± 8.76	28.12 ± 10.88
	Week 8	19.60 ± 8.66	23.08 ± 12.08
General Psychopathology subscale	Week 0	50.44 ± 9.92	47.52 ± 6.46
	Week 2	43.56 ± 9.30	41.88 ± 9.76
	Week 8	34.56 ± 10.78	37.84 ± 11.89

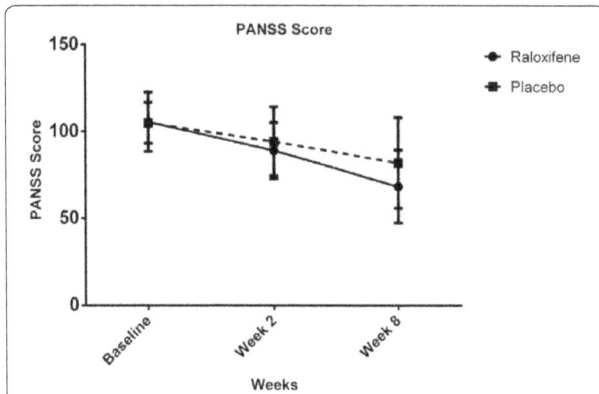

Figure 2 PANSS scores for the intervention type across three time periods (Raloxifene group: solid line, Placebo group: dashed line).

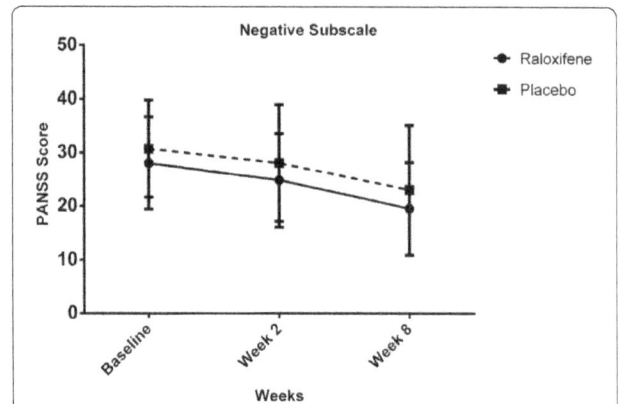

Figure 4 Negative subscale scores for the intervention type across three time periods (Raloxifene group: solid line, Placebo group: dashed line).

(60 mg/d) to regular antipsychotic treatment significantly reduced negative, positive, and general psychopathology symptoms compared to the placebo group.

In a randomized clinical trial [4], 35 postmenopausal women with schizophrenia received 120 mg/day adjunctive raloxifene compared to either adjunctive raloxifene HCl (60 mg/day) or placebo. A significantly greater recovery of total and general PANSS symptoms was noted in patients receiving 120 mg/day adjunctive raloxifene compared to either 60 mg/day adjunctive raloxifene HCl or placebo. In addition, adjunctive Raloxifene has been successfully used in single case reports for menstruating women suffering from resistant schizophrenia. A 29-year-old woman, with drug-resistant schizophrenia, experienced significant improvement in socio-occupational functioning, with reduction in symptom severity, over a 7-month follow-up period, [18].

It is significant that we encountered no adverse effects in the raloxifene group compared to the placebo group. The safer raloxifene profile compared with estrogenic compounds, makes it a preferred drug when adjunctive

hormonal therapy of schizophrenia for post-menopausal women is considered. The lack of adverse effects on breast and uterine tissue is an imperative advantage of Raloxifene over estrogen [19].

The ovarian hormone 17β-estradiol acts in the central nervous system to regulate neuroendocrine events and reproduction. Estradiol controls gene expression, neuronal survival, neuronal and glial differentiation, and synaptic transmission and has anti-inflammatory, protective and reparative properties in the brain [20,21]. A number of studies seem to indicate that raloxifene acts on brain dopamine and serotonin systems in a way that is similar to that of conjugated estrogens [22].

It is proposed that conjugated estrogens may exercise their therapeutic potential either by modulating brain neurotransmission or through neuroprotective effects. On the other hand, the incidence of schizophrenia in men is consistently observed to be approximately 1.5 times higher than its in women [23] and there is a male predominance in incidence in the early twenties, but a

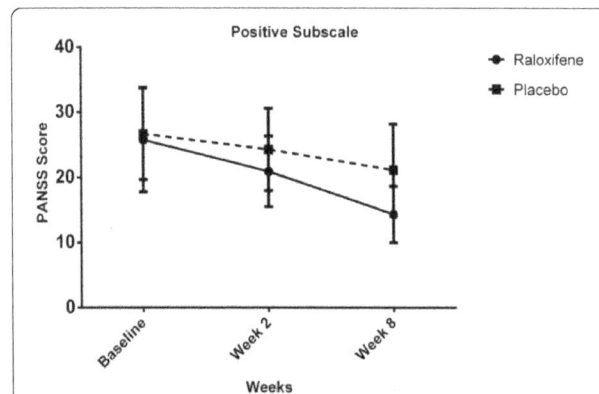

Figure 3 Positive subscale scores for the intervention type across three time periods (Raloxifene group: solid line, Placebo group: dashed line).

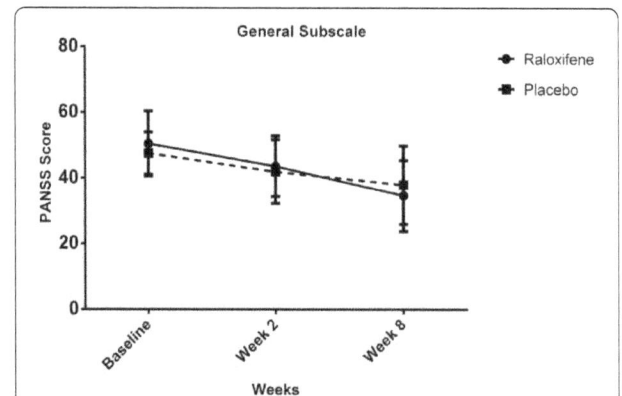

Figure 5 General Psychopathology subscale scores for the intervention type across three time periods (Raloxifene group: solid line, Placebo group: dashed line).

female predominance in older middle age [24]. Estrogen may have an impact on schizophrenia by several mechanisms. Short-term, it seems to have fast membrane effects by modifying functional activity in the dopaminergic synapse; for longer periods, it may appear to have genomic effects by altering synthesis at dopamine receptors. There is also evidence to suggest that estrogen alters serotonergic systems. Estrogen can also promote neuronal regeneration and block mechanisms of neuronal death [4]. In addition, numerous studies have described association between serotonin 1A receptor and major psychiatric disorders, such as schizophrenia and bipolar disorder [25]. Both serotonin and estrogen have been involved in modulation of mood and cognition. Even though substantial functional relations between estrogen and serotonin are recognized, the nature of their relationship has not been fully illuminated [26]. This study has some limitations which should be considered. The sample size was relatively small and the study course and follow-up period were relatively short. We did not measure the effect of raloxifene on menopausal symptoms as well. Furthermore, lack of cognitive assessments is another limitation of the present study.

Conclusions

In conclusion, it seems that according to our findings, raloxifene as an adjunctive treatment was shown to be superior to placebo in improving the positive symptoms in patients receiving risperidone. However, this drug did not show a benefit in treating the negative and general symptoms of schizophrenia when was added to risperidone therapy.

Abbreviations
SERMs: Selective estrogen receptor modulators; PNASS: Positive and negative syndrome scale.

Competing interests
No conflict of interest exists for any of the authors associated with the manuscript and there was no source of extra-institutional commercial funding. The funding organization had no role in the design and conduct of the study; in the collection, analysis, and interpretation of the data; or in the preparation, review, or approval of the manuscript and the decision to submit the paper for publication.

Authors' contributions
GK, SH and AN: Sample collection, FF: Statistical Analysis, Article writing, SA, LK, MK and FR: Designer and project manager, Article writing. All authors read and approved the final manuscript.

Acknowledgments
This study was supported by a grant from Tehran University of Medical Sciences to Prof. Shahin Akhondzadeh (Grant No: 17215). This study was Dr. Gilda Kianimehr's postgraduate thesis toward the Iranian Board of Psychiatry.

Author details
[1]Psychiatric Research Center, Roozbeh Hospital, Tehran University of Medical Sciences, Tehran 13337, Iran. [2]Shariati Hospital, Neurology Department, Tehran University of medical Sciences, Tehran, Iran. [3]Razi Psychiatric Hospital, University of Social Welfare and Rehabilitation, Tehran, Iran. [4]Qods Hospital, Kurdistan University of Medical Sciences, Sanandaj, Iran. [5]Infertility Ward, Arash Hospital, Tehran University of Medical Sciences, Tehran, Iran. [6]Psychiatric Research Center, Roozbeh Psychiatric Hospital, Tehran University of Medical Sciences, South Kargar Street 13337, Tehran, Iran.

References
1. Kulkarni J, Gavrilidis E, Worsley R, Hayes E: Role of estrogen treatment in the management of schizophrenia. *CNS Drugs* 2012, **26**(7):549–557.
2. Mortimer AM: Relationship between estrogen and schizophrenia. *Expert Rev Neurother* 2007, **7**(1):45–55.
3. Begemann MJ, Dekker CF, van Lunenburg M, Sommer IE: Estrogen augmentation in schizophrenia: a quantitative review of current evidence. *Schizophr Res* 2012, **141**(2–3):179–184.
4. Kulkarni J, Gurvich C, Lee SJ, Gilbert H, Gavrilidis E, de Castella A, Berk M, Dodd S, Fitzgerald PB, Davis SR: Piloting the effective therapeutic dose of adjunctive selective estrogen receptor modulator treatment in postmenopausal women with schizophrenia. *Psychoneuroendocrinology* 2010, **35**(8):1142–1147.
5. Akhondzadeh S, Nejatisafa AA, Amini H, Mohammadi MR, Larijani B, Kashani L, Raisi F, Kamalipour A: Adjunctive estrogen treatment in women with chronic schizophrenia: a double-blind, randomized, and placebo-controlled trial. *Prog Neuropsychopharmacol Biol Psychiatry* 2003, **27**(6):1007–1012.
6. Akhondzadeh S, Mokhberi K, Amini H, Larijani B, Kashani L, Hashemi L, Nejatisafa AA, Shafaei AR: Is there a relationship between estrogen serum level and symptom severity throughout the menstrual cycle of patients with schizophrenia? *Therapy* 2005, **2**(5):745–751.
7. Wu YC, Hill RA, Gogos A, van den Buuse M: Sex differences and the role of estrogen in animal models of schizophrenia: interaction with BDNF. *Neuroscience* 2013, **239**:67–83.
8. Velazquez-Zamora DA, Garcia-Segura LM, Gonzalez-Burgos I: Effects of selective estrogen receptor modulators on allocentric working memory performance and on dendritic spines in medial prefrontal cortex pyramidal neurons of ovariectomized rats. *Horm Behav* 2012, **61**(4):512–517.
9. Usall J, Huerta-Ramos E, Iniesta R, Cobo J, Araya S, Roca M, Serrano-Blanco A, Teba F, Ochoa S: Raloxifene as an adjunctive treatment for postmenopausal women with schizophrenia: a double-blind, randomized, placebo-controlled trial. *J Clin Psychiatry* 2011, **72**(11):1552–1557.
10. Huerta-Ramos E, Iniesta R, Ochoa S, Cobo J, Miquel E, Roca M, Serrano-Blanco A, Teba F, Ochoa S: Effects of raloxifene on cognition in postmenopausal women with schizophrenia: A double-blind, randomized, placebo-controlled trial. *Eur Neuropsychopharmacol* 2014, **24**(2):223–231.
11. Kay SR, Fiszbein A, Opler LA: The positive and negative syndrome scale (PANSS) for schizophrenia. *Schizophr Bull* 1987, **13**(2):261–276.
12. Farokhnia M, Azarkolah A, Adinehfar F, Khodaie-Ardakani MR, Hosseini SM, Yekehtaz H, Tabrizi M, Rezaei F, Salehi B, Sadeghi SM, Moghadam M, Gharibi F, Mirshafiee O, Akhondzadeh S: N-acetylcysteine as an adjunct to risperidone for treatment of negative symptoms in patients with chronic schizophrenia: a randomized, double-blind, placebo-controlled study. *Clin Neuropharmacol* 2013, **36**(6):185–192.
13. Farokhnia M, Sabzabadi M, Pourmahmoud H, Khodaie-Ardakani MR, Hosseini SM, Yekehtaz H, Tabrizi M, Rezaei F, Salehi B, Akhondzadeh S: A double-blind, placebo controlled, randomized trial of riluzole as an adjunct to risperidone for treatment of negative symptoms in patients with chronic schizophrenia. *Psychopharmacology (Berl)* 2014, **231**(3):533–542.
14. Khodaie-Ardakani MR, Mirshafiee O, Farokhnia M, Tajdini M, Hosseini SM, Modabbernia A, Rezaei F, Salehi B, Yekehtaz H, Ashrafi M, Tabrizi M, Akhondzadeh S: Minocycline add-on to risperidone for treatment of negative symptoms in patients with stable schizophrenia: Randomized double-blind placebo-controlled study. *Psychiatry Res* 2014, **215**(3):540–546.
15. Hosseini SM, Farokhnia M, Rezaei F, Gougol A, Yekehtaz H, Iranpour N, Salehi B, Tabrizi M, Tajdini M, Ghaleiha A, Akhondzadeh S: Intranasal desmopressin as an adjunct to risperidone for negative symptoms of schizophrenia: A randomized, double-blind, placebo-controlled, clinical trial. *Eur Neuropsychopharmacol* 2014, **24**(6):846–855.
16. Chouinard G, Margolese HC: Manual for the Extrapyramidal Symptom Rating Scale (ESRS). *Schizophr Res* 2005, **76**(2–3):247–265.
17. Kulkarni J, Gavrilidis E, Wang W, Worsley R, Fitzgerald PB, Gurvich C, Van Rheenen T, Berk M, Burger H: Estradiol for treatment-resistant

schizophrenia: a large-scale randomized-controlled trial in women of child-bearing age. *Mol Psychiatry* 2014, doi:10.1038/mp.2014.33.

18. Raveendranathan D, Shivakumar V, Jayaram N, Rao NP, Venkatasubramanian G: **Beneficial effects of add-on raloxifene in schizophrenia.** *Arch Womens Ment Health* 2012, **15**(2):147–148.

19. Chua WL, de Izquierdo SA, Kulkarni J, Mortimer A: **Estrogen for schizophrenia.** *Cochrane Database Syst Rev* 2005, **4**: CD004719.

20. Spencer JL, Waters EM, Romeo RD, Wood GE, Milner TA, McEwen BS: **Uncovering the mechanisms of estrogen effects on hippocampal function.** *Front Neuroendocrinol* 2008, **29**(2):219–237.

21. Vegeto E, Benedusi V, Maggi A: **Estrogen anti-inflammatory activity in brain: a therapeutic opportunity for menopause and neurodegenerative diseases.** *Front Neuroendocrinol* 2008, **29**(4):507–519.

22. Usall J, Coromina M, Araya S, Ochoa S: **Effect of raloxifene (a Selective Estrogen Receptor Modulator (SERM)) as coadjuvant to antidepressant treatment: a case report.** *Actas Esp Psiquiatr* 2011, **39**(5):334–336.

23. Welham J, Isohanni M, Jones P, McGrath J: **The antecedents of schizophrenia: a review of birth cohort studies.** *Schizophr Bull* 2009, **35**(3):603–623.

24. Abel KM, Drake R, Goldstein JM: **Sex differences in schizophrenia.** *Int Rev Psychiatry* 2010, **22**(5):417–428.

25. Kishi T, Okochi T, Tsunoka T, Okumura T, Kitajima T, Kawashima K, Yamanouchi Y, Kinoshita Y, Naitoh H, Inada T, Kunugi H, Kato T, Yoshikawa T, Ujike H, Ozaki N, Iwata N: **Serotonin 1A receptor gene, schizophrenia and bipolar disorder: an association study and meta-analysis.** *Psychiatry Res* 2011, **185**(1–2):20–26.

26. Amin Z, Canli T, Epperson CN: **Effect of estrogen-serotonin interactions on mood and cognition.** *Behav Cogn Neurosci Rev* 2005, **4**(1):43–58.

12

Opportunities and obstacles to the development of nanopharmaceuticals for human use

Nasser Nassiri Koopaei[1] and Mohammad Abdollahi[2,3,4*]

Abstract: Pharmaceutical nanotechnology has generated breakthrough developments in improving health care and human life from its emergence. The biomaterials employed mainly aim at improving drug delivery systems, imaging and diagnostic technologies while the nanoscale materials are in widespread use in other industries such as electronics and optics. Such advancement may revolutionize the drug development and therapy with new and more efficient treatments. Although, nanotechnology assists humankind in improving its well being, it has certain limitations that entail thorough investigation by the regulatory and scientific authorities. To address concerns regarding the safety and toxicity profile of the nanopharmaceuticals, we have reviewed the challenges and solutions of nanopharmaceuticals use in human health and the related health risks. In this regard, regulatory and scientific bodies such as countries' Food and Drug Administration (FDA), Organization for Economic Co-operation and Development (OECD), European Medicine Agency (EMA), Environmental Protection Agency (EPA), National Institute for Occupational Safety and Health (NIOSH), and World Health Organization (WHO) can participate in developing and reinforcing safety measures and regulatory frameworks to insure the public health. The regulatory authorities may enforce the nanopharmaceutical industries to conduct comprehensive toxicity tests and monitor the adverse drug reaction reports in close collaboration with the scientific community to act accordingly and inform the public as the implementation of the strategy.

Keywords: Human Use, Nanopharmaceuticals, Toxicity Profile, Regulatory Framework

Introduction

Pharmaceutical nanotechnology deals with the scope of pharmaceutical compounds that emerge from a multidisciplinary field of science entailing the development and application of molecular structures with dimensions smaller than 100 nm [1]. The nanoscale feature of these products and devices render them special capabilities that can be used to produce devices and products as therapeutic agents and other purposes [1, 2]. Pharmaceutical nanotechnology has generated breakthrough developments in health care and human life [3]. The biomaterials employed in this field mainly aim at improving drug delivery systems, imaging and diagnostic technologies while the nanoscale materials are of widespread use in other industries such as electronics and optics [4]. In 1995 with the approval of Doxil® (liposomal doxorubicin) by the US FDA, the pharmaceutical nanotechnology passed its first evolutionary milestone with the subsequent approval of other products but the approvals are in their early stage with less than 50 US FDA approved drug formulations while more are in the pipeline [1, 5, 6]. However, nanotechnology applications in the treatment of some of most critical metabolic and genetic diseases and cancer, delivery systems, genetic tests, as well as imaging and diagnostics are promising enough to absorb huge amounts of investment into research and development efforts both in the academia and the industry [1, 4, 5]. Noteworthy, nanotechnology provides humankind with exceptional opportunities to improve its wellbeing, but it also has certain limitations that entail thorough investigation by the regulatory and

* Correspondence: Mohammad@TUMS.Ac.Ir;
Mohammad.Abdollahi@UToronto.Ca
[2]Department of Toxicology & Pharmacology, Faculty of Pharmacy and Pharmaceutical Sciences Research Center, Tehran University of Medical Sciences, Tehran, Iran
[3]Endocrinology and Metabolism Research Center, Endocrinology and Metabolism Clinical Sciences Institute, Tehran University of Medical Sciences, Tehran, Iran
Full list of author information is available at the end of the article

scientific authorities [6, 7]. The present study reviews the literature on the pharmaceutical application of nanomaterials and then raises the question regarding the possible health risks associated with nanopharmaceuticals use in humans. Concerns about human use of nanomaterials become overwhelming when we know that these nanostructures do not completely abide by the scientific principles that form the basis for our knowledge about how human physiologic system deals with exogenous compounds and toxicity tests also fail to adequately address the nanotoxicity issues for human beings, animals and the environment. Moreover, the research strives to bring the toxicological aspect of nanopharmaceuticals and pending health risks to top agenda in regulatory bodies as well as scientific community.

Nanopharmaceuticals: advantageous applications and toxicological concerns

Liposomes, niosomes, polymer based micelles, nanostructured vaccines, polymersomes, dendrimeric nanostructures are nanoparticulate structures used as novel and targeted drug delivery systems. These nanostructures have special structural and functional capabilities and aspects that offers specific applications when engineered like the composition and percentage of components, size distribution and physical structure. In the sense, the nanoparticles could be responsive to the environment, targeted or assume other specificities [8, 9].

Special characteristics of nanostructures make them useful agents for both diagnosis and imaging agents (Fig. 1) [10]. Nanochips and nanoarrays employ different

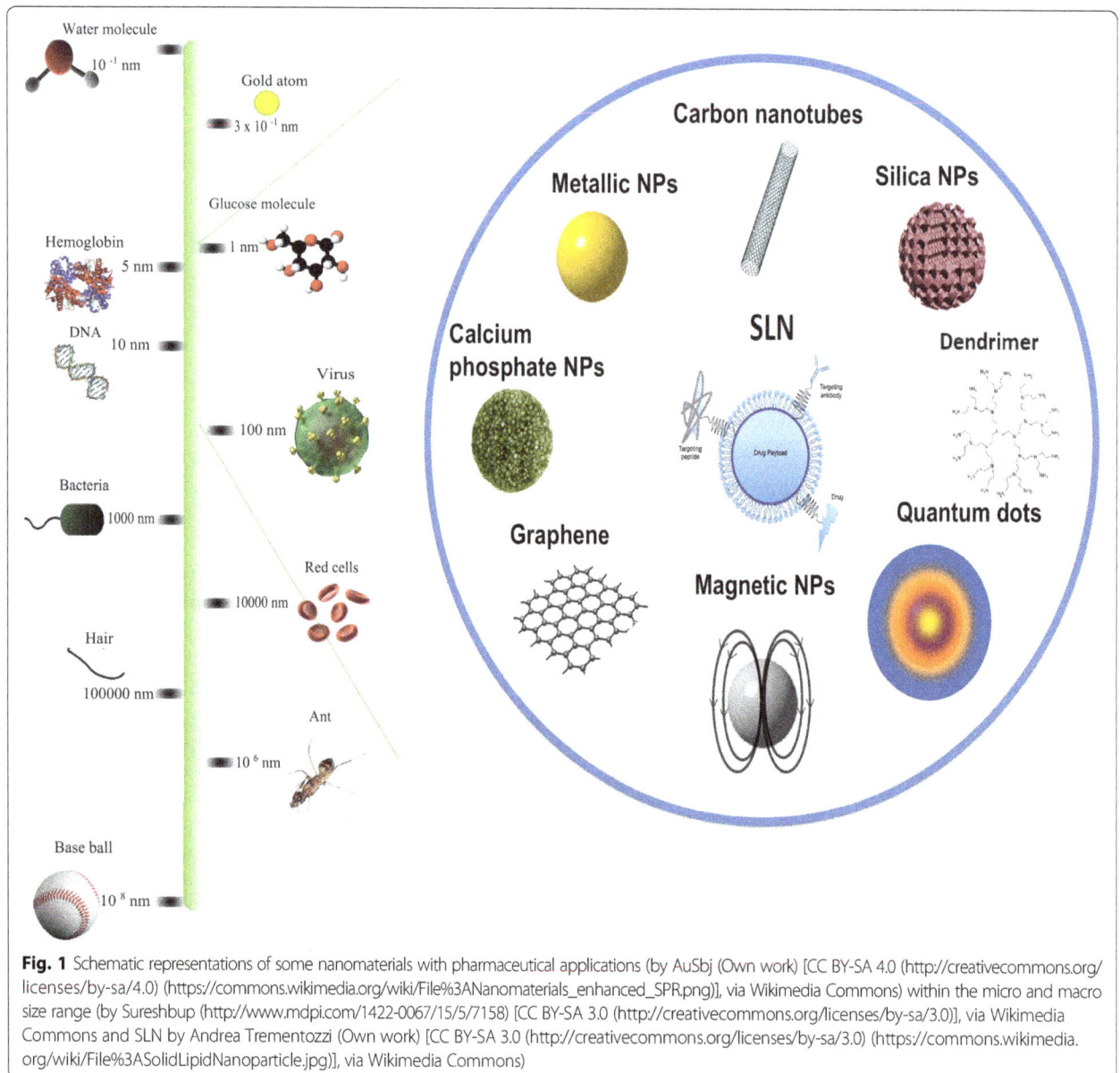

Fig. 1 Schematic representations of some nanomaterials with pharmaceutical applications (by AuSbj (Own work) [CC BY-SA 4.0 (http://creativecommons.org/licenses/by-sa/4.0) (https://commons.wikimedia.org/wiki/File%3ANanomaterials_enhanced_SPR.png)], via Wikimedia Commons) within the micro and macro size range (by Sureshbup (http://www.mdpi.com/1422-0067/15/5/7158) [CC BY-SA 3.0 (http://creativecommons.org/licenses/by-sa/3.0)], via Wikimedia Commons and SLN by Andrea Trementozzi (Own work) [CC BY-SA 3.0 (http://creativecommons.org/licenses/by-sa/3.0) (https://commons.wikimedia.org/wiki/File%3ASolidLipidNanoparticle.jpg)], via Wikimedia Commons)

methods to measure various biomarkers within biologic samples to monitor disease formation and progression. Moreover, nanotheranostics contain both diagnostic and pharmacotherapeutic agents in one formulation to attain various purposes. They may be aimed at drug delivery, drug release, drug efficacy and therapeutic drug monitoring. In addition, different nanoparticles have been developed to improve the diagnostic capabilities of nuclear magnetic resonance imaging (Fig. 2) [11, 12].

With all the features in mind, there are certain concerns with regards to nanoparticulate structure for human use [13]. Nanoparticles toxicity has attracted the most vital criticism because they represent exceptional characteristics such as size, size distribution, surface charge and properties, expanded surface area, self-assembly and stability [4].

These features influence the nanoparticles' ADME (Adsorption, Distribution, Metabolism and Excretion) properties like cellular uptake, distribution within the body fluids, and transport through biological barriers. For instance, the tiny molecular size of the nanoparticles enables them to cross the natural biological barriers in the brain and eye or other cells. Route of administration also determines the toxicity profile to a lesser extent as for example, nanopharmaceuticals may trigger neurotoxicity and inflammatory responses or even the systemic circulation when applied in inhalation forms through their penetration into the CNS via posterior nasal mucosal layer [14]. However, our knowledge is yet scant enough not to be sure about the mechanistic toxicology of nanoparticles since the currently available toxicity tests are not fully

assuring and data obtained from in vitro or animal studies are not always extrapolatable to human [15, 16].

Exposure to nanopharmaceuticals may affect manufacturing personnel, healthcare professionals and the patients. However, when the nanopharmaceuticals are disposed or excreted via waste water, the general public will also be at exposure. Therefore, elaborate monitoring systems based on physicochemical characterization are required [1, 15]. As the nanoparticles enter the body, they penetrate the epithelial and endothelial barriers and then undergo cellular uptake processes like diffusion, different endocytosis pathways such as receptor mediated endocytosis dictated by their physicochemical and surface properties. Then their biodistribution also follows relatively unknown patterns rather than those of other conventional pharmaceuticals, though such organ deposition in the Central Nervous System (CNS) and growing fetus would be of dramatic concern along with other organs like liver, kidney and spleen. Although nanopharmaceuticals cytotoxicity mechanisms are not well defined, but oxidative stress, proinflammatory effects and genotoxicity are theocratized via Reactive Oxygen Species (ROS) formation, GSH/GSSG ratio alteration, upregulation of transcription factors and signaling kinases, DNA damage and mutation [1, 17]. Cytotoxicity and genotoxicity have been seen with nanodrugs containing metallic ions like aluminum oxide, gold, copper oxide, silver, zinc oxide, titanium oxide, iron oxide and carbon based nanomaterials. Although silica and polymer based nanomaterials have been deemed to be more

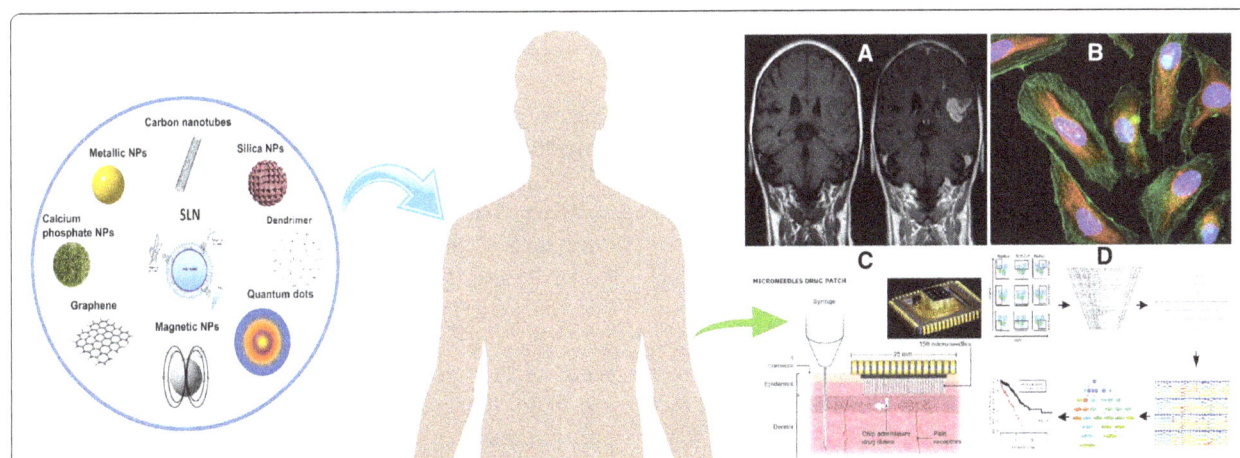

Fig. 2 Applications of nanomaterials as (A) MRI contrast agents adapted from Wikimedia Commons [by Hellerhoff (own work); CC BY-SA 3.0 (http://creativecommons.org/licenses/by-sa/3.0) (https://commons.wikimedia.org/wiki/File%3ABluthirnschranke_nach_Infarkt_nativ_und_KM.png)], via Wikimedia Commons), (B) drug delivery targeting using antibody (by Gerry Shaw [GFDL (http://www.gnu.org/copyleft/fdl.html) or CC BY-SA 3.0 (http://creativecommons.org/licenses/by-sa/3.0) (https://commons.wikimedia.org/wiki/File%3AHeLa_cells_stained_with_antibody_to_actin_(green)_%2C_vimentin_(red)_and_DNA_(blue).jpg)], via Wikimedia Commons), (C) novel drug delivery devices (by National Health Federation [CC BY-SA 3.0 (http://creativecommons.org/licenses/by-sa/3.0) (https://commons.wikimedia.org/wiki/File%3ATransdermal_microneedles.png)], via Wikimedia Commons) and (D) treatment optimization by developing marker based cell characterization (by Nima Aghaeepour et al. [Public domain], via Wikimedia Commons (https://commons.wikimedia.org/wiki/File%3AFlowType-RchyOptimyx.png))

biocompatible and relatively nontoxic, they may also involve ROS formation and cytotoxicity [9]. Some toxicity tests have been proposed for the nanopharmaceuticals before their approval both in vitro and in vivo. In vitro tests may include but not limited to uptake and transport characterization, cytotoxicity assays (Lactate Dehydrogenase, tetrazolium, Alamar Blue, OECD developed Neutral Red dye assays that are based upon Neutral Red dye cellular uptake), genotoxicity (Ames test, comet assay, micronucleus and chromosomal aberration assays) and carcinogenotoxicity (SHE test, BALB/c 3 T3 and C3H10T1/2 assays). Validated in vivo tests should include at least ADME studies and acute and chronic organ toxicity tests; however, these in vivo tests are time and cost consuming and entail ethical compromises [1, 9, 18]. OECD guidelines provide a wealth of technical documents for the toxicity testing of nanomaterials, but the OECD is yet developing the standard materials critical for the testing, working on the development of carcinogenotoxicity tests like SHE test, BALB/c 3 T3 and C3H10T1/2 assays. The OECD guideline for the tests on routine chemicals are useful in this regard to some extent, but they need more detailed discussion on the biohazards and physicochemical characterizations [1].

Regulatory framework for nanopharmaceuticals

Concerns regarding the safety and toxicity profile of the nanopharmaceuticals involve active participation of regulatory and scientific bodies, including but not limited to FDA, EMA, EPA, NIOSH, WHO to develop and reinforce safety measures and regulatory frameworks to insure the public health [7, 19].

In this venue, scientific associations as well as the scientific committees within regulatory authorities like US FDA and EMA release technical documents and recommendations for the industry and regulators that lead mostly the evaluation and approval of the products and devices as per the postulation of the public health and quality of life. US FDA has recently updated its regulatory approach to the nanopharmaceuticals through guidelines and denoted that for products that contain nanoscale materials or properties attributable to the dimensions, may require premarket review or where not applicable, urges the industry to consult the FDA very early in the product development phase to address the product's regulatory status and concerns with regards to its safety, effectiveness or public health impact [20]. Moreover, the FDA declared its regulatory policy towards the nanopharmaceuticals earlier. It stated that the body would be scientifically focused on the product filing and applies for premarket review or consultation approach as per the rules and regulations. The FDA already keeps the industry responsible for its products meet all the legal requirements like safety, effectiveness

and other product quality attributes. Nevertheless, the authority continues to run post-market monitoring surveys to protect the consumers while maintaining its role in preparing technical documents and advisory guidelines [21]. The bioequivalent versions of the nanotechnology derived products or nanosimilars compose a new era of extensive regulatory burden. In addition, regulatory authorities of other countries have to keep in pace with the market trend and mobilize their capacities for the oncoming nanosimilars. Overall, the nanoparticulate biomaterials such as liposomes and dendrimers involve more elaborate investigations caused by their modified formulations and ADME [3, 22].

Nanopharmaceuticals approval should contain close characterization of physicochemical properties as they have size and size distribution that may increase the chance of thromboembolic complications via facilitating the thrombosis cascade. On the other hand, nanopharmaceuticals require sophisticated stability and ADME studies because most of the critical parameters of their safety and efficacy may evade during shelf life and cause morbidities and fatalities. Moreover, FDA has approved some liposomal, dendrimer based, PEGylated and albumin bound compounds while the overwhelming number of candidates are on their way to market [23–26].

It should not be forgotten that discovery of new medicines has been always expensive, time-consuming, competitive, with unknown outcome to pass all preclinical and clinical phases of approval. Therefore, to reduce the attrition rate in further steps, investigators must pay enough attention to safety of medicines, development risks, dose ranging, early proof of concept/principle, and patient stratification based on biologically and/or clinically validated biomarkers [27].

Future prospects of nanopharmaceuticals in human health

With the advent of nanosized structures and their special characteristics, many fields of science started to take advantage of these extraordinarily modifiable and functional features based on their special needs. Medical and pharmaceutical experts also employed these capabilities to develop new drugs, medical devices and therapeutic methods. Cancer is a major cause of mortality and morbidity that has benefited from nanopharmaceuticals and promising progress is also on the way. In spite of the currently approved drugs for cancer chemotherapy, there are more than twenty candidates in clinical trials for approval process. These candidates either improve therapeutic/toxicity profile of existing drugs or contain novel molecules [28, 29]. Dermatology is also applying nanostructures for different diseases treatment because of the special structure of skin and natural barriers that could be simply overcome through noninvasive methods using the nanosized structures [30]. Drug delivery system, nanotherapeutics, nanobots, nanoshells, nanotubes, gene therapy, and vaccination and immunization improvement rank among the functional structures that pharmaceuticals will borrow from nanotechnology while chip technology, quantum dots and sensor nanobots emerge advantageous for diagnostic purposes [31, 32]. However, reconstructive medicine and tissue engineering look forward to applying nanotechnology to cover the gap in clinical practice by providing biodegradable and biocompatible tissues [33]. Radiation enhancers are also under investigation to increase the usability of radiotherapy in war against cancer [34]. Personalized medicine is the other field of interdisciplinary medical science that is enjoying the nanomaterials like theranostics and data management to improve patient care based on certain patient's needs, genetic and health status [35].

Concluding remarks

In conclusion, it should be stated that nanopharmaceuticals may pave the way for new therapies for unmet medical needs and optimization of the existing therapies with their promising features. But, in the meanwhile their limitations should also be considered since adverse events may come out during their use in the populations with metabolic variations as well as health status. The nanodrugs modified biokinetics necessitate well established toxicology profiling through in vitro and especially in vivo tests since the lab tests mostly cover their toxicity in cell lines with different physiological properties rather than the healthy people and patients. The test endpoints may include oxidative stress burden, inflammatory system, genotoxicity, carcinogenicity, respiratory, cardiovascular, central and peripheral nervous system, hematopoietic and lymphatic system, developmental and reproductive toxicity. To achieve this goal, validated and standard test protocols as well as reference standards seem critical. Nonetheless, Quality by Design (QbD) approach adopted by the FDA gains importance to manufacture nanodrugs in reliable and reproducible processes. Therefore, it would be advisable for the regulatory authorities to enforce the nanopharmaceutical industries to conduct comprehensive toxicity tests and monitor the adverse drug reaction reports closely to act accordingly and inform the public. Proper collection of possible toxicities and adverse events from the medical and public community is recommended.

Abbreviations

ADME: Adsorption, Distribution, Metabolism and Excretion; CNS: Central Nervous System; EMA: European Medicine Agency; EPA: Environmental Protection Agency; FDA: Food and Drug Administration; NIOSH: National Institute for Occupational Safety and Health; QbD: Quality by Design; ROS: Reactive Oxygen Species; WHO: World Health Organization

Authors' contributions

Both authors have made substantive equal contributions to the paper and read and approved the final manuscript.

Competing interests

The authors have no commercial associations or sources of support that might pose a competing interest. MA is the Editor-in-Chief of DARU Journal of Pharmaceutical Sciences.

Author details

[1]Department of Pharmaceutics, School of Pharmacy, University of Florida, Orlando, USA. [2]Department of Toxicology & Pharmacology, Faculty of Pharmacy and Pharmaceutical Sciences Research Center, Tehran University of Medical Sciences, Tehran, Iran. [3]Endocrinology and Metabolism Research Center, Endocrinology and Metabolism Clinical Sciences Institute, Tehran University of Medical Sciences, Tehran, Iran. [4]Toxicology Interest Group, Universal Scientific Education and Research Network, Tehran University of Medical Sciences, Tehran, Iran.

References

1. Demetzos C. Pharmaceutical Nanotechnology: Fundamentals and Practical Applications. Singapore: Springer; 2016.
2. Ge Y, Li S, Wang S, Moore R. Nanomedicine: Principles and Perspectives. New York: Springer; 2014.
3. Chang EH, Harford JB, Eaton MAW, Boisseau PM, Dube A, Hayeshi R, Swai H, Lee DS. Nanomedicine: past, present and future–a global perspective. Bioch Bioph Res Co. 2015;468(3):511–7.
4. Pourmand A, Abdollahi M. Current opinion on nanotoxicology. DARU. 2012;20(1):1.
5. Weissig V, Pettinger TK, Murdock N. Nanopharmaceuticals (part 1): products on the market. Int J Nanomed. 2014;9:4357.
6. Weissig V, Guzman-Villanueva D. Nanopharmaceuticals (part 2): products in the pipeline. Int J Nanomed. 2015;10:1245.
7. Bawa R, Barenholz Y, Owen A. The challenge of regulating nanomedicine: Key issues, in nanomedicines. In: Braddock M, editor. Nanomedicines: design, delivery and detection. Cambridge: Royal Society of Chemistry; 2016. p. 290–314.
8. Ogris M, Oupicky D. Nanotechnology for nucleic acid delivery. New York: Humana Press; 2013.
9. Bahadar H, Maqbool F, Niaz K, Abdollahi M. Toxicity of nanoparticles and an overview of current experimental models. Iran Biomed J. 2016;20(1):1.
10. Bawa R. Handbook of Clinical Nanomedicine From Bench to Bedside. Boca Raton: Pan Stanford Publishing; 2015.
11. Lammers T, Aime S, Hennink WE, Storm G, Kiessling F. Theranostic nanomedicine. Accounts Chem Res. 2011;44(10):1029–38.
12. Abdelkader H, Alany RG. Controlled and continuous release ocular drug delivery systems: pros and cons. Curr Drug Deliv. 2012;9(4):421–30.
13. Zhang XQ, Xu X, Bertrand N, Pridgen E, Swami A, Farokhzad OC. Interactions of nanomaterials and biological systems: Implications to personalized nanomedicine. Adv Drug Deliv Rev. 2012;64(13):1363–84.
14. Zolnik BS, Sadrieh N. Regulatory perspective on the importance of ADME assessment of nanoscale material containing drugs. Adv Drug Deliver Rev. 2009;61(6):422–7.
15. Mostafalou S, Mohammadi H, Ramazani A, Abdollahi M. Different biokinetics of nanomedicines linking to their toxicity; an overview. DARU. 2013;21(1):1.
16. Saeidnia S, Manayi A, Abdollahi M. From in vitro Experiments to in vivo and Clinical Studies; Pros and Cons. Curr Drug Discov Technol. 2015;12(4):218–24.
17. Shvedova A, Pietroiusti A, Kagan V. Nanotoxicology ten years later: lights and shadows. Toxicol Appl Pharm. 2016;299:1–2.
18. Shetab-Boushehri SV, Abdollahi M. Current concerns on the validity of in vitro models that use transformed neoplastic cells in pharmacology and toxicology. Int J Pharmacol. 2012;8(6):594–5.
19. Berkner S, Schwirn K, Voelker D. Nanopharmaceuticals: Tiny challenges for the environmental risk assessment of pharmaceuticals. Environ Toxicol Chem. 2015;35(4):780–7.
20. http://www.fda.gov/RegulatoryInformation/Guidances/ucm257698.htm. Accessed 13 Sept 2016.

21. http://www.fda.gov/ScienceResearch/SpecialTopics/Nanotechnology/ucm301114.htm. Accessed 13 Sept 2016.

22. Dawidczyk CM, Kim C, Park JH, Russell LM, Lee KH, Pomper MG, Searson PC. State-of-the-art in design rules for drug delivery platforms: lessons learned from FDA-approved nanomedicines. J Control Release. 2014;187:133–44.

23. Haynes CL. The emerging field of nanotoxicology. Anal Bioanal Chem. 2010;398(2):587–8.

24. Monteiro-Riviere NA, Tran CL. Nanotoxicology: progress toward nanomedicine. Boca Raton: CRC press; 2014.

25. Srikumaran M. Nanopharmaceuticals patenting issues and FDA regulatory challenges. Sci Tech Lawyer. 2008;5(2):10.

26. Lee CC, MacKay JA, Fréchet JMJ, Szoka FC. Designing dendrimers for biological applications. Nat biotechnol. 2005;23(12):1517–26.

27. Safavi M, Sabourian R, Abdollahi M. The development of biomarkers to reduce attrition rate in drug discovery focused on oncology and central nervous system. Expert Opin Drug Discov. 2016;11(10):939–56.

28. Bregoli L, Movia D, Gavigan-Imedio JD, Lysaght J, Reynolds J, Prina-Mello A. Nanomedicine applied to translational oncology: a future perspective on cancer treatment. Nanomedicine. 2016;12(1):81–103.

29. Lloyd-Hughes H, Shiatis AE, Pabari A, Mosahebi A, Seifalian A. Current and future nanotechnology applications in the management of melanoma: a review. J Nanomed Nanotechnol. 2015;6:6.

30. Landriscina A, Rosen J, Friedman AJ. Nanotechnology, inflammation and the skin barrier: innovative approaches for skin health and cosmesis. Cosmetics. 2015;2(2):177–86.

31. Kumar M, Verma D, Yadav R. Nanomedicine: future prospective in disease diagnosis and preventions. World J Clin Pharmacol Microbiol Toxicol. 2015;1(1):3–8.

32. Anderson D, Sydor MJ, Fletcher P, Holian A. Nanotechnology: The Risks and Benefits for Medical Diagnosis and Treatment. J Nanomed Nanotechnol. 2016; doi:10.4172/2157-7439.1000e143

33. Gardner J. Nanotechnology in medicine and healthcare: Possibilities, progress and problems. SAJBL. 2015;8(2):50–3.

34. Pottier A, Borghi E, Levy L. The future of nanosized radiation enhancers. Br J Radiol. 2015; doi:10.1259/bjr.20150171

35. Herrmann IK, Rösslein M. Personalized medicine: the enabling role of nanotechnology. Nanomedicine. 2016;11(1):1–3.

13

Determination of stress-induced degradation products of cetirizine dihydrochloride by a stability-indicating RP-HPLC method

Paloma Flórez Borges[1,2*†], Pilar Pérez Lozano[1†], Encarna García Montoya[1†], Montserrat Miñarro[1†], Josep R Ticó[1†], Enric Jo[2†] and Josep M Suñe Negre[1†]

Abstract

Background: A new, simple and accurate stability-indicating reverse phase high performance liquid chromatography method was developed and validated during the early stage of drug development of an oral lyophilizate dosage form of cetirizine dihydrochloride.

Methods: For RP-HPLC analysis it was used an Eclipse XDB C8 column 150 mm × 4.6 mm, 5 μm (Agilent columns, Barcelona, Spain) as the stationary phase with a mobile phase consisted of a mixture of 0.2 M K_2HPO4 pH 7.00 and acetonitrile (65:35, v/v) at a flow rate of 1 mL min^{-1}. Detection was performed at 230 nm using diode array detector. The method was validated in accordance with ICH guidelines with respect to linearity, accuracy, precision, specificity, limit of detection and quantification.

Results: The method results in excellent separation between the drug substance and its stress-induced degradation products. The peak purity factor is >950 for the drug substance after all types of stress, which confirms the complete separation of the drug substance peak from its stress induced degradation products.
Regression analysis showed $r^2 > 0.999$ for cetirizine dihydrochloride in the concentration range of 650 μg mL^{-1} to 350 μg mL^{-1} for drug substance assay and a $r^2 > 0.999$ in the concentration range of 0.25 μg mL^{-1} to 5 μg mL^{-1} for degradation products. The method presents a limit of detection of 0.056 μg mL^{-1} and a limit of quantification of 0.25 μg mL^{-1}. The obtained results for precision and accuracy for drug substance and degradation products are within the specifications established for the validation of the method.

Conclusions: The proposed stability-indicating method developed in the early phase of drug development proved to be a simple, sensitive, accurate, precise, reproducible and therefore useful for the following stages of the cetirizine dihydrochloride oral lyophilizate dosage form development.

Background

In the early stage of drug development, forced degradation studies are used to facilitate the development of an analytical methodology, in order to obtain a better understanding of the drug substance (DS) studied and the final drug product (DP) stability, providing data regarding degradation pathways and degradation products (DE) [1]. Such studies are needed to assure that all the regulatory requirements of a drug are fulfilled, such as the identification of possible DE, degradation pathways and intrinsic stability of the drug molecule. Part of the study is the development and validation of the stability indicating analytical method involved [2,3]. The overall objective of this work is to develop a new formulation with the drug substance ($C_{21}H_{27}Cl_3N_2O_3$) cetirizine dihydrocloride (CTZ; the dihydrochloride of a 2-[4-chlorobenzhydryl) piperazin-1-yl] ethoxyacetic acid). CTZ is a non-sedative H_1 antihistaminic drug, a piperazine derivative and metabolite of hydroxyzine (Figure 1) [4]. CTZ presents an increased degree of polarity, which makes it less capable of crossing the blood brain barrier, hence reducing the sedative side effects in comparison

* Correspondence: pflorezb@gmail.com
†Equal contributors
[1]Pharmacy and Pharmaceutical Technology Department, Faculty of Pharmacy, University of Barcelona, Avda Joan XXIII s/n 08028, Barcelona, Spain
[2]Reig Jofre Group, c. Gran Capitá 6 08970, Sant Joan Despi, Barcelona, Spain

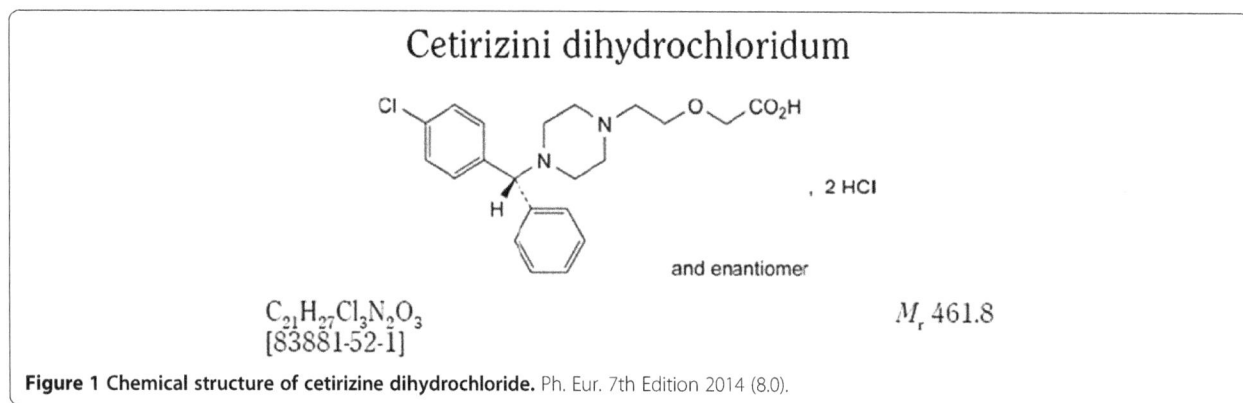

Figure 1 Chemical structure of cetirizine dihydrochloride. Ph. Eur. 7th Edition 2014 (8.0).

with first generation antihistamines, such as diphenhydramine and hydroxyzine [5-7]. CTZ is administrated generally in tablets and liquid forms orally to promote the relief of symptoms related to allergic rhinitis, chronic idiopathic urticaria and other rashes [8,9].

This new formulation consists of an oral lyophilized dosage form, whose aim is to facilitate swallowing (in the case of patients with dysphagia, such as children and elderly, for instance), easy to administer, effective, safe and stable over time.

Several HPLC methods have been reported in literature for the determination of CTZ alone [10-13] and also determining CTZ simultaneously with other drug substances, as in multicomponents preparations [14-16]. In order to develop a new chromatographic method for the determination and quantification of CTZ and its DE generated after a forced degradation study, several chromatographic methods for CTZ were investigated in the literature. Among them, was the Ph. Eur. method for CTZ [17]. However, the latter was discarded due to the use of a normal phase chromatographic column and mobile phase that used much organic solvent (acetonitrile, not very cost-effective). Also, the Ph. Eur. method presents a very acid mobile phase pH (pH <0.5), which is known to diminish the life span of the chromatographic column [18]. Also, some chromatographic analytical methods [12,13] used chromatographic columns of reverse phase, usually C18 and C8. Depending on the type of separation pursued (as for instance, CTZ combined with another DS), isocratic or gradient methods were used, and also mobile phases with ionic pairing. We have developed a reverse-phase high performance liquid chromatography (RP-HPLC) method by studying the effect of the stationary phase (C18 or C8 analytical columns) on peak resolution, the influence of pH -mobile phase-when adjusting the desired retention time (t_R) for the DS. Plus, by using a reverse-phase column, we reduced the amount of organic solvent (acetonitrile) used for the

identification of the DS, in comparison to the analytical method validated by Ph. Eur. [17], which uses a normal phase chromatographic column, requiring more organic solvent due to its characteristics [18-25]. Therefore the aim of this study is to determine all possible DE generated under stress conditions, by developing and validating a stability-indicating RP-HPLC method for cetirizine dihydrochloride in the early stage of drug development of an oral lyophilizate.

Methods
Chemicals and reagents
All chemicals were analytical grade and used as received. All solutions were prepared in Milli-Q deionized water from a Milli Q gradient A10 water purification system (Molsheim, France). CTZ bulk powder (Cetirizine dihydrochloride, Ph. Eur) was purchased from Jubilant Lifesciences Ltd (Mysore, India) and kindly provided by Reig Jofre Group (Barcelona, Spain). HPLC grade acetonitrile was obtained from Panreac (Barcelona, Spain). Ortho-phosphoric acid 85% was purchased from Panreac (Barcelona, Spain). Potassium phosphate dibasic Ph. Eur. (K_2HPO_4) was purchased from Fagron (Terrassa, Spain). Hydrochloric acid 37%, sodium hydroxide and hydrogen peroxide (H_2O_2) at 33% were purchased from Panreac (Barcelona, Spain).

Equipment and chromatographic conditions
Samples were analyzed on Dionex Ultimate 3000 HPLC Thermo Fisher Scientific (California, USA), equipped with data system Chromeleon version 6.8 SP2 Build 2284, with degasifier SR3000, LPG-3400 quaternary pump, injector WPS3000, oven 6P TCC-3100, UV–vis detector PDA-3000. For initial development studies it was used an analytical chromatographic column Kromasyl 100-5C18 150 mm × 4.6 mm, 5 μm particle size (Tecnokroma Akzonobel, Terrasa, Spain). For final development and method validation, it was used an analytical

chromatographic column Eclipse XDB-C8 150 mm × 4.6 mm, 5 μm particle size (Agilent columns, Barcelona, Spain). An isocratic mobile phase consisting of acetonitrile and 0.2 M potassium phosphate dibasic Ph. Eur. buffer solution at pH 7.00 (35:65 v/v) was used, and the analysis was carried out at a flow rate of 1 mL min^{-1}. All determinations were performed at 30°C. The injection volume was 25 μL. The detector was set at λ 230 nm. The peak homogeneity was expressed in terms of peak purity factor and was obtained directly from spectral analysis report using the above mentioned software. Other apparatus included a Crison micropH 2002 pH

meter (Barcelona, Spain) and Heraeus oven T5028 for thermal degradation (dry heat at 105°C) (Hanaus, Germany).

Forced degradation studies and preparation of samples

The forced degradation studies were carried out by preparing several standard solutions of CTZ at 500 μg mL^{-1}, for each degradation study. Each sample was analyzed according to the previous procedures described under the proposed analytical method. In order to determine whether the analytical method is suitable to be a stability-indicating

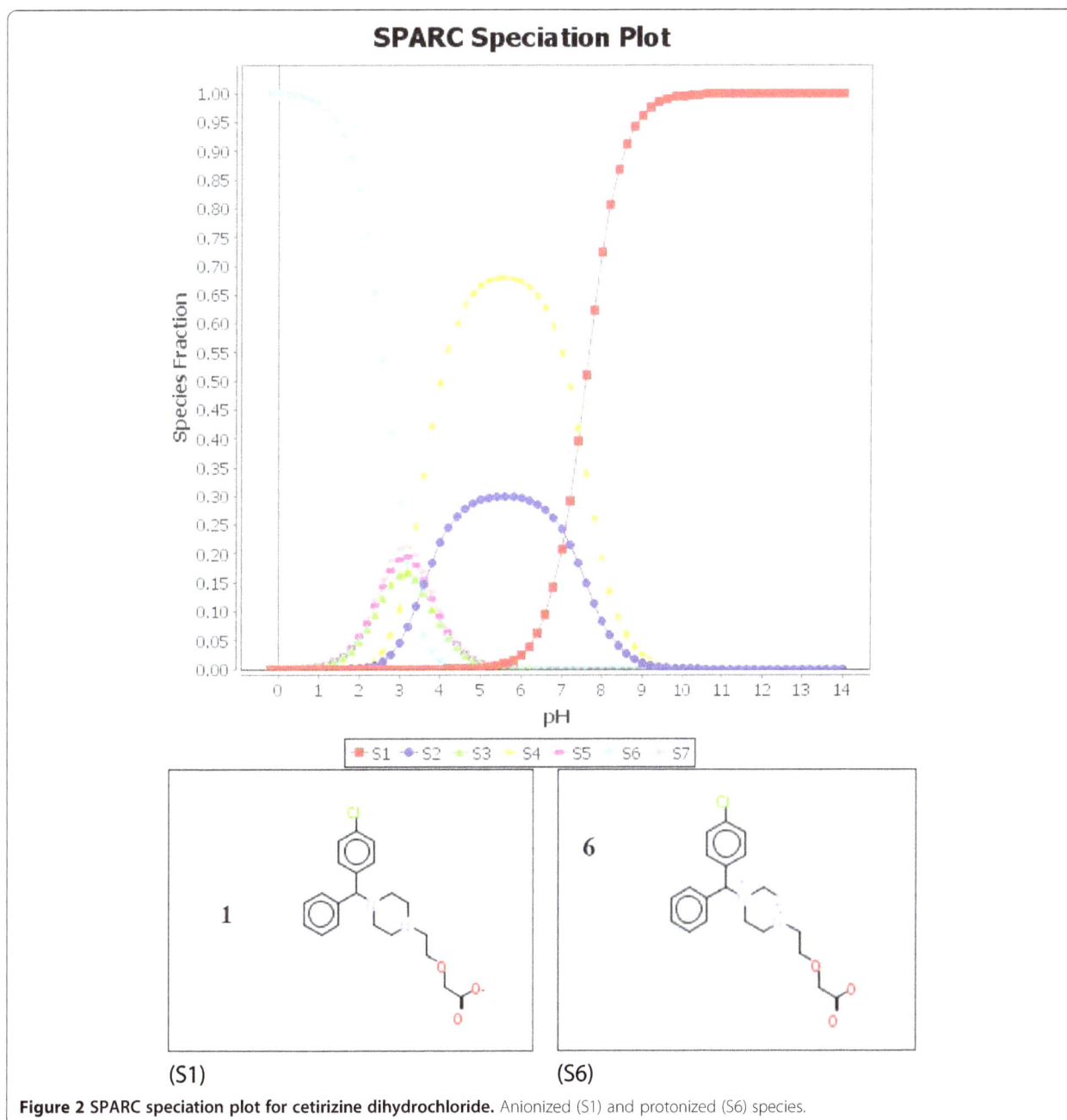

Figure 2 SPARC speciation plot for cetirizine dihydrochloride. Anionized (S1) and protonated (S6) species.

assay, forced degradation studies under different conditions were carried out according to the following procedure:

a) Acid and basic hydrolysis: 5 mg of bulk powder was treated with 5 mL of 0.1 M HCl and 0.1 M NaOH. The flasks were placed in a dry air oven at 105°C. Another 5 mg of bulk powder was also treated with 5 mL of 0.1 M HCl and 0.1 M NaOH at room temperature, for 24 hours.

b) Oxidation with H_2O_2 at 33%: 5 mg of bulk powder was exposed to 5 mL of hydrogen peroxide at 33% (W/v). The vial was kept at room temperature for 24 hours.

c) Infrared (IR) and Ultraviolet (UV) light: 5 mg of bulk powder was exposed under an infrared lamp and another 5 mg of bulk powder was exposed under an ultraviolet lamp, for 24 hours.

d) Humidity HR 79%: the 5 mg bulk powder sample was placed inside a humidifier with HR 79%, for 24 hours.

e) Heat at 105°C: 5 mg of bulk powder sample was placed inside a 105°C dry air oven for 24 hours.

f) Shed sunlight for 15 days: 5 mg of bulk powder was kept in a vial for 15 days, at room temperature and exposed to direct sunlight.

Once the stress conditions were complete, 10 mL of 0.2 M phosphate buffer (pH 7.00) was added to the samples in order to achieve the standard solution concentration of 500 μm mL-1. Moreover, all the solutions and blanks were filtered with a 0.45 μm syringe filtration disk PVDF. Results were compiled in terms of relative retention times (rtR) found during the analysis.

Validation of the analytical method

In order to validate the RP-HPLC method developed, ICHQ2B guideline recommendations were followed, in terms of selectivity, linearity, range, accuracy, precision, limit of detection (LOD) and limit of quantification (LOQ) [26]. In order to fulfill ICH specifications in terms of linearity and range for the analytical method (content uniformity and assay of DS and finished product), a linear range within 70-130% was studied, by analyzing a series of three replicates, i.e., three independent sets (k = 3), each with seven different concentrations (n = 6): 350 μg ml^{-1} - 650 μg ml^{-1}, considering 500 μg ml^{-1} as 100% (standard solution), in order to provide information on the variation in peak area values between samples of the same concentration. For evaluation of the precision estimates, repeatability and intermediate precision were performed at three concentration levels (650, 500 and 350 μg ml^{-1}, corresponding to 130, 100 and 70%), and 10 injections of each sample (K = 10), per day. Mean average, standard deviation (SD) and relative standard deviation (RSD) of t_R and the peak area achieved individually of day 1 and 2 were calculated. After the HPLC analysis, the response factor (RF) was calculated between the response (Y) and concentration achieved (X), as Y/X. Therefore, mean average, SD and RSD were calculated using the response factors obtained with an Excel 2007 spread sheet. The response factors results must comply with a RSD ± 2%. For accuracy the concentration found expressed by function of repeatability of the standard

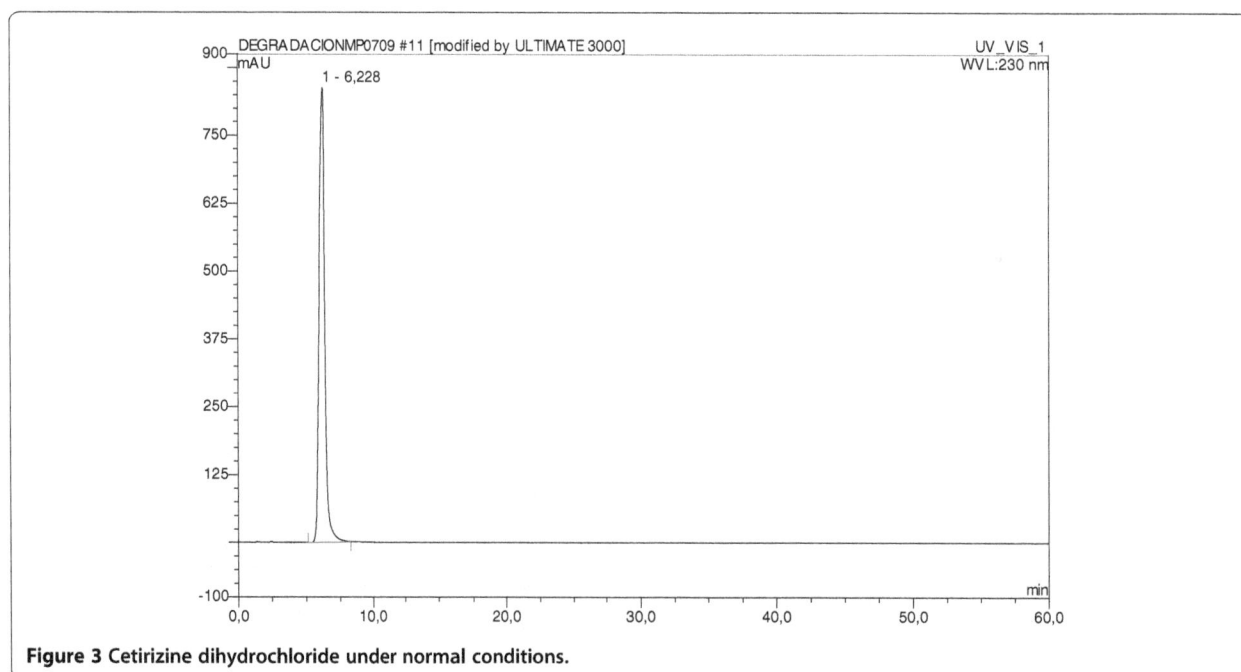

Figure 3 Cetirizine dihydrochloride under normal conditions.

Table 1 Summary of product degradation peaks in relative retention time (rt_R)

Stress conditions	rt_R (min)								CTZ								
Humidity HR79%									1.00								
Acid hydrolysis *RT			0.51					0.81	0.87	1.00								
Acid hydrolysis at 105°C	0.46		0.50		0.64				0.87	1.00						5.00		
Ultraviolet light (UV)			0.52	0.59				0.81		1.00		2.00			4.30			
Infrared light (IR)			0.51	0.60	0.66			0.81		1.00								
Basic hydrolysis *RT			0.53					0.81	0.87	1.00								
Basic hydrolysis at 105°C	0.46	0.48	0.51	0.58		0.71		0.86		1.00	1.60	2.00	2.80	3.40		5.00		9.10
Dry heat at 105°C			0.50			0.72	0.80	0.90		1.00					4.30	5.00		
Shed sunlight 15 days				0.60						1.00								
H_2O_2 at 33%			0.51							1.00		1.90	2.60		4.40		5.70	
Normal conditions										1.00								

*RT: Room temperature.

solution, relative error in percentage and the percentage of recovery, with mean average, SD and RSD deviation of each of the three concentrations studied (650, 500 and 350 μg ml $^{-1}$, was considered of three replicates) were calculated. For the DS, 98-102% percentage of recovery was considered as being acceptable [27].

For the determination and quantification of the DE, linearity, precision, accuracy and LOD and LOQ were calculated. In order to carry out this validation, further dilutions from a stock solution of 500 μg ml $^{-1}$ with the specified mobile phase were carried out in order to achieve the correspondent concentrations: 5 μg mL^{-1}, 2.5 μg mL^{-1}, 1.25 μg mL^{-1}, 0.5 μg mL^{-1}, 0.25 μg mL^{-1}, 0.125 μg mL^{-1}. A total of seven independent calibration curves, i.e., seven replicates (k = 7) were prepared. The LOD and LOQ were calculated by the ratio between the standard deviation of y-intercepts of regression lines of the seven calibration curves mentioned before by averaging the slopes of calibration curve multiplied by 3.3 and

10, respectively [26,27]. Each serial dilution (k = 7) was analyzed, with n = 6 (level of concentrations).

In terms of relative error and percentage of recovery three concentrations (5, 1.25 and 0.25 μg mL^{-1}) from the range of DE were evaluated. All the solutions prepared were filtered with a 0.45 μm syringe filtration disk PVDF to the vials for injection in the HPLC system.

Results and discussion

HPLC method development

As an early stage study of drug development, our goal was to acknowledge all possible DE generated under stress conditions for CTZ. The information acquired in the early stage of the study will lead us to a better understanding of the DS itself and also the possible DE that we may find during the next step of the oral lyophilized development study. Therefore it was not our objective the development of a fast analytical method for the DS per se, but actually the development of an analytical

Table 2 Peak purity determination by diode-array UV–vis spectra of CTZ and stress studies results

Forced degradation conditions	[a]Peak purity index match	Decomposition (%)	Extent of decomposition
Humidity HR79%	952	0	None
Acid hydrolysis *RT	990	0	None
Acid hydrolysis at 105°C	998	19	Substantial
Ultraviolet light (UV)	962	9	Substantial
Infrared light (IR)	962	8	Substantial
Basic hydrolysis *RT	972	0	None
Basic hydrolysis at 105°C	986	15	Substantial
Dry heat at 105°C	953	3	Substantial
Shed sunlight 15 days	996	10	Substantial
Oxidative medium *RT	998	79	Substantial
CTZ (phosphate buffer solution)	990	0	Normal conditions

[a]indicates the value for peak purity index match of CTZ above 950, considering 1000 as 100% match; *RT: Room temperature.

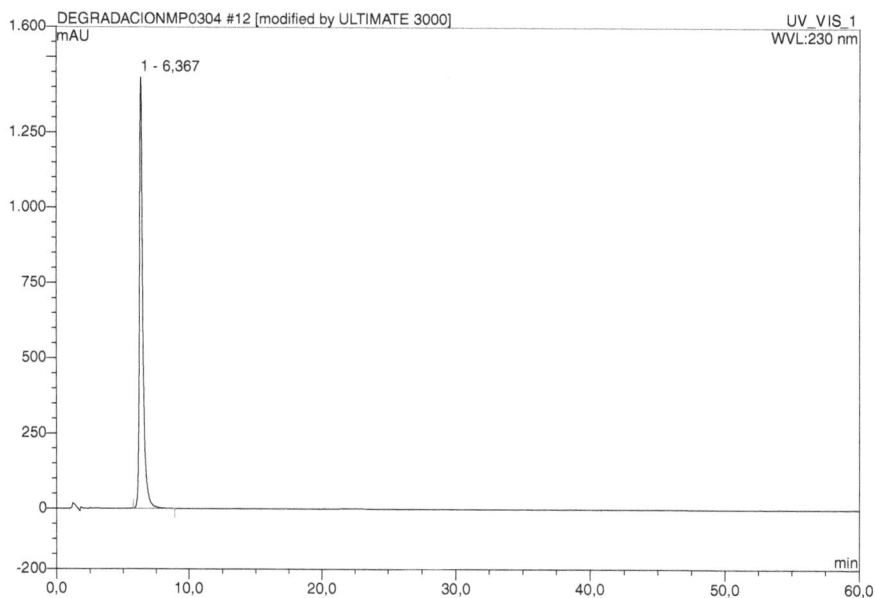

Figure 4 Cetirizine dihydrochloride under humidity HR79%.

method that could detect a complete profile of DE for this DS, leaving for the following studies of drug development the aim of reducing run time, for instance.

CTZ is freely soluble in water, and practically insoluble in acetone and metilen chlorate [17]. Considering its hydrophilic nature, reverse phase columns were chosen in order to investigate the chromatographic profile with two types of packing material for stationary phases: C18 (more hydrophobic, octadecylsilyl), and C8 (intermediate hydrophobicity, octylsilyl). We also studied the molecule

of CTZ using the physicochemical calculator SPARC (Sparc Performs Automated Reasoning in Chemistry) developed by the United States Environmental Protection Agency (EPA) for the purpose of predicting which pH would suit best for CTZ ionization [28]. The speciation plot for CTZ (Figure 2) shows that pH3 is not recommended for the ionization of CTZ due to the existence of six different species of ionized CTZ with no clear definition among them, whereas at pH2 we can find the protonated CTZ (S6) and at pH7 the anionized

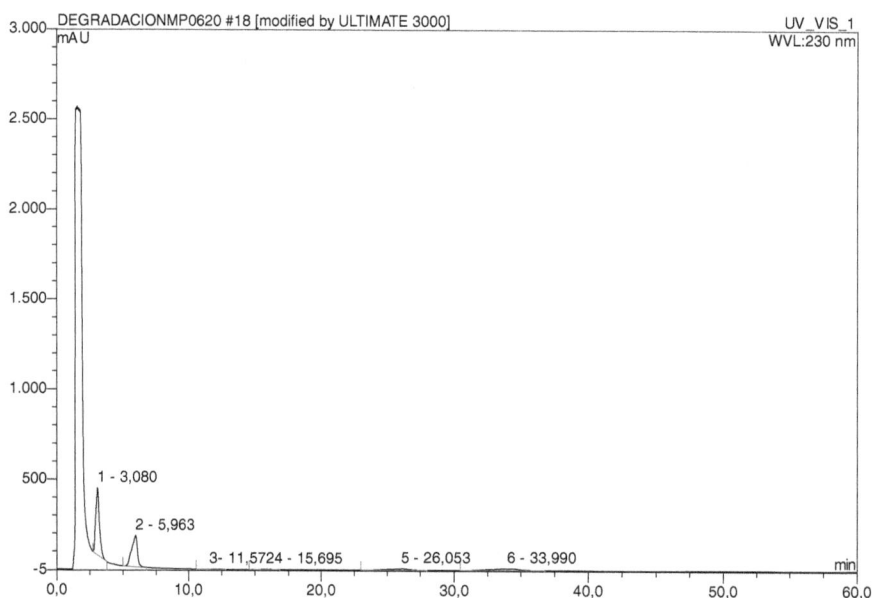

Figure 5 Cetirizine dihydrochloride under H_2O_2 at 33%.

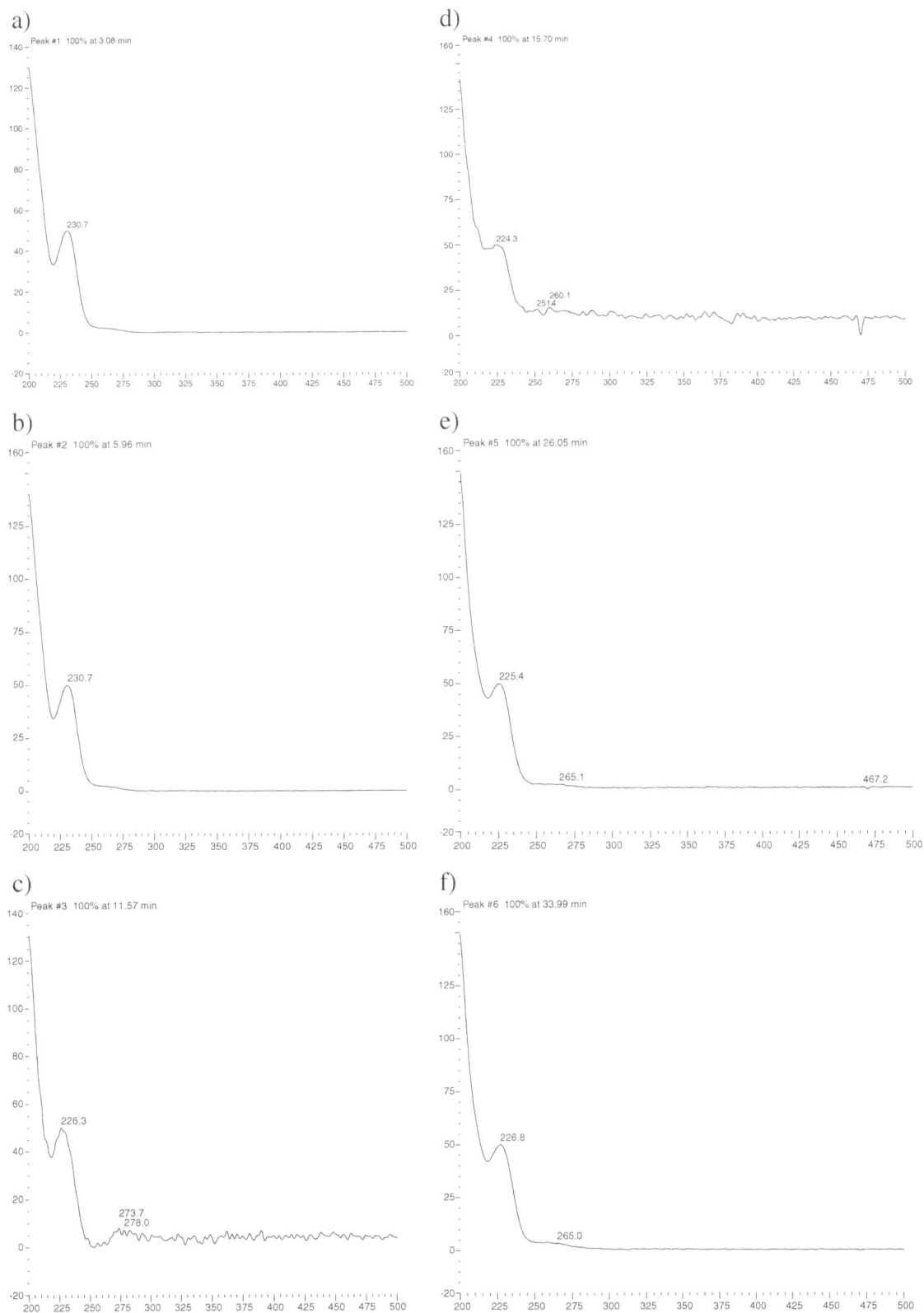

Figure 6 Chromatographic spectra of cetirizine dihydrochloride (b) and its degradation products (a, c, d, e and f) under H_2O_2 at 33%, in nm.

Table 3 Repeatability and intermediate precision according to retention time (t_R) and peak area for CTZ assay

Day	t_R				Peak area	
	µg mL^{-1}	Mean average ± [a]SD (min) [b]K = 10	[c]RSD (%)		Mean average ± [a]SD (mAU.min) [b]K = 10	[c]RSD (%)
1	650	5.79 ± 0.0274	0.4747		512.54 ± 1.7865	0.5365
	500	5.79 ± 0.0327	0.5646		399.69 ± 1.9090	0.4777
	350	5.80 ± 0.0228	0.3929		281.21 ± 1.7867	0.6353
2	650	5.77 ± 0.0195	0.3384		511.75 ± 2.2059	0.4310
	500	5.78 ± 0.0149	0.2584		399.54 ± 1.5972	0.3997
	350	5.80 ± 0.0248	0.4279		281.63 ± 1.0483	0.3722

[a]SD (Standard deviation); [b]K (number of injections); [c]RSD (Relative standard deviation).

CTZ (S1) (Figure 3). The pKa values estimated for CTZ are: 2.7 (pKa1), 3.6 (pKa2) and 7.6 (pKa 3) [29]. However, due to the finding of chromatographic methods that used buffer solutions at pH3 or around 3 (2.8, 3.5, for instance) we decided to considered pH3 in our study [10-12,14]. During the preliminary studies of the analytical method development, we have combined different proportions of acetonitrile and aqueous solution at pH3 (MilliQ water acidified at pH3 with orto-phosphoric acid 85%). The preliminary studies were carried out by the injection of a 500 µg mL^{-1} solution of CTZ, using a C18 analytical chromatographic column, flow rate of mobile phase of 1 mL min^{-1}, an injection volume of 25 µL, oven temperature of 30°C, 230 nm of wavelength, in isocratic mode. The effects of the optimum eluent composition were studied, obtaining a retention time (t_R) of eight minutes for CTZ with a 35:65 (v/v) of acetonitrile and aqueous solution at pH3. Also, we tried to adjust the mobile phase –studying the effect of the proportion between the organic solvent and buffer solution pH– in order to achieve a t_R of approximately 6–7 for CTZ. To diminish the t_R, we finally tried to use a buffer solution of 0.2 M K$_2$HPO$_4$ pH7. We observed that maintaining the same proportions of organic solvent and buffer solution, but changing the pH from 3 to 7, using potassium phosphate dibasic buffer solution at 0.2 M

solution at pH7, we achieved a t_R of 5–6 minutes. However, CTZ peak shape presented tail broadening. Therefore, in order to avoid using ion pair to improve peak resolution, we have changed the analytical chromatographic column C18 (Kromasyl 100–5 C18) to a C8 (Eclipse XDB C8), and tested with the same conditions as before: acetonitrile and phosphate buffer solution pH 7 (35:65, respectively), injection volume 25 µL, flow rate 1 mL min^{-1}, temperature 30°C, 230 nm of wavelength. This resulted in eliminating tail broadening. Having determined the eluent proportions of the isocratic mobile phase and the pH of the aqueous solution as pH7, obtaining the desired t_R, we have established the stability-indicating method to carry out the forced degradation studies.

Results of forced degradation study

CTZ was degraded up to 19% under acid hydrolysis at 105°C, presenting five degradation peaks. Under basic hydrolysis at 105°C, CTZ was degraded up to 15%, presenting twelve degradation peaks, followed by shed sun light (10%, one degradation peak), UV (9%, four degradation peaks), IR (8%, four degradation peaks) and dry heat at 105°C (3%, 6 degradation peaks). CTZ under photolytic stress -shed sunlight during 15 days, IR and UV light- presented degradation peaks with two, four

Table 4 Concentrations found, relative error in percentage, percentage of recovery and estimates for CTZ assay

[a]Theoretical concentration (µg mL^{-1})	Concentration found (µg mL^{-1})	Relative error%	[b]Recovery%	Mean recovery	[c]SD of recovery
650	641.29	1.25	98.75	98.66	0.09
650	641.27	1.36	98.65		
650	640.67	1.45	98.56		
500	500.96	0.19	100.19	100.49	0.57
500	500.71	0.14	100.14		
500	505.80	1.14	101.16		
350	352.16	0.61	100.61	100.95	0.43
350	352.77	0.78	100.79		
350	355.05	1.42	101.44		

[a]650 µg mL^{-1} = 130%, 500 µg mL^{-1} = 100%, 350 µg mL^{-1} = 70%; [b]recovery limits (98-102%); [c]SD (Standard deviation).

Table 5 Mean average, standard deviation (SD) and relative standard deviation (RSD%) of peak area mAU (5 – 0.125 μ mL⁻¹)

Theoretical concentration (μg mL⁻¹)	Mean concentration average ± [a] SD (μg mL⁻¹) ([b] k = 7)	[c]RSD (%)
5.000	4.0495 ± 0.1040	2.5701
2.500	2.0121 ± 0.0251	1.2502
1.250	1.0012 ± 0.0326	3.2622
0.500	0.4021 ± 0.0327	8.1334
0.250	0.1818 ± 0.0111	6.1605

[a]SD (Standard deviation); [b]k (number of replicates); [c]RSD (relative standard deviation).

and five peaks, respectively (Table 1). CTZ presented DE peaks under acid (three DE peaks) and basic hydrolysis at room temperature (three DE peaks). However, degradation was not substantial in both cases (Table 2). Comparing the chromatographic profile of CTZ dissolved in buffer solution (Figure 3) with no stress conditions (normal conditions) with CTZ under Humidity HR79% (Figure 4), it is observed that CTZ showed no substantial degradation under Humidity HR79%, presenting a similar chromatographic profile with CTZ dissolved in buffer solution at the same concentration. Under oxidative stress, CTZ presented 79% of degradation, showing five degradation peaks (Figure 5) and in Figure 6 it can be visualized by the chromatographic spectra of each DE and CTZ. Furthermore, the peak purity value for CTZ under oxidative stress was of 998 (considering 1000 as 100% match), indicating a homogenous peak (Table 2). However, in the beginning of the elution process, the diode-array assay detects DE higher that its threshold, demonstrating a possible saturation of the chromatographic column with H_2O_2 at 33%. There is also the hypothesis that 79% of decomposition can also be the result of the degradation of DE, which would generate more DE, due to the exposure of CTZ during 24 hours under oxidative condition. This leads to the conclusion that may be necessary to change the oxidative stress condition procedure, by reducing the concentration of peroxide (33%) or reducing the time of exposure of the DS with H_2O_2 (24 hours), or both. Satisfactory results were obtained studying the peak purity

Table 6 Relative error (%) and percentage of recovery

Concentration (μg mL⁻¹)	Mean concentration found (μg mL⁻¹) ([a]k = 7)	[b]Relative error% (mean)	[c]Mean Recovery%	[d]SD of recovery%
5	5.000	0.620	100.070	0.74
1.25	1.248	3.310	99.840	4.10
0.25	0.235	9.390	94.210	10.00

[a]k = 7 (number of replicates); [b]mean relative error% ; [c]mean recovery%; [d]standard deviation.

index for CTZ under stress conditions, which confirms the high specificity of the analytical method for CTZ (Table 2).

Method validation

The developed method was validated using ICH guidelines [26]. Validation parameters included linearity, precision, accuracy, precision, and specificity, LOD and LOQ [26,27].

Assay for drug substance method

Linearity for CTZ assay was verified by triplicate analysis of seven different concentrations, i.e., three sets of 130-70% range of CTZ. As a result, the linear regression equation was found to be Y = 769.56 X + 14.573 (r^2 = 0.9994, k = 3 (number of replicates), n = 7 (level of concentrations), 650 μg mL⁻¹ to 350 μg mL⁻¹) for CTZ. In which, Y was the dependent variable, X was independent variable, 769.56 was the slope and which showed change in dependent (Y) variable per unit change in independent (X) variable; 14.573 was the Y-intercept i.e., the value of Y variable when X = 0.

As for the analytical method precision (Table 3), three concentration levels (650, 500 and 350 μg ml⁻¹, corresponding to 130, 100 and 70%), and 10 injections of each sample, per day were prepared. The results have shown the repeatability and intermediate precision presenting a RSD inferior to 2.7% according to AOAC [27] (1.43% and 1.03%, respectively). In terms of accuracy, according to the obtained results (Table 4), the percentage of recovery ranges from 98.56 to 101.44, from being within the limits established according to AOAC [27] (98-102%), which indicates the accuracy of the method for CTZ.

It was studied seven independent sets of dilutions, i.e., seven replicates (k =7), each set with six different concentrations (n = 6) in the range of 5–0.125 μg mL⁻¹. Calculating LOD and LOQ by the ratio between the SD of y-intercepts of regression lines of the seven serial dilutions of six different concentrations mentioned before by averaging the slopes of calibration curve multiplied by 3.3 and 10, respectively, the analytical method presented a LOD of 0.056 μg mL⁻¹ and a LOQ of 0.17 μg mL⁻¹. However, it was demonstrated that the LOQ value of 0.17 μg mL⁻¹ was not lineal. Therefore, taken into account the range defined in ICH guidelines to the DE, for linearity reasons it was considered the range around a suggested (probable) limit [26]. Therefore, the linearity should be established from the LOQ to 120%. So a new LOQ (SD (μg mL⁻¹) = 0.0111, RSD (%) = 6.1605) was established (0.25 μg mL⁻¹). The linear regression equation was found to be Y = 0.8125X-0.014 (r^2 = 0.9999, n = 5 (level of concentrations), k = 7 (number of replicates), 0.25-5 μg mL⁻¹) (Table 5).

In reference to the results of the analytical method validation, in both Table 5 (repeatability) and Table 6 (recovery), the RSD and the range complies with RSD permitted (2.7%) and the range (90-110%) according to AOAC [27], assuring the applicability of the developed analytical method for the determination and quantification of DE.

Conclusions

A new and simple RP-HPLC method was developed for the determination of CTZ and its DE during the early stage of drug development of an oral lyophilized dosage form. The proposed method was demonstrated to be linear, precise, accurate and specific, based on method validation. Satisfactory results were obtained in separating the peak of CTZ from the DE produced by forced degradation. Plus, it is a cost-effective method that requires a simple mobile phase (phosphate buffer solution and acetonitrile, 65:35 v/v) and also does not require the use of ion pairing, which can result in difficulty in recovering initial column properties. It was also able to separate with good specificity the DS peak from the entire DE generated during the stress condition study, which help us in the next step of the drug development of the oral lyophilizate, by adapting the validated method considering further aspects, such as the interactions between CTZ and the excipients chosen for the final medicinal product. The proposed analytical method proved to be stability-indicating and therefore useful in the following stages of drug development.

Abbreviations

DS: Drug substance; DP: Drug product; DE: Degradation products; CTZ: Cetirizine dihydrochloride; RP-HPLC: Reverse phase high performance liquid chromatography; t_R: Retention time; rt_R: Relative retention time; LOD: Limit of detection; LOQ: Limit of quantification; IR: Infrared light; UV: Ultraviolet light.

Competing interests

The authors declare that they have no competing interests.

Authors' contributions

PFB, PPL and EGM: participate in method development and optimization, perform the experiments for forced degradation studies and method validation, collect experimental data and write the manuscript. JMSN and EJ: propose and supervise the implementation of various experiments and revised the manuscript. JRT and MM: revised data and supervised the manuscript. All authors read and approved the final manuscript.

References

1. Ahuja S: Overview of HPLC Method Development for Pharmaceuticals. In *HPLC Method Development for Pharmaceuticals*. Edited by Ahuja S, Rasmussen HT. Amsterdam: Academic Press; 2007:1–17.
2. Rasmussen HT, Swinney KA, Gaiki S: HPLC Method Development in Early Phase Pharmaceutical Development. In *HPLC Method Development for Pharmaceuticals*. Edited by Ahuja S, Rasmussen HT. Amsterdam: Academic Press; 2007:353–371.
3. Alsante KM, Ando A, Brown R, Ensing J, Hatajik TD, Kong W, Tsuda Y: The role of degradant profiling in active pharmaceutical ingredients and drug products. *Adv Drug Deliv Rev* 2007, 59(1):29–37.
4. Sweetman SC: Martindale: the complete drug reference: [https://www.medicinescomplete.com/mc/martindale/current/]
5. Simons FER: Advances in H1-antihistamines. *N Engl J Med* 2004, 351:2203–2217.
6. Atkins PC, Zweiman B, Moskowitz A, von Allmen C, Ciliberti M: Cellular inflammatory responses and mediator release during early developing late-phase allergic cutaneous inflammatory responses: effects of cetirizine. *J Allergy Clin Immunol* 1997, 99:806–811.
7. Walsh GM, Annunziato L, Frossard N, Knol K, Levander S, Nicolas JM, Tagliatela M, Tharp MD, Tillemant JP, Tillemant H: New insights into the second generation antihistamines. *Drugs* 2001, 61:207–236.
8. Ortonne JP: Urticaria and its subtypes: the role of second-generation antihistamines. *Eur J Intern Med* 2012, 23:26–30.
9. Komarow HD, Metcalfe DD: Office-based management of urticaria. *Am J Med* 2008, 121:379–384.
10. Kim CK, Yeong KJ, Ban E, Hyun MJ, Kim JK, Jin SE, Park JS: Narrow-bore high performance liquid chromatographic method for the determination of cetirizine in human plasma using column switching. *J Pharm Biomed Anal* 2005, 37:603–609.
11. Zaater MF, Tahboub YR, Najib NM: RP-LC method for the determination of cetirizine in serum. *J Pharm Biomed Anal* 2000, 22:739–744.
12. El Walily AFM, Korany MA, El Gindy A, Bedair MF: Spectrophotometric and high performance liquid chromatographic determination of cetirizine dihydrochloride in pharmaceutical tablets. *J Pharm Biomed Anal* 1998, 17:435–442.
13. Macek J, Ptáček P, Klíma J: Determination of cetirizine in human plasma by high-performance liquid chromatography. *J Chromatogr B* 1999, 736:231–235.
14. Dharuman J, Vashudevan M, Ajithlal T: High performance liquid chromatographic method for the determination of cetirizine and ambroxol in human plasma and urine— a boxcar approach. *J Chromatogr B* 2011, 879:2624–2631.
15. Likar MD, Mansour HL, Harwood JW: Development and validation of a dissolution test for a once-a-day combination tablet of immediate-release cetirizine dihydrochloride and extended-release pseudoephedrine hydrochloride. *J Pharm Biomed Anal* 2005, 39:543–551.
16. Hadad GM, Emara S, Mahmoud WMM: Development and validation of a stability-indicating RP-HPLC method for the determination of paracetamol with dantrolene or/and cetirizine and pseudoephedrine in two pharmaceutical dosage forms. *Talanta* 2009, 79:1360–1367.
17. European Pharmacopoeia 7th Edition 2014 (8.0): [http://online6.edqm.eu/ep801/]
18. Jaber AMY, Al Sherife HA, Al Omari MM, Badwan AA: Determination of cetirizine dihydrochloride, related impurities and preservatives in oral solution and tablet dosage forms using HPLC. *J Pharm Biomed Anal* 2004, 36:341–350.
19. Karakuş S, Küçükgüzel I, Küçükgüzel SG: Development and validation of a rapid RP-HPLC method for the determination of cetirizine or fexofenadine with pseudoephedrine in binary pharmaceutical dosage forms. *J Pharm Biomed Anal* 2008, 46:295–302.
20. Neue UD, Alden BA, Grover R, Grumbach ES, Iraneta PC, Méndez A: HPLC Columns and Packings. In HPLC Method Development for Pharmaceuticals. In *HPLC Method Development for Pharmaceuticals*. Edited by Ahuja S, Rasmussen HT. Amsterdam: Academic Press; 2007:45–83.
21. Visky D: Column Characterization and Selection. In *HPLC Method Development for Pharmaceuticals*, Volume 8. Edited by Ahuja S, Rasmussen HT. Amsterdam: Academic Press; 2007:85–109.
22. Bosch E, Espinosa S, Rosés M: Retention of ionizable compounds on high-performance liquid chromatography III. Variation of pK values of acids and pH values of buffers in acetonitrile-water mobile phases. *J Chromatogr A* 1998, 824:137–146.
23. Bosch E, Espinosa S, Rosés M: Retention of ionizable compounds in high-performance liquid chromatography IX. Modelling retention in reversed-phase liquid chromatography as a function of pH and solvent composition with acetonitrile-water mobile phases. *J Chromatogr A* 2002, 947:47–58.
24. Espinosa S, Bosch E, Rosés M: Retention of ionizable compounds in high-performance liquid Chromatography 14. Acid–base pK values in acetonitrile–water mobile phases. *J Chromatogr A* 2002, 964:55–66.
25. Agrafiotou P, Ràfols C, Castells C, Bosch E, Rosés M: Simultaneous effect of pH, temperature and mobile phase composition in the chromatographic retention of ionizable compounds. *J Chromatogr A* 2011, 1218:4995–5009.

26. International Conference on Harmonization, ICH Q2B: Validation of Analytical Procedures: Terms and Definitions. Step 5 (1996) [http://www.ich.org/products/guidelines/quality/article/quality-guidelines.html]

27. Official methods of analysis of AOAC [http://www.eoma.aoac.org/]

28. Sparc Performs Automated Reasoning in Chemistry [http://archemcalc.com/sparc]

29. Pubchem Open chemistry database [http://pubchem.ncbi.nlm.nih.gov/compound/2678?from=summary#section=Top]

14

Epidural administration of neostigmine-loaded nanofibers provides extended analgesia in rats

Masoomeh Yosefifard and Majid Hassanpour-Ezatti[*]

Abstract

Background: In this study, neostigmine-loaded electrospun nanofibers were prepared and then their efficacy and duration of analgesic action were studied after epidural administration in rats by repeated tail flick and formalin tests.

Methods: The neostigmine poly vinyl alcohol (PVA) nanofibers were fabricated by electrospinning methods. The nanofibers (1 mg) were injected into the lumbar epidural space (L5-L6) of rats (n = 6). Cerebrospinal fluid samples of rats were collected 1, 5 and 24 hours after injection and then were sampled once weekly for 4 weeks. Free-neostigmine concentration was measured in the samples spectrophotometrically. Rat nociceptive responses were evaluated by repeated tail-flick and formalin tests for 5 weeks after the nanofibers (1 mg) injection. Locomotor activity of rats was measured in the open-field at the same period.

Results: The cerebrospinal fluid concentration of free neostigmine reached 5 µg/ml five hours after injection and remained constant until the end of the experiments. The tail-flick latency of treated rats was significantly (p < 0.01) increased and remained constant up to 4 weeks. Pain scores of the rats in both phases of formalin test were significantly (p < 0.01) reduced during the same periods, Epidural injection of the nanofibers had no effect on locomotor activity of rats in an open-field.

Conclusions: Our results indicate that the neostigmine nanofibers can provide sustained release of neostigmine for induction of prolonged analgesia after epidural administration. High tissue distribution and penetration of the nanofibers in dorsal horn can increase thermal and chemical analgesia duration without altering locomotor activity in rats for 4 weeks.

Keywords: Neostigmine, Nanofibers, Analgesia, Epidural, Electrospinning

Background

Recently, researchers have been employing new techniques to improve both the efficacy and duration of analgesic effect of some drugs. Epidural administration of neostigmine could reduce pain in patients with uncontrolled pain [1]. It has been reported that intrathecally administered neostigmine could also provide effective analgesia in both phases of formalin test in rat [2]. Although, in clinical studies intrathecal neostigmine infusion is used for induction of prolonged analgesia in chronic patients [3], the application of a catheter for drug infusion would increase the risk of infection in patients and also requires complicated surgery. An alternative procedure for increasing the duration of neostigmine action after epidural injection is its combination with other

drugs [4]. However, this method might induce side effects such as nausea, vomiting, sedation and respiratory depression in patients. It is shown that elevation of endogenous acetylcholine level at spinal cord synapses mediate neostigmine analgesia following epidural injection [5]. Also, intrathecal co-administered of neostigmine with local anesthetic can increase its duration of action [6]. Liposomal neostigmine for epidural application is another approach being used for control release of neostigmine, but unfortunately this formulation has short duration of action [7]. In recent years, incorporation of drugs in electrospun nanofibers has been used for making sustained and controlled-release drugs; Tseng and coworkers could fabricate lidocaine biodegradable nanofiber and showed a sustain delivery of lidocaine into the epidural space in rats [8]. On the other hand, it has been shown that intratecal administration of a dose of an analgesic drug could

* Correspondence: hassanpour@Shahed.ac.ir
Department of Biology, Sciences School, Shahed University, Tehran, IRAN

produce different results in the tail-flick and formalin tests [9]. Therefore, scientists compared the epidural or intrathecal anesthetic efficacy of same doses of an analgesic compound with two kinds of nociceptive stimulus such as tail flick and formalin test. Thus, it is certain that the selected dose of the drug is effective for different kinds of pain.

The aims of present study were: (1) fabrication of neostigmine-loaded poly vinyl alcohol (PVA) nanofibers by electrospinning methods; (2) *in-vitro* evaluation of neostigmine release from the nanofibers; (3) assessment of free-neostigmine concentration in the cerebrospinal fluid of rats after the nanofiber injection for 4 weeks; and (4) evaluation of the efficacy and duration of analgesia in thermal and chemical pain model by consecutive tail-flick and formalin test during 5 weeks after the injection of nanofibers.

Materials and methods
Chemical
Neostigmine methylsulfate was obtained as a gift sample from the laboratory of Dr. Sayyed Omid Ranaei Syadat, Tehran, Iran. In our experiment, all chemicals were of analytical grade purchased from Sigma-Aldrich.

Preparation of nanofibers using electrospinning
The neostigmine-loaded poly vinyl alcohol nanofibers were prepared according to the procedure of Arecchi et al. [10]. Briefly, poly vinyl alcohol solution was prepared by dissolving 6 gram of poly vinyl alcohol powder in 100 ml of deionized water. The mixture was slowly heated to 95°C for 8 hours. To compensate for the loss of water due to evaporation during heating and stirring, deionized water was added to the solution to return it to the original volume. Thus, the final concentration of poly

vinyl alcohol in solution was kept at 6 wt% [10]. Neostigmine 1.25% (w/w) was dissolved in double distilled deionized water and was added to the poly vinyl alcohol solution and stirred for 25 minutes before electrospinning. For preparing neostigmine-loaded electrospinning nanofibers, the 6% PVA solutions were mixed by volumetric ratios of 50:50 with neostigmine solution. Then, the mixture was pumped at a constant rate using a syringe pump toward a needle tip. The utilized electrical potential for electrospinning was 25 kV and the distance between the collector and the needle tip was 15 cm. The electrospinning was performed at room temperature and the resulting neostigmine-loaded nanofibers were collected on an aluminum foil. The schematic figure of electrospinning set up is shown in Figure 1. Then, the nanofibers were incubated at 150°C for 5 minutes, treated with ethanol for 1 hour and dried overnight at room temperature [11]. Final neostigmine-loaded nanofibers contained %1.25 (w/w) neostigmine/poly(vinyl alcohol). Finally, the structure of free and neostigmine-loaded nanofibers was studied using scanning electron microscopy.

In vitro Acetylcholinesterase (AChE) inhibition assay by nanofibers containing different ratios of neostigmine/poly (vinyl alcohol)
The measurement of AChE inhibitory activity of neostigmine released from the nanofibers was carried out in a vial using spectrophotometric method proposed by Ellman et al. [13]. The percent of AChE inhibition was compared among the nanofibers that were made from different proportions of poly vinyl alcohol (5, 6, 7, 8%w/w) and contained different concentrations of neostigmine (0.000125 and 0.00125w/w). Acetylcholinesterase, AChE (E.C 3.1.1.7) was expressed with the baculovirus system

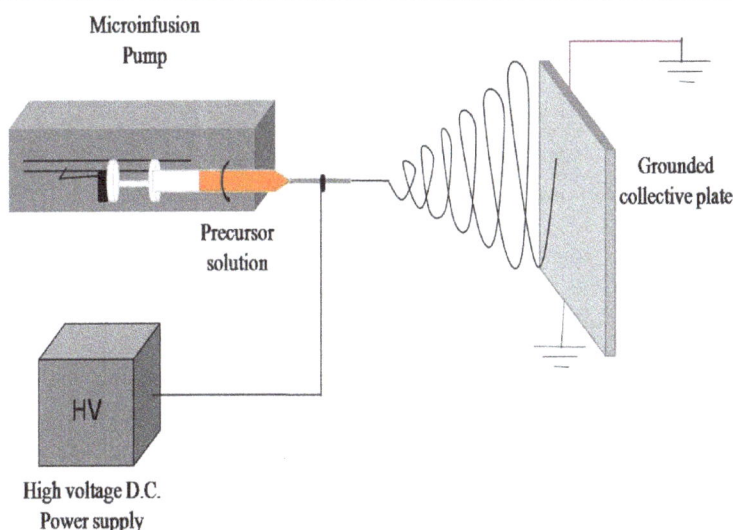

Figure 1 Schematic representation of an electrospinning setup for production of neostigmine-PVA loaded nanofibers [12].

[14]. A typical run consisted of 5 μL of AChE solution at final assay concentrations of 0.03 U/mL; 200 μL of 0.1 M phosphate buffer (pH 7.4); 5 μL of DTNB at a final concentration of 0.3 mM, prepared in 0.1 M phosphate buffer (pH 7.4) with 0.12 M of sodium bicarbonate. Then, the nanofibers containing neostigmine were added to each mixture reaction (1 mL) in vials, vortexed for 1 min, and then centrifuged rapidly at 16 000 g for 1 min. The intensity of the yellow solution in the resulting supernatants were determined spectrophotometrically at 412 nm every 5 min, three times consecutively. Percent of remaining activity of AChE was determined after incubation with the neostigmine-loaded nanofibers which were fabricated by different concentrations of poly vinyl alcohol and loaded with different doses of neostigmine.

Encapsulation efficiency and in vitro release

To determine the encapsulation efficiency, 10 mg of the neostigmine-loaded nanofibers were stored in 1 ml of PBS (pH 7.4). The solution was incubated for 1 min at 37°C. At 5 min intervals, a sample was withdrawn and centrifuged at 16,000 g for 10 min. The precipitated samples were taken and resuspended in 10 ml fresh release medium to keep a complete sink condition and placed back to the shaker. The supernatant solution was retained for HPLC analysis. A mixture of acetonitrile and ammonium acetate (75:25 v/v) was added to the solution after the PBS had been removed. The resulting solution was analyzed using HPLC, in which a C-18 column was used and the mobile phase was delivered at a rate of 1 ml/min. One hundred microliters of sample was injected by an autosampler and the column effluent was detected at 248 nm.

Morphologies of electrospun nanofibers

The surface morphology of the nanofibers was observed by scanning electron microscopy (S-4800, Hitachi, Japan). The free poly vinyl alcohol and neostigmine-loaded nanofibers were placed on a stage and sputter-coated with carbon.

Animals

Adult male Sprague–Dawley rats (200–250 g) were purchased from Razi Institute of Iran. The rats were kept at 22°C, 12 hour night/day cycle, and received tap water and food Ad libitum. The present study followed the ethical guidelines for investigation of experimental pain in conscious animals as well as the Institutional Animal Ethical Committee of Shahed University, formed under Committee for Purpose of Control and Supervision of Experiments on Animals (CPCSEA, Reg. No. PRC-115), approved by the pharmacologic protocols [15].

The experimental groups

The experimental groups consisted of six rats. Rats were divided into: (a) control group in which, the rats received epidural injection of 5 μl normal saline solution; (b) sham group in which, the rats were treated with epidural injection of 1 mg poly vinyl alcohol nanofibers and flushed by 5 μl saline solution; (c) neostigmine-loaded nanofiber group in which, the rats were treated with epidural injection of neostigmine-loaded nanofibers (1 mg) and flushed by 5 μl saline solution. Epidural injection was done at L5-L6 intervertebral space.

Lumbar epidural injection of the neostigmine-loaded nanofibers

Rats were anesthetized briefly with ether and shaved at the lower back, then placed in the prone position with lower back elevated and flexed ventrally. A lumbar puncture was performed at L5–L6 intervertebral space, perpendicular to the skin, using a 30-gauge needle attached to a 50-μl Hamilton syringe. A catheter of a PE10 polyethylene tube, which was pre-filled with 1 mg neostigmine-loaded nanofibers isolated from 5 μl of saline using a small air bubble, was placed into the needle and advanced 4 cm from the tip of the needle up to the lumber enlargement, which was confirmed by a tail-twitch. The nanofibers were slowly injected and flushed with saline. Three minutes later, the catheter and the needle were respectively removed.

Methylene blue injections

Pilot experiments were performed to evaluate the spread of injected solution in the spinal subarachnoid space. Using the same technique and injection volumes described above, the rats received spinal injections of 5 μl methylene blue 1 mg/ml solution. The area of spread of the methylene blue was examined upon animal necropsy 10 min after intrathecal injections. Besides, all intrathecal solutions contained 5% methylene blue and the included data were only from the animals in which intrathecal placement was confirmed postmortem.

CSF sampling

CSF samples were collected based on procedures described by Haddadi et al. Rats anesthetized by i.p. injection of a mixture of ketamine (80 mg/kg) and xylazine (10 mg/kg) [16]. Then, each rat was placed in a stereotaxic apparatus and its neck was flexed so that a 29-gauge needle could be lowered between the base of the skull and the first cervical vertebra into the cisterna magna. Needle placement was verified by drawing a small amount of CSF into the needle and observing the clear CSF in the polyethylene tube connecting the needle to a 100 μl syringe (Hamilton). CSF (50 μl) was collected in polypropylene test tubes that were put immediately on dry ice and then stored at −80°C until the determination of neostigmine concentration. Samples of CSF of rats were taken 1, 5 and 24 h after the injection of neostigmine nanofibers. The sampling procedure continued once a week for 4 weeks.

Measurement of neostigmine concentration in CSF of rats

Neostigmine concentration in CSF sample of rats (n = 6) was estimated by ultraviolet visible spectrophotometer at 261 nm (Shimadzu UV-1700, Japan) [17]. Aqueous standard solutions of neostigmine methylsulfate were prepared in phosphate buffer (pH 7.4) and their absorbance was measured by applying the same procedures. The method was validated with respect to precision and linearity. To determine the precision of the method, neostigmine concentration in CSF samples was analysed six times a day (intra-day precision) and during six continuous days (inter-day precision). The linearity of measurement was evaluated by analyzing different concentrations of the standard solution of neostigmine. Beer-Lambert's concentration range was found to be 0.01-0.001 μg/ml [17].

Behavioral tests

In the present study, two methods were simultaneously used for evaluating anesthetic effect of a single dose of neostigmine-loaded nanofibers against thermal and chemical types of nociceptive stimuli after epidural injection. Some scientists have claimed that the analgesic effect due to the activation of cholinergic mechanisms also depends on the experimental pain model that is utilized for its evaluation [18].

Tail-flick test

The repeated tail-flick method was used for measuring the analgesic responses of rats after epidural treatment with the neostigmine-loaded nanofibers to a high intensity thermal nociceptive stimulus. Some researchers have also suggested that changes in tail-flick latency may be interpreted in terms of central sensitization and that the repeated tail-flick latency might be considered as a useful marker of chronic nociception [19]. Thus, the tail-flick latencies were repeatedly measured in rats before and on 1st, 15th and 21st days after epidural injection based on the methods proposed by Kríz et al. [19]. The average time interval between the onset of light stimuli and the tail-flick response was measured and defined as tail-flick latency. Since the test should be conducted in triplicates, the tail was marked in three places: proximal, middle, distal. The intensity of radiant heat was adjusted to establish the baseline latencies for 3–5 seconds. The heat stimulus was discontinued after 20 seconds to avoid tissue damages. (Cut off point = 20 s). Each rat was tested 3 times with a 3-second interval. Data were expressed as mean ± SEM (n = 6).

Formalin test

The formalin test is usually used for evaluation of antinociceptive drugs which are administrated intrathecally against the high intensity of chemical pain stimulus. In order to avoid interaction of both techniques' effects on the same animals, it is better to evaluate the formalin test at least 7 days after the tail-flick test, because the tail-flick test has no impact on the formalin test results after this period [20]. Therfore, in this study the formalin test was performed 7 days after the tail flick test. In practice, formalin (2.5%, 50 μl) was injected subcutaneously into the intraplantar surface of different feet of rats after treatment with nanofibers. Then, the rats were gently placed in plexiglass chambers. The pain behavior within the first 15 min of intraplantar formalin injection was recorded as the early phase scores, while the pain behavior between 20 and 60 min of the formalin injection was recorded as the late phase. The behavioral rating scale was as follows: 0 = the injected paw is not favored; 1 = the injected paw rests lightly on the floor and little or no weight is placed on it; 2 = the injected paw is elevated and is not in contact with any surface; 3 = the injected paw is licked, bitten and shaken. Pain scores were calculated by using this formula:

$$\text{Pain score} = 0T0 + 1T1 + 2T2 + 3T3/\text{Time block(s)}$$

where T0-T3 is the number of seconds spent in each of the behavioral categories. All tests were conducted between 9:00 AM and 5:00 PM. Pain scores were expressed as mean ± SEM. A probability of $p < 0.01$ was considered significant.

Measurement of locomotor activity in open field

Locomotor activity was measured using an open field test. The rats were individually placed in one corner of the open field ($100 \times 100 \times 48$ cm). Movement of each rat in the field during 15 min of testing session was recorded. After 15 min, the rat was removed to the home cage, and the open field area was cleaned. The total distance and the average velocity of each rat in the field were recorded.

Statistical analyses

The results were expressed as mean ± S.E.M., and statistical significance was evaluated by a two-way repeated measure analysis of variance (ANOVA) followed by Bonferroni tests. The statistical significance criterion (P-value) was 0.05. All data calculations and statistical analyses were done by using Prism version 5 (GraphPad Software Inc., San Diego, CA).

Results
Morphology of electrospun nanofibers

According to the SEM micrograph shown in Figure 2, electrospun free poly vinyl alcohol nanofibers (A) and the neostigmine-loaded nanofibers (B) were circular in cross-section with an average diameter ranging from 500 nm up to 1,000 nm. The drug encapsulation in vesicular-like reservoirs along the nanofibers was confirmed by the scanning electron microscopy.

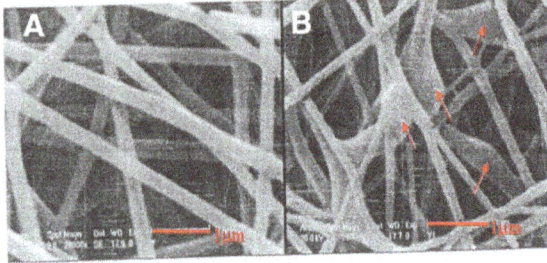

Figure 2 The Scanning electron microscope photomicrograph of Polyvinyl Alcohol nanofibers before (A) and after neostigmine loading (B). In this figure the arrows show the loading position of neostigmine in the core of nanofibers. Magnification: 20,000 × .

In vitro AChE inhibition

The percent of AChE inhibition changed with proportions of PVC (Figure 3A) and the concentration of neostigmine (Figure 3B) that were used in fabrication of the loaded-nanofibers. All neostigmine-loaded nanofibers contained some levels of inhibitory activity against AChE. However, the nanofibers containing 6% poly vinyl alcohol and 0.00125w/w neostigmine showed more effective inhibitory effect on AChE activity compared to others in vitro.

Verification of epidural injection

The spread of methylene blue dye into the epidural space indicated that the dye was only distributed in lumbar segments of rat spinal cord (Figure 4).

Neostigmine concentration in CSF of rats

The time course of neostigmine concentrations in CSF is shown in Figure 5. The results of this study showed that

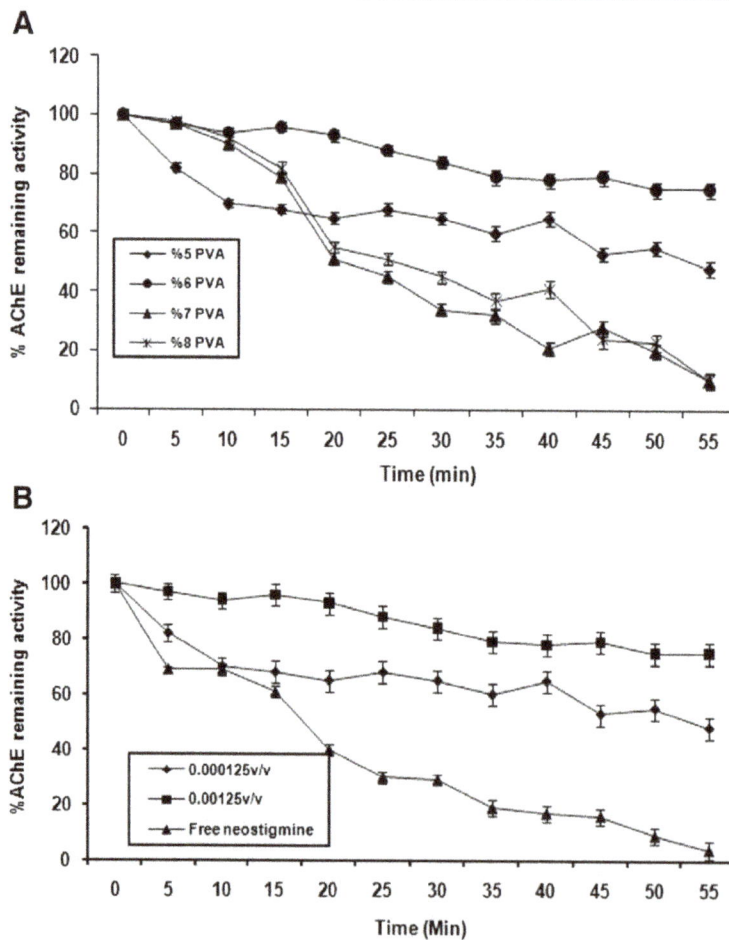

Figure 3 Percentage activity remaining during inhibition of acetylcholinesterase after addition of nanofibers. (A) The measurement of acetylcholinesterase activity following addition of the nanofibers were fabricated with different proportions of poly vinyl alcohol and neostigmine (0.00125 v/v); **(B)** the acetylcholinesterase activity after addition of the neostigmine nanofibers that fabricated by %6 PVA and two different concentrations of neostigmine (pH = 7/4, 22°C).

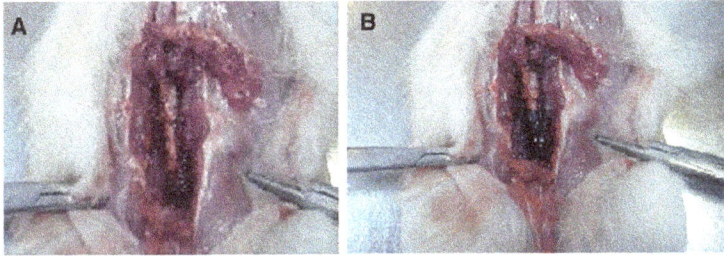

Figure 4 Verification of injection site and evaluation the distribution of methylene blue injected into the epidural space. (A) The exposed lumbar spinal cord region of control rats and **(B)** drug extension evaluation by epidural injection of 50 μL 1% methylene blue.

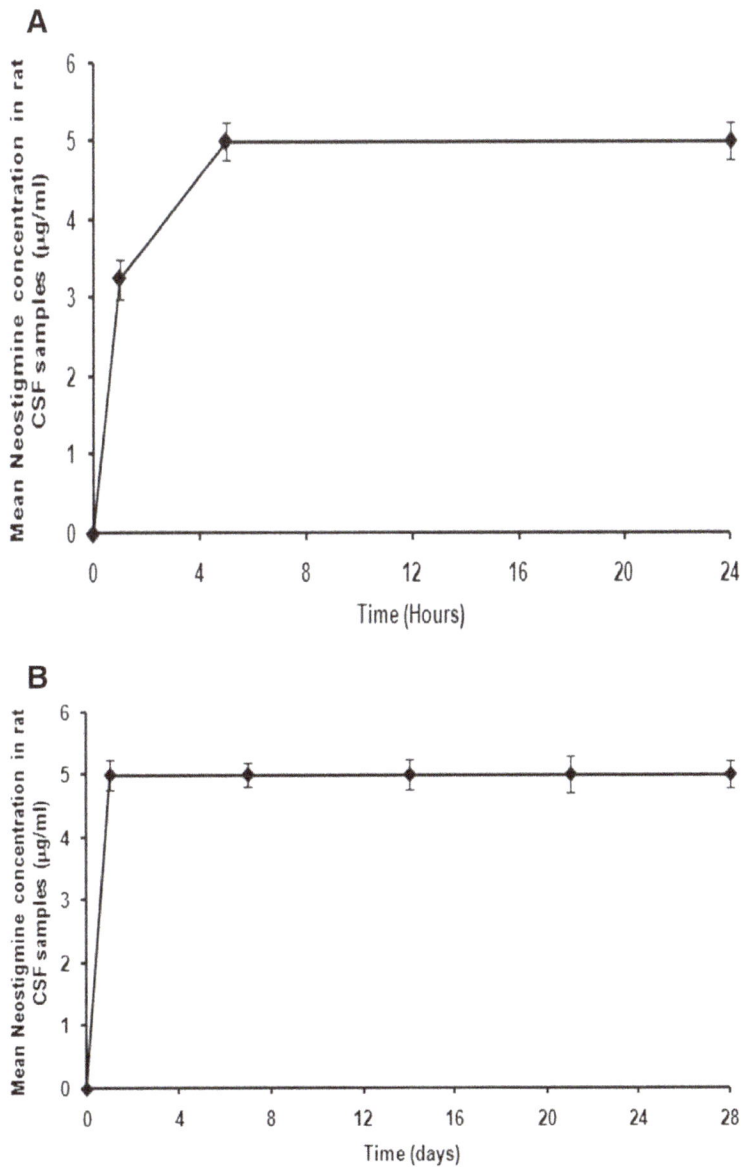

Figure 5 Measurement of neostigmine concentration in CSF in rats. CSF concentrations of neostigmine were measured, **(A)** up to 24 hours and **(B)** for 4 weeks after epidural injection of neostigmine loaded nanofibers. Values presented are means ± SEM.

neostigmine concentrations in CSF were significantly increased from baseline to a maximum concentration (5 ± 0.1 µg/ml) during 5 hours after epidural administration (Figure 5-A). The concentration of free neostigmine in CSF of rats remained constant at 5 ± 0.1 µg/ml during 4 weeks after injection of the nanofibers (Figure 5-B).

Formalin test

The epidural administration of neostigmine-loaded nanofibers decreased the pain score significantly ($p < 0.001$) in early (Figure 6A) and late (Figure 6B) phases of the formalin test in rats for five weeks after injection of the neostigmine nanofibers.

Tail-flick test

The duration of analgesia after epidural injection of neostigmine-loaded nanofibers is shown in Figure 7. The

tail-flick latency of rats was significantly ($p < 0.01$) increased and remained stable for four weeks after injection of the neostigmine nanofibers.

Locomotor activity in open-field

The mean traveling distance (Figure 8A) and the velocity (Figure 8B) of rats in the open-field in 7, 14 and 21 days post-injection were not affected by epidural administrations of the nanofibers in comparison with the sham group.

Discussion

The results of the present investigation revealed that neostigmine was successfully loaded into the poly vinyl alcohol nanofibers using the electrospinning technique. The SEM images confirmed the incorporation of neostigmine in the nanofibers. As seen in Figure 2, no drug crystals

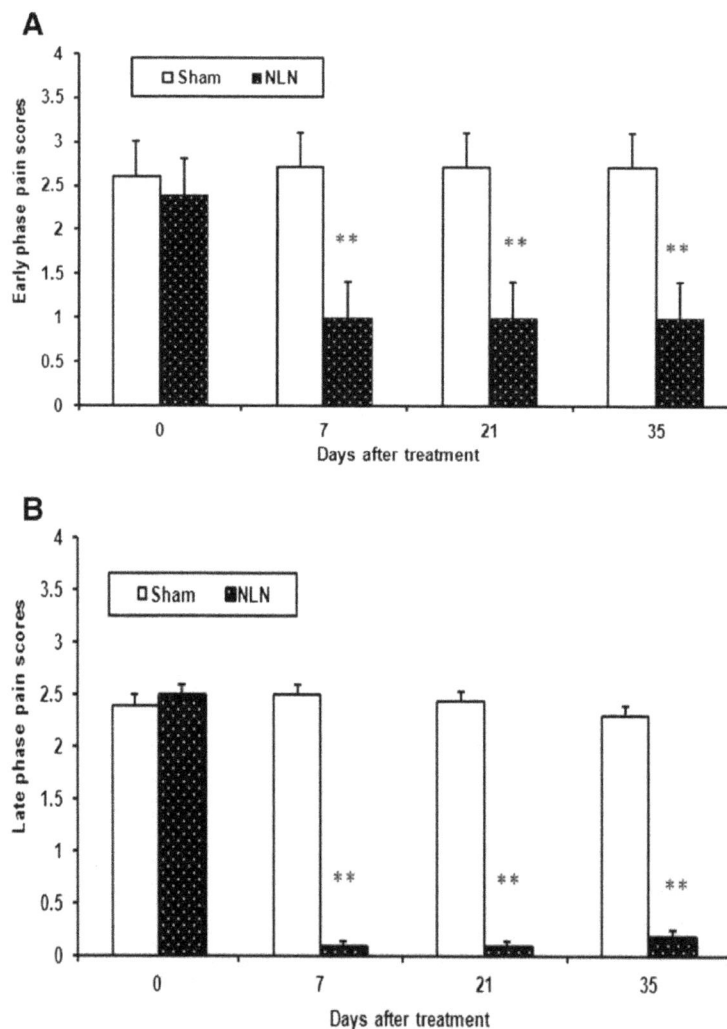

Figure 6 The effect of epidural injection of neostigmine loaded nanofibers (NLN) on the cumulative nociceptive scores of rats in the early phase (A) the late phase (B) of formalin test. Sham group treated with free PVA nanofibers (Mean ± SEM, n = 6, **p < 0.01, Repeated-two way ANOVA followed by Bonferroni test).

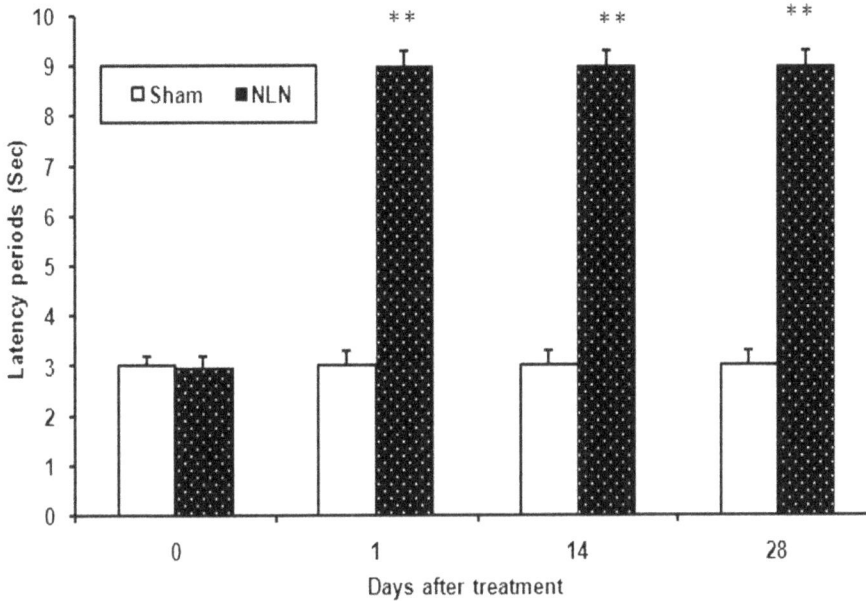

Figure 7 Effect of epidural neostigmine loaded nanofibers (NLN) administration on tail-flick latencies of rats (Mean ± SEM, n = 6, **p < 0.01, repeated two way ANOVA followed by Bonferroni test), Sham group treated with epidural free PVA nanofibers.

were detected by electron microscopy on the surface or outside of the loaded nanofibers. The electrospinning technique has been already used effectively to produce other drug-loaded nanofibers. The poly vinyl alcohol nanofibers have proven their performance in controlled release of antinociceptive drugs [21]. PVA nanofibers prepared by electrospinning technique also provide a suitable matrix for sustain release of drugs based on available evidence [22]. Therefore, it seems that the electrospinning method and poly vinyl alcohol nanofibers are appropriate choices for encapsulation of neostigmine.

The in vitro study of AChE inhibition after injection of the nanofibers indicated that the neostigmine released from the nanofibers can inhibit AChE effectively and the loading of neostigmine within the nanofibers did not compromise the inherent of AChE inhibitory activity. The results of enzyme activity assay also indicated that

the change in the ratio of PVA- neostigmine can influence the amount of neostigmine release and percent of AChE inhibition. Measurement of neostigmine concentrations in cerebrospinal fluid (CSF) has suggested that the profile of the neostigmine release from the loaded nanofibers follows a biphasic pattern characterized by an initial fast release during 5 hours and following sustained release phase. A similar biphasic behavior has also been reported for ethyl cellulose nanofibers fabricated by using electrospinning process [23]. This form of drug release is an ideal situation for the rapid relief of symptoms which optimizes the therapy and avoids repeated administration for the patients' convenience. Furthermore, the researchers treated the nanofibers with ethanol in order to reduce the drug release rate. It is reported that the burst release of drug from nanofibers was eliminated after treatment with alcohol. In practice, the use of

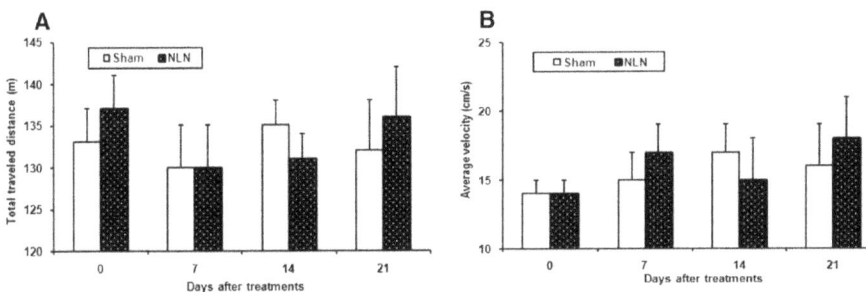

Figure 8 Measurement of rats total traveled distance (A) and average velocity (B) for 3 weeks after epidural injection of neostigmine loaded nanofibers (NLN). Sham group treated with free PVA nanofibers (Mean ± SEM, n = 6, **p < 0.01, Repeated-two way ANOVA followed by Bonferroni test).

such drug-loaded nanofibers for spinal cord drug delivery can increase the duration of drug efficacy. For example, Schmidt and co-workers enhanced epidural liposome-encapsulated hydromorphone's duration of analgesia action from 2 to 72 hours in rats [24]. Based on the above reports, a combination of all these mechanisms can provide explanation for stable concentration of neostigmine in in vitro situation.

The results of the present study indicated that the thermal pain threshold was increased in rats after single epidural injection of the neostigmine-loaded nanofibers and persisted for as long as 28 days. Consecutive formalin test in rats also showed that the pain scores decreased in both phases and remained stable up to 35 days after injection. The early phase response of the formalin test was considered to be the result of direct effects of formalin on nociceptive fibers. It may be modulated by cholinergic spinal inhibitory interneurons [25]. The late phase was caused by tissue damage as well as inflammation and reflecting a state of central sensitization. Park and co-workers demonstrated that intratecal administration of atropine, a muscarinic antagonist, could decrease rat hindpaw persistent pain after formalin injection into the hindpaw [26]. Moreover, the intrathecal injection of neostigmine could reduce the pain in both phases of the formalin test.

The high sensitivity of tail flick technique for measurement of pain threshold after manipulation of spinal cholinergic system has been reported [27]. In addition, consecutive evaluation of tail-flick latency was considered as a marker of chronic nociception. Comparing the antinociceptive effect of the neostigmine loaded nanofibers in these two pain models showed that the effective analgesic dose of neostigmine was chosen for pain relief in our experiments.

In support of the present findings it can be said that after being release from nanofibers, the free neostigmine increased the level of endogenous acetylcholine at dorsal horn of spinal cord. Following mechanisms have been proposed to explain the anti-nociception action of acetylcholine at the dorsal horn level. It is shown that acetylcholinesterase inhibition increased acetylcholine level at spinal cord and then it caused (i) the activation of presynaptic nicotinic acetylcholine receptors and decrease in glutamate release from C-fiber terminals in the dorsal horn [28]; (ii) the inhibition of presynaptic release of glutamate from primary afferent axons by stimulation of GABAergic interneurons via activation of muscarinic acetylcholine receptors [29]; (iii) the stimulation of the nicotinic acetylcholine receptors on GABA-ergic inhibitory interneurons that triggered the firing of spinothalamic pain transmission neurons [30]; and (iv) the reduction of neuroinflammation by blocking microglial cell activity via stimulation of the nicotinic receptors [31]. Furthermore, neostigmine could stimulate GABA release from dorsal horn neurons [32] and its stimulatory effect on GABA release continued even after drug clearing from the CSF [33]. All of these mechanisms can play a significant role in effective analgesia induced by epidural application of neostigmine nanofibers.

In addition, loading of drugs in nanostructures increased its tissue penetration power [34], which probably makes them activate more inhibitory interneurons in deeper layers of dorsal horn of spinal cord. This property could provide an additional advantage for neostigmine-loaded nanofibers.

Comparison of the present findings with previous results [3,35] showed that the duration of analgesia after administration of the neostigmine-loaded nanofiber was longer than all previous neostigmine-containing mixture in animal or human studies. A relation was shown between concentrations of a drug in cerebrospinal fluid and its analgesic effect [36]. It can be concluded that the loaded amount of neostigmine in the nanofibers was sufficient to produce and maintain a relatively constant concentration of free neostigmine in CSF for induction of long-term analgesia. Also, the low rate of drug biotransformation in CSF could be another possible factor to increase the duration of neostigmine effect after epidural injection [37].

In spite of the free neostigmine side effects on locomotor activity after epidural administration in human [38], injection of the neostigmine-loaded nanofibers had no adverse effects on rats. Furthermore, the epidural administration of neostigmine-loaded nanofibers did not significantly alter locomotor activity in rats. Probably, the lack of side effects is due to the restricted release of neostigmine from nanofibers in dorsal horn of spinal cord. In support of this idea, it was shown that no adverse effects were noted after the epidural administration of neostigmine when the drug spread was restricted into lower part of the spinal cord [39].

Conclusion

In this study, electrospun polyvinyl alcohol nanofibers were used as a controlled release matrix for the incorporation of neostigmine. The findings suggested that the nanofibers made from poly vinyl alcohol can easily be loaded with neostigmine. The SEM image confirmed loading of drug in nanofibers. The lumbar epidural administration of the nanofibers can reduce acute and chronic thermal and chemical pain in rats for 5 weeks. Also, its application had no significant effect on locomotor activity of rats.

Abbreviations
AChE: Acetylcholinesterase; PBS: Phosphate Buffer Saline; CSF: Cerebrospinal Fluid; NLN: Neostigmine Loaded Nanofibers.

Competing interests
The authors declare that they have no competing interests.

Acknowledgments
The authors would like to thank Dr. Sayyed Omid Ranaei for her preparation of neostigmine nanofibers.

References

1. Mahajan R, Grover VK, Chari P: Caudal neostigmine with bupivacaine produces a dose-independent analgesic effect in children. *Can J Anaesth* 2004, **51**:702–6.
2. Yoon MH, Choi JI, Kwak SH: Characteristic of interactions between intrathecal gabapentin and either clonidine or neostigmine in the formalin test. *Anesth Analg* 2004, **98**:1374–1379.
3. Jain A, Jain K, Bhardawaj N: Analgesic efficacy of low-dose intrathecal neostigmine in combination with fentanyl and bupivacaine for total knee replacement surgery. *J Anaesthesiol Clin Pharmacol* 2012, **28**:486–490.
4. Owen MD, Ozsarac O, Sahin S, Uckunkaya N, Kaplan N, Magunaci I: Low-dose clonidine and neostigmine prolong the duration of intrathecal bupivacaine-fentanyl for labor analgesia. *Anesthesiology* 2000, **92**:361–366.
5. Greig NH, Utsuki T, Ingram DK, Wang Y, Pepeu G, Scali C, Yu QS, Mamczarz J, Holloway HW, Giordano T, Chen D, Furukawa K, Sambamurti K, Brossi A, Lahiri DK: Selective butyrylcholinesterase inhibition elevates brain acetylcholine, augments learning and lowers Alzheimer beta-amyloid peptide in rodent. *Proc Natl Acad Sci U S A* 2005, **102**:17213–17218.
6. Kumar P, Rudra A, Pan AK, Acharya A: Caudal additives in pediatrics: a comparison among midazolam, ketamine, and neostigmine coadministered with bupivacaine. *Anesth Analg* 2005, **101**:69–73.
7. Grant GJ, Piskoun B, Bansinath M: Intrathecal administration of liposomal neostigmine prolongs analgesia in mice. *Acta Anaesthesiol Scand* 2002, **46**:90–94.
8. Tseng YY, Liao JY, Chen WA, Kao YC, Liu SJ: Biodegradable poly ([D, L]-lactide-co-glycolide) nanofibers for the sustainable delivery of lidocaine into the epidural space after laminectomy. *Nanomedicine (Lond)* 2014, **9**:77–87.
9. Lv S1, Yang YJ, Hong S, Wang N, Qin Y, Li W, Chen Q: Intrathecal apelin-13 produced different actions in formalin test and tail-flick test in mice. *Protein Pept Lett* 2013, **20**:926–231.
10. Arecchi A1, Mannino S, Weiss J: Electrospinning of poly (vinyl alcohol) nanofibers loaded with hexadecane nanodroplets. *J Food Sci* 2010, **75**:N80–88.
11. Kenawy ER, Abdel-Hay FI, El-Newehy MH, Wnek GE: Controlled release of ketoprofen from electrospun poly (vinyl alcohol) nanofibers. *Mater Sci Eng A* 2007, **459**:390–396.
12. Welcome Z, Wu H, Nyairo E, Rogers C, Dean D, Wekesa K, Gunn K, Villafane R: Cytotoxicity and cell adhesion properties of human mesenchymal stem cells in electrospun nanofiber polymer scaffolds. *Int J Adv Biotec Bioinform* 2012, **1**:41–47.
13. Ellman GL, Courtney KD, Andres V Jr, Feather-stone RM: A new and rapid colorimetric determination of acetylcholinesterase activity. *Biochem Pharmacol* 1961, **7**:88–95.
14. Chaabihi H, Fournier D, Fedon Y, Bossy JP, Ravallec M, Devauchelle G, Cérutti M: Biochemical characterization of *Drosophila melanogaster* acetylcholinesterase expressed by recombinant baculoviruses. *Biochem Biophys Res Commun* 1994, **203**:734–742.
15. Zimmermann M: Ethical guidelines for investigations of experimental pain in conscious animals. *Pain* 1983, **16**:109–110.
16. Haddadi R, Nayebi AM1, Farajniya S, Brooshghalan SE, Sharifi H: Silymarin improved 6-OHDA-induced motor impairment in hemi-parkisonian rats: behavioral and molecular study. *Daru* 2014, **22**:38–46.
17. Thatte AA, Kadam RJ, Pramila T, Bhoi UA, Deshpande KB: Development, validation and application of UV spectrophotometric method for the determination of oseltamivir phosphate in bulk and pharmaceutical dosage. *Int J ChemTech Res* 2011, **3**:569–573.
18. Prado WA, Gonçalves AS: Antinociceptive effect of intrathecal neostigmine evaluated in rats by two different pain models. *Braz J Med Biol Res* 1997, **30**:1225–1231.
19. Kríz N, Yamamotová A, Tobiás J, Rokyta R: Tail-flick latency and self-mutilation following unilateral deafferentation in rats. *Physiol Res* 2006, **55**:213–20.
20. Afolabi AO, Mudashiru SK, Alagbonsi IA: Effects of salt-loading hypertension on nociception in rats. *J Pain Res* 2013, **6**:387–392.
21. Taepaiboon P, Rungsardthong U, Supaphol P: Drug loaded electrospun mats of poly(vinyl alcohol) fibres and their release characteristics of four model drugs. *Nanotechnology* 2006, **17**:2317–2329.
22. Yu DG, Zhu LM, White K, Branford-White C: Electrospun nanofiber-based drug delivery systems. *Health* 2009, **1**:67–75.
23. Li C, Wang ZH, Yu DG, Williams GR: Tunable biphasic drug release from ethyl cellulose nanofibers fabricated using a modified coaxial electrospinning process. *Nanoscale Res Lett* 2014, **9**:258–268.
24. Schmidt JR, Krugner-Higby L, Heath TD, Sullivan R, Smith LJ: Epidural administration of liposome-encapsulated hydromorphone provides extended analgesia in a rodent model of stifle arthritis. *J Am Assoc Lab Anim Sci* 2011, **50**:507–512.
25. Yu D, Thakor DK, Han I, Ropper AE, Haragopal H, Sidman RL, Zafonte R, Schachter SC, Teng YD: Alleviation of chronic pain following rat spinal cord compression injury with multimodal actions of huperzine A. *Proc Natl Acad Sci U S A* 2013, **110**:E746–55.
26. Park P, Schachter S, Yaksh T: Intrathecal huperzine A increases thermal escape latency and decreases flinching behavior in the formalin test in rats. *Neurosci Lett* 2010, **470**:6–9.
27. Lograsso M, Nadeson R, Goodchild CS: The spinal antinociceptive effects of cholinergic drugs in rats: receptor subtype specificity in different nociceptive tests. *BMC Pharmacol* 2002, **2**:20–29.
28. Young T, Wittenauer S, McIntosh JM, Vincler M: Spinal alpha3beta2 nicotinic acetylcholine receptors tonically inhibit the transmission of nociceptive mechanical stimuli. *Brain Res* 2008, **1229**:118–124.
29. Cai YQ, Chen SR, Han HD, Sood AK, Lopez-Berestein G, Pan HL: Role of M2, M3, and M4 muscarinic receptor subtypes in the spinal cholinergic control of nociception revealed using siRNA in rats. *J Neurochem* 2009, **111**:1000–1010.
30. Rashid MH, Ueda H: Neuropathy-specific analgesic action of intrathecal nicotinic agonists and its spinal GABA-mediated mechanism. *Brain Res* 2002, **953**:53–62.
31. Shytle RD, Mori T, Townsend K, Vendrame M, Sun N, Zeng J, Ehrhart J, Silver AA, Sanberg PR, Tan J: Cholinergic modulation of microglial activation by alpha 7 nicotinic receptors. *J Neurochem* 2004, **89**:337–343.
32. Baba H, Kohno T, Okamoto M, Goldstein PA, Shimoji K, Yoshimura M: Muscarinic facilitation of GABA release in substantia gelatinosa of the rat spinal dorsal horn. *J Physiol* 1998, **508**:83–93.
33. Perucca E: Extended-Release Formulations of Antiepileptic Drugs: Rationale and Comparative Value. *Epilepsy Curr* 2009, **9**:153–157.
34. Khanbabaie R, Jahanshahi M: Revolutionary Impact of Nanodrug Delivery on Neuroscience. *Curr Neuropharmacol* 2012, **10**:370–392.
35. Yoon MH, Park HC, Kim WM, Lee HG, Kim YO, Huang LJ: Evaluation for the interaction between intrathecal melatonin and clonidine or neostigmine on formalin-induced nociception. *Life Sci* 2008, **83**:845–850.
36. Natalini CC: Plasma and cerebrospinal fluid alfentanil, butorphanol, and morphine concentrations following caudal epidural administration in horses. *Ciência Rural* 2006, **36**:1436–1443.
37. Suto T, Obata H, Tobe M, Oku H, Yokoo H, Nakazato Y, Saito S: Long-term effect of epidural injection with sustained-release lidocaine particles in a rat model of postoperative pain. *Br J Anaesth* 2012, **109**:957–967.
38. Alkan M, Kaya K: Postoperative analgesic effect of epidural neostigmine following caesarean section. *Hippokratia* 2014, **18**:44–49.
39. Omais M, Lauretti GR, Paccola CAJ: Epidural morphine and neostigmine for postoperative analgesia after orthopedic surgery. *Anesth Analg* 2002, **95**:1698–1701.

15

Preliminary investigation of the effects of topical mixture of *Lawsonia inermis* L. and *Ricinus communis* L. leaves extract in treatment of osteoarthritis using MIA model in rats

Atousa Ziaei[1], Shamim Sahranavard[1], Mohammad Javad Gharagozlou[2] and Mehrdad Faizi[3*]

Abstract

Background: Many plants have been introduced in Iranian traditional medicine for treatment of different joint problems including knee pain. Topical application of the mixture of *Lawsonia inermis* L. leaves (Henna) with aqueous extract of *Ricinus communis* L. leaves have been mentioned to have significant effects on reducing knee pain. The present study was designed to evaluate the analgesic and anti-inflammatory effects of the mixture of these two herbs in male rats.

Methods: We induced knee osteoarthritis as a model of chronic pain by intra-articular injection of mono sodium iodoacetate (MIA). Mechanical allodynia, hotplate latency test, spontaneous movements and gait analysis were used for the evaluation of analgesic activity. Anti-inflammatory activity was evaluated by measuring the diameter and the volume of the injected paw compared to contralateral paw. These tests were monitored at days 1, 3, 7, 14 and 21 of MIA administration. Histopathological evaluations were also used to assess the efficacy of the treatment on inflammation and lesions in knee tissue. In all tests, diclofenac topical gel was used as a positive control. The herbal extracts, their mixture, and vehicle or diclofenac gel were administered daily for 14 days by topical route.

Results: The mixture of these two extracts significantly reduced the knee joint width and volume of the injected paws and also improved foot prints in gait analysis after 3 days of MIA injection. Analysis of mechanical allodynia (after 21 days), hotplate latency test (after 10 days), spontaneous movements (after 7 days) and in positive control group (after 3 days in all tests and in mechanical allodynia after 14 days) compared to the vehicle group, showed significant effects. Topical usage of the selected formulation made significant histopathological changes on the knee of the rats. Compared to the vehicle group, the tests and diclofenac groups showed less reactions characterized by negligible edema and a few scattered inflammatory lymphoid cells.

Conclusion: The present findings showed that the present formulation not only was able to mitigate pain and inflammation in the paws but also made significant histopathological changes on the knee of the rats. Further studies are necessary to confirm the effect of the formulation.

Keywords: *Lawsonia inermis* L, Leaves, MIA, Osteoarthritis, Rats, *Ricinus communis* L

* Correspondence: m.faizi@sbmu.ac.ir
[3]Department of Pharmacology and Toxicology, School of Pharmacy, Shahid Beheshti University of Medical Sciences, Tehran, Iran
Full list of author information is available at the end of the article

Background

Pain is a major symptom in many medical conditions and it is the most common reason for medical consultation. Approximately half of all licensed drugs that had been registered worldwide in a 25 years period prior to 2007 were natural products or synthetic derivatives of natural products [1]. For thousands of years, natural products derived from plants, animals and microorganisms have been used as treatments for human diseases. Knowledge of the medical use of natural products has been transmitted from generation to generation over the years [2]. It seems that drugs, especially those which have plant origin and have been used in the Iranian traditional medicine (ITM) could be an appropriate initiative in research projects aiming at development of new analgesic drugs.

A formula containing the mixture of *Lawsonia inermis* L. and *Ricinus communis* L. was chosen for evaluation of knee pain reduction from the Iranian traditional medicine books such as: *Makhzan-ol Advieh* [3], *Gharabadin-e-kabir* [4] and *Tohfat al-mu'minin* [5]. In these books, the mixture of mentioned plants has been recommended for knee pain treatment.

Osteoarthritis (OA) is a degenerative joint disease characterized by joint pain and progressive loss of articular cartilage [6]. Mono sodium iodoacetate (MIA) is a chemical substance that induced OA as a model of knee pain. This model is used for the study of pain and analgesic drug effects because it is reproducible and mimics the pathological changes and the pain of osteoarthritis in humans [7]. Injection of MIA, an inhibitor of glycolysis, into the femorotibial joint of rodents, promotes loss of articular cartilage similar to that observed in human OA [6]. The joint problem induced in this way, is called induced MIA hereafter.

Lawsonia inermis L. (Lythraceae) is used in the treatment of diseases such as leprosy and headache and has cosmetic purposes like accelerating the growth and dying hair and nails [8] and has also been reported to have anti-inflammatory, antinociceptive and antipyretic effects [9]. The natural constituents of *L.inermis* are Lawsone (2-hydroxy-1,4-naphthoquinone), mucilage, essential oils, tannic acid, gallic acid, fats, glucose, mannitol, and resin [10].

Ricinus communis L. (Euphorbiaceae) is used for the treatment of swelling, gout and skin diseases [11]. Polyphenols and flavonoids are the major compounds found in this plant and have anti-inflammatory and antioxidant activities [11, 12].

The present study was designed to evaluate the analgesic and anti-inflammatory effects of the mixture of topical extracts of *L.inermis* and *R.communis* according to the Iranian traditional manuscripts. The efficacy of the used formulation in reducing knee pain was evaluated by inducing osteoarthritis. All of the pharmacological experiments were also performed to determine the effects of *L.inermis* or *R.communis* extract separately.

Methods
Preparation of the extracts

Dry leaves of *Lawsonia inermis* L. were gathered from Yazd, Iran and identified and authenticated by a plant taxonomist at the herbarium of School of Traditional Medicine, Shahid Beheshti University of Medical Sciences, Tehran, Iran. The voucher specimen was deposited with number of HMS 331 in the herbarium. The dried leaves were powdered coarsely with a mechanical grinder (Desktop mill, 8300, Iran). The powder was passed through sieve No.40 and stored in an airtight container for further use. The powdered leaves were macerated in ethanol and water (80:20) and allowed to shake for 24 h and then were filtered through a filter paper (Whatman filter paper No.1). The maceration process was repeated 3 times. The filtered extract was concentrated in a rotary evaporator (Heidolph, HB digital, Germany) at 40 °C and then used freeze drier (Benchtop, SLC Virtis, USA) to remove water (the herbal extract ratio was 19 %). The dry extract was stored in cool place until used.

Fresh leaves of *Ricinus communis* were gathered from Tehran, Iran and identified and authenticated and deposited similar to *L.inermis* with voucher number of 3577. Subsequently, leaves were dried in shade and powdered by a mechanical grinder. The powdered leaves were macerated in water and allowed to shake for 24 h, same as described for *L.inermis* (the herbal extract ratio was 22 %). The herbal extracts were added at the same concentrations as mentioned in ITM references [3–5] and we did not perform comparative evaluation of different doses of the extracts.

Drug administration

The dry extracts were mixed with the same percentage, suspended in water (0.2 g/0.3 ml). This is the maximum amount of the mixture of extracts that solved in the lowest amount of the vehicle and cover all of the animal 's knee and administered topically on the left hind paw of the animal in all groups, from day 1 to 14 (once a day dosing) respectively. The control group (Vehicle) received the same volume of vehicle (water) by the same route. 0.4 g of diclofenac 1 % gel (Razak Pharmaceutical Company) was used topically in the positive control group [13].

Animals and experimental groups

Wistar male rats (160–180 g body weight) were purchased from the Pasteur Institute of Iran. They were housed in standard polypropylene rat cages and kept in a room with controlled condition (temperature 25 ± 2 °C and relative humidity 40–50 %) in a 12 h light-dark cycle. The rats were given a standard laboratory diet and have free access to food and water. Each rat was only used once. All procedures for the treatment of animals were approved by the Research Committee of Shahid Beheshti University of Medical Sciences and institutional animal care and use committee with approval code SBMU.REC.1392.343.

For induction of OA, rats were anesthetized with ketamine-xylazine (100 and 10 mg/kg) intra-peritoneally [14, 15]. Osteoarthritis was induced by an injection of mono sodium iodoacetate (MIA, Sigma-Aldrich, USA) at a dose of 3 mg/50 μL normal saline to intra articular space of the left hind limb [16–18].

In this study, 36 adult male wistar rats were used. They were randomly divided in to 6 groups including sham group (S; $n = 6$) that received saline instead of MIA, negative control group (N; $n = 6$) with OA induction and treating by vehicle, combination group (T; $n = 6$) with OA induction and treating by topical mixture of the plant extracts, *L.inermis* group (L; $n = 6$), *R.communis* group (R; $n = 6$) and positive control group (P; $n = 6$) with OA induction and treating by diclofenac topical gel. On day 21, after performing behavioral tests, rats of all groups were sacrificed by overdosing ether [19]. To evaluate the histological changes, rats were sacrificed on day 14 after 3 h of the formulation or diclofenac gel administration and left knee was collected for histological examination.

Behavioral tests
Mechanical allodynia (Von Frey test)
Von Frey filaments (North Coast Medical, Inc. CA, USA) have been used to assess the mechanical sensitivity of the hind paw of the animals with knee joint arthritis. Typically, paw withdrawal threshold (PWT) is measured in response to increasing pressure stimuli applied to the plantar surface by von Frey filaments. Rats were removed from their home cages and placed in a Plexiglass cage with a wire mesh bottom [20]. The rats were allowed to acclimate for 15 min (or until exploratory and grooming behavior declined to a level compatible with behavioral testing). Von Frey monofilaments were applied at a 90° to the mid-plantar of the left hind paw of the rats (ipsilateral side of MIA injection) with a series of monofilaments that ranged from 0.6 to 26 g in stiffness. Filaments were held in place and then removed; they were applied at the same location; 5 times for 1.5 s with inter stimulus intervals of 1 min. Rats were tested using the up-down method. A positive response was defined as a rapid withdrawal of the left hind paw or licking of the paw (three out of five were considered positive). The first day of the testing provided a baseline measure of tactile sensitivity. Rats in each group were then tested with von Frey monofilaments on post-injection days 1, 3, 7, 10, 14 and 21.

Spontaneous locomotor activity (Open field test)
This method has been used to evaluate the locomotor activity of rodents [21]. The test was performed in a Plexi glass box of $40 \times 40 \times 40$ cm with transparent walls and black floor (in contrast with the color of the rat). Each rat was initially placed in the center of the box and its activity was recorded by a video camera for 10 min (at the same temperature and light conditions). Locomotor activity was measured in the square arena. The behavior was recorded by a video camera mounted on the ceiling, relayed to a monitor and total distance moved of the rat was analyzed by tracking software (EthoVision, Noldus, The Netherlands). Spontaneous locomotion was assessed on six consecutive days. On each day, each rat was placed in the center of the arena and allowed to explore it for 10 min. In this period, the rat's movements were recorded with a video camera. The computer software calculated the distance that the rat moved and the total distance during 10 min period was measured. At the end of each test, the box was removed and the entire test chamber was cleaned with a damp cloth and subsequently dried [22].

Gait analysis test (Footprint)
Analyzing the walking patterns of the rat by recording its footprints is a well-established and widely employed method for the assessment of motor nerve recovery after nerve injury [23]. We used the software image J to analyze the rat's footprints. Analysis footprints by image J 1.37 software is extremely useful and reduces intervention results such as operator subjectivity which can limit the statistical significance of the numerical data generated.

Tracking tunnels are basically rectangular, designed to allow the target animal to walk through unhindered. A tracking paper made of an absorbent white paper was used. Rats were stained with the ink-foot stump then each animal attracted into the tunnel after walking across the ink leaves footprints on the absorbent paper. The ink is absorbed into the paper leaving tracks which can be analyzed by the software image J [24].

Hotplate test
The analgesic response was the latency observed from the time the rat was placed on the heated surface until the first overt behavioral sign of nociception such as (a) the rat licking a hind paw, (b) vocalization or (c) an escape response [25].

Animals were placed individually on a hotplate with the temperature adjusted to 52 °C (UgoBasile, Varese, Italy). Exposure to heat continued until a nociceptive reaction in either of the hind paws occurred. The latency of the withdrawal response of each of the hind paws was determined at 1, 3, 7, 10, 14 and 21 days after injection of MIA. The heat source was maintained at constant intensity, which produced a stable withdrawal latency of approximately 8–10s in vehicle group. The animals were tested in only one series of measurements and the typical responses were hind paw shaking and/or lifting and the rat was immediately removed from the hotplate after the response was observed. The latency to the response was recorded manually with a chronometer and the maximum permanence permitted on the hot surface was 60s. The experiments were performed in a sound-attenuated and air-conditioned (25–30 °C) laboratory.

Inflammatory tests
Measuring paw diameter
The paw diameter was measured at intervals of 1, 3, 7, 10, 14 and 21 days after the injection of MIA using Colis (Helios, Germany) after MIA injection. The difference between inflamed and right knee's joint width at 6 time points was calculated (indicating the degree of inflammation) and was compared to the amount for vehicle group (N) [26].

Measuring paw edema using mercury
This method was done by the method previously reported by Fereidoni and his colleagues [27]. A cylinder filled with mercury was placed on a sensitive digital balance. The values on the digital balance were recorded. According to the gravity of mercury, the expected measures were calculated and compared with the observed value. The formula used for this measurement is $V = W/p$, in which V stands for volume, W for weight and p for gravity [27]. Measurements of the inflamed paw were continued for 21 days after MIA injection and performed five times on each rat and the average of middle three values was calculated.

Histological evaluation
Histological studies were performed to ensure the responses obtained from the pharmacological experiments. On MIA post day 14, rats were sacrificed and MIA or saline injected knee joints (including distal femur and proximal tibia) were fixed in 10 % buffered formaldehyde solution, decalcified using formic acid-sodium citrate method [28]. This method is superior to other decalcification techniques, since preserves the histological and staining properties of tissues very well. The formalin-fixed specimens were washed properly by distilled water to remove the residues of formaldehyde from the tissues. Then, the specimens were transferred into a jar containing sufficient volume of formic acid–sodium citrate solution, prepared as follows [28].

Solution A: 50 g of sodium citrate was dissolved in 250 ml of distilled water.
Solution B: 125 ml of 90 % formic acid were added to 125 ml of distilled water.
To make a working solution, equal volumes of the solutions A and B were mixed before use. Due to higher volume of the bone tissue of the specimens, the decalcifying solution was changed every single day until decalcification was completed. The decalcified specimens were washed very well with distilled water in order to remove decalcified residues.

A longitudinal section was made at the extensor site in such a manner that divided the specimen into two equal pieces. The tissue samples were processed in a tissue processor, paraffin blocks were made and 5–6 μm thick sections were made with a microtome. Sections were stained with the Harris haematoxylin and eosin method [28]. The histology was evaluated through double-blind observations following the method described previously.

Scoring of the severity of the articular or periarticular tissue lesions including acute or chronic inflammatory lesions in the tissue sections stained with Harris haematoxylin and eosine method was done by using a magnification of X100-X400 as follows:

0: **Negative;** Normal tissue architecture.
1: **Mild;** A very mild tissue edema accompanied by a few scattered mononuclear cells including lymphocytes.
2: **Moderate;** Many mononuclear or polymorphonuclear leukocytes accompanied by hyperemia and edema or beginning of granulation tissue formation.
3: **Severe;** Marked acute or chronic inflammation characterized by fibrinopurulent exudates or granulation tissue formation accompanied by mononuclear infiltration with or without tendinal adhesions to the adjacent tissues.
4: **Very severe;** Marked severe acute or chronic inflammation accompanied by tissue necrosis and tendinal adhesions.

The number of pathology sections that were used: three sections in the Sham group, four sections in rats, a day after they were injected with MIA(Inflammation peak), four sections in group (P), four sections in group (T), five sections in group (N) with no treatment.

Histological studies were done on five groups: 1-Sham injected by Saline (group S). 2- One day after injection of MIA that substantial inflammation of the synovial joints was observed in the model. Some days later, the inflammatory response in the synovium subsides, necrotic cartilage collapse, and chondrocytes are lost [29, 30]. 3- Diclofenac gel or group (P) as positive group 4-Mixture of the extracts or group (T) 5- Vehicle or no treatment or group (N).

Statistical analysis

The obtained data were analyzed by the statistical program Prism 5. Results launched by Average ± SEM. Due to the two interventions (different groups on different days), we used two-way ANOVA to determine the differences between the experimental groups and the mean obtained in the presence of interference interaction between groups. To evaluate the significant differences between the groups, the post hoc Bonferroni test was used. Amounts of $p < 0.05$ were considered as the minimum level of significance. Asterisks indicate a statistically difference from group (N); * $p < 0.05$, ** $p < 0.01$, *** $p < 0.001$.

Results

Mechanical allodynia

Results are expressed as pain threshold measurements with von Frey filament stimulation of the area. A decrease in pain threshold compared to group (N) was demonstrated in all of the groups on the ipsilateral side (Fig. 1).

Treatment was initiated 1 day after the MIA injection and pain was assessed on the days 1, 3, 7, 10, 14 and 21. Paw withdrawal threshold significantly increased (indicating less pain) in the test group and the diclofenac gel group compared with vehicle and sham groups. The pain threshold specifically increased in group (P) after 10 days and in group (T) after 21 days compared to group (N) ($p < 0.05$) (Fig. 1).

Spontaneous locomotor activity

Total distance traveled in the arena during 10 min showed a significant effect after 7 days compared to group (N). Topical administration of diclofenac gel also

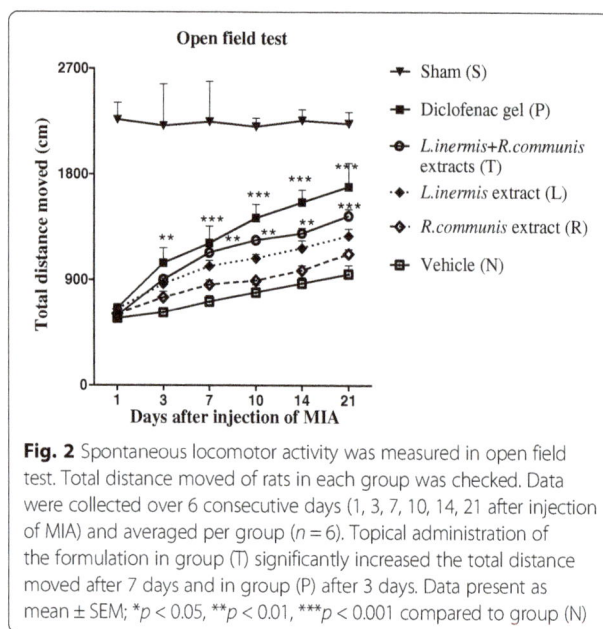

Fig. 2 Spontaneous locomotor activity was measured in open field test. Total distance moved of rats in each group was checked. Data were collected over 6 consecutive days (1, 3, 7, 10, 14, 21 after injection of MIA) and averaged per group (n = 6). Topical administration of the formulation in group (T) significantly increased the total distance moved after 7 days and in group (P) after 3 days. Data present as mean ± SEM; *$p < 0.05$, **$p < 0.01$, ***$p < 0.001$ compared to group (N)

significantly increased the total distance moved after 3 days (Fig. 2).

Footprint

Images of footprint patterns enabled the observation of abnormalities in the foot placing (Fig. 3). The rats in group MIA presented measurable foot placing for 21 days. These animals loaded their weight on the medial part of their affected foot. In group sham, no changes were developed. Significant changes were seen in group (T) and group (P) after 3 days compared to group (N). They were measured both in the affected and in the non affected hind legs (Fig. 4).

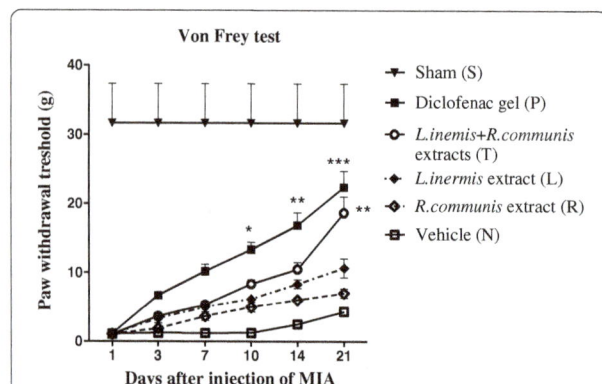

Fig. 1 Paw withdrawal threshold (PWT) was measured by von Frey monofilaments. At days 1, 3, 7, 10, 14, 21 after injection of MIA (n = 6), von Frey testing on the inflamed paw showed significant effect compared to group (N); after 21 days in test group (T) and after 10 days in positive control or group (P) of MIA injection. Data present mean ± SEM; *$p < 0.05$, **$p < 0.01$, ***$p < 0.001$ compared to group (N)

Fig. 3 Walking tracks

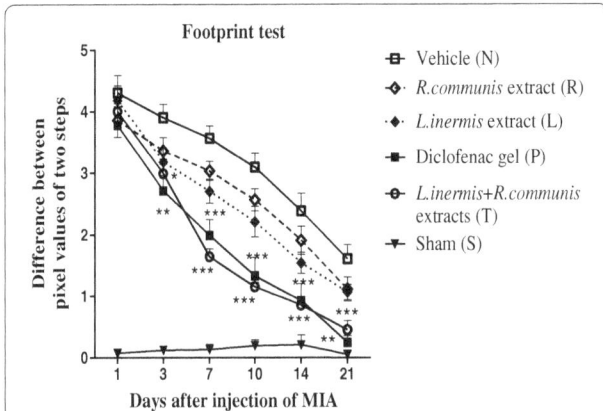

Fig. 4 MIA injection affected weight bearing of the paws during locomotion. Comparing the differences between pixel values of right and left hind paw tracks on the paper which obtained by image J software in different days. Significant reduction between pixel values of two steps were seen in group (T) and group (P) after 3 days compared to group (N). Data presented as mean ± SEM; *$p < 0.05$, **$p < 0.01$, ***$p < 0.001$ compared to group (N)

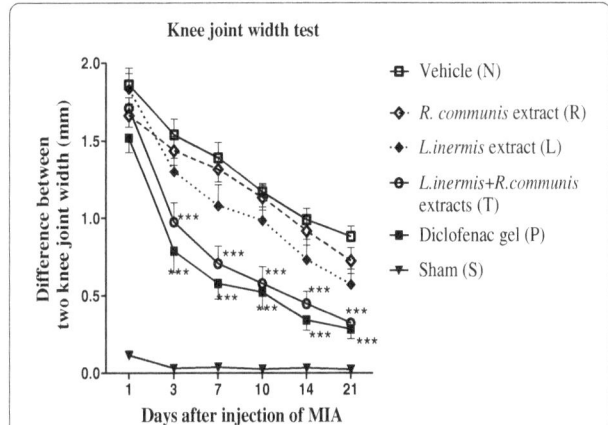

Fig. 6 Comparison the differences between the inflamed and right knee's joint width. The knee's joint width was measured by colis in different days 1, 3, 7, 10, 14, 21 for each group. Treatments were continued for 14 days. Compared to group (N), differences between two knee joint widths were significantly reduced in group (T) and group (P) after 3 days. Data are expressed as mean ± SEM; *$p < 0.05$, **$p < 0.01$, ***$p < 0.001$

Hotplate

As illustrated in Fig. 5, the Intra- articular injection into the left hind paw of the rats caused a reduction in the latency of the withdrawal response to heat stimulation compared to sham group (S). The latency values as compared to group (N), was increased after 10 days and in group (P) after 3 days compared to group (N) (Fig. 5).

Measuring paw diameter

In Fig. 6, Data of anti-inflammatory activity of the extracts in MIA induced paw edema are shown. The left paw diameter after different day s intervals was used as criteria for evaluation of inflammation. Generally, data indicated that the extracts possessed anti-inflammatory

activity compared to the vehicle group and it showed after 3 days significant effect as compared to group (N) can be seen and it was as the same as the effect of group (P) (Fig. 6).

Measuring paw volume

Chronic pain suffering rats were given daily topical administration of extracts, diclofenac and vehicle for 14 days. The volume of the left hind paw was measured with mercury column in different days. The effect was observed after 3 days as the same as diclofenac gel and the paw volume was reduced compared to the vehicle group (Fig. 7).

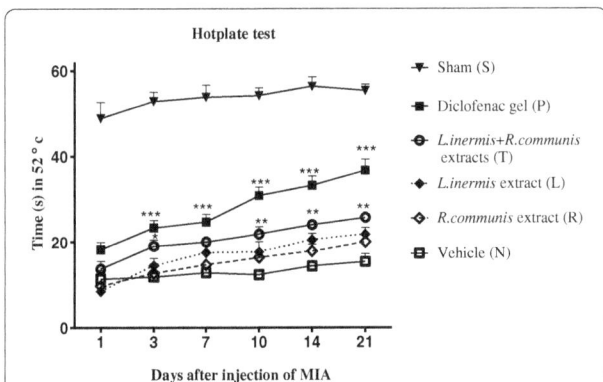

Fig. 5 The response latency time of the paws to heat stimulation in hotplate test. The response latency time of the paws was measured at 1, 3, 7, 10, 14, 21 days after injection MIA compared to group (N) in each group. The latency values were increased after 10 days in group (T) and after 3 days in group (P). Data are expressed as mean ± SEM; *$p < 0.05$, **$p < 0.01$, ***$p < 0.001$ compared to group (N)

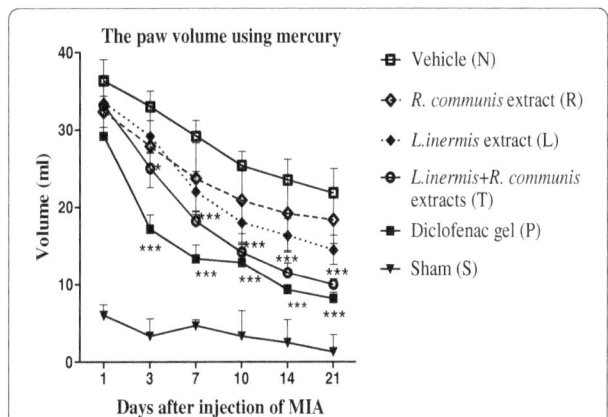

Fig. 7 The volume of the inflamed paw was measured with mercury coloumn in different days. The paw volume significantly reduced after 3 days in group (T) and group (P) compared to group (N). Data are showed as mean ± SEM of edema volume induced by MIA; *$p < 0.05$, **$p < 0.01$, ***$p < 0.001$ compared to group (N)

Topically using *L.inermis* (henna) extract on each paw was effective in reducing the OA pain and inflammation, compare to vehicle but p value was not less than the accepted level of significance ($p > 0.05$) therefore it did not achieve complete pain remission. Topically using *R. communis* was not effective as *L. inermis* and showed little antinociceptive and anti-inflammatory activities in pharmacological tests.

Histology

The results of the pathological findings and scoring of the lesions are depicted in Table 1. As seen in Table 1, the Sham group received saline and was euthanized 14 days later. The articular tissue structures including synovium, synovial tissue, adjacent ligaments, tendons and tendinal sheath and subcutaneous tissues and muscles had normal tissue architecture and were intact (score0) (Fig. 8).

Rats that received MIA and were euthanized 24 h later showed severe acute fibrinopurulent inflammatory reaction. Fibrinopurulent exudates were affected synovial tissues, ligaments, tendons, tendinal sheath, muscles and subcutaneous tissues (score 4) (Fig. 9).

In those groups treated by diclofenac gel group (P) or group (T) that received the mixture of the extracts remedy and euthanized 14 days later the same results were obtained. A very mild edema and presence of a few scattered lymphocytes were observed. Articular tissue structure, including synovium, ligament, tendons and subcutaneous tissue were histologically normal (score1) (Fig. 10).

In the vehicle group that only received MIA and euthanized 14 days later, chronic inflammatory reactions accompanied by tendinal adhesion were noticed. Formation of granulation tissue with neovascularization, edema, infiltration of mononuclear leucocytes including lymphocytes and adhesion of tendons to its tendinal sheath were observed (score 3) (Fig. 11).

According to the obtained data, topical use of the mixture extracts showed anti-inflammatory and analgesic effects on osteoarthritis induced by MIA.

Discussion

Previous studies have shown that lawsone, isoplumbagin and lawsaritol isolated from *Lawsonia inermis* exhibit anti-inflammatory and analgesic effects in rats [8, 31]. Besides, experiments showed that methanolic extract of *Ricinus communis* leaves, contain flavonoids: rutin, quercetin, epicatechin and polyphenols and gentisic acid have anti-inflammatory activity in rats when administered orally [12] but the topical usage of their combination has not yet been investigated.

Studies showed that intra- articular injection of MIA in rats produces chronic osteoarthritis pain, pharmacological tests were performed in the early (up to 1 week after MIA) versus late (between 2 and 4 weeks after MIA) phase of the rat MIA model [32]. In the present study, six time points 1, 3, 7, 10, 14 and 21 days were taken for determining pain and inflammation to see the effect of the formulation on both acute and chronic phases.

In this study mixture of *Lawsonia inermis* L. and *Ricinus communis* L. extracts were used as a topical medication to relief induced joint pain and diclofenac gel which has analgesic and anti-inflammatory effects and has been shown to be effective in the treatment of a variety of acute and chronic pains and inflammatory conditions such as osteoarthritis [33], was used as positive control.

The mixture of extracts showed analgesic effect by reducing mechanical allodynia measured by von Frey filaments increased from a baseline of 0.6 g to 26 g. Comparing the rats of group (N), the significant effect was seen in group (T) after 21 days and in group (P) after 10 days. The responses after day 10, 21 showed that the formulation affected the late inflammatory reactions to painful mechanical stimuli.

Table 1 Comparison of the histological effects of different groups and their scores

Groups	Pathological finding	Score
Sham or group (S)	The articular tissue structures including synovium, synovial tissue, adjacent ligaments, tendons and tendinal sheath and subcutaneous tissues and muscles had normal tissue architecture.	0
A day after injected MIA (Inflammation peak day)	Severe acute fibrinopurulent inflammatory reaction. Fibrinopurulent exudates were affected synovial tissues, ligaments, tendons, tendons sheath, muscles and subcutaneous tissues.	4 sharp
Diclofenac gel or group (P)	A very mild edema and presence of a few scattered lymphocytes. Articular tissue structure, including synovium, ligament, tendons, subcutaneous tissue were histologically normal	1
The mixture of extracts or group (T)	As the same as diclofenac.	1
No treatment or group (N)	Chronic inflammatory reactions accompanied by tendinal adhesion were noticed. Formation of granulation tissue with neo vascularization, edema, infiltration of mononuclear leucocytes including lymphocytes and adhesion of tendons to its tendinal sheath were observed.	3

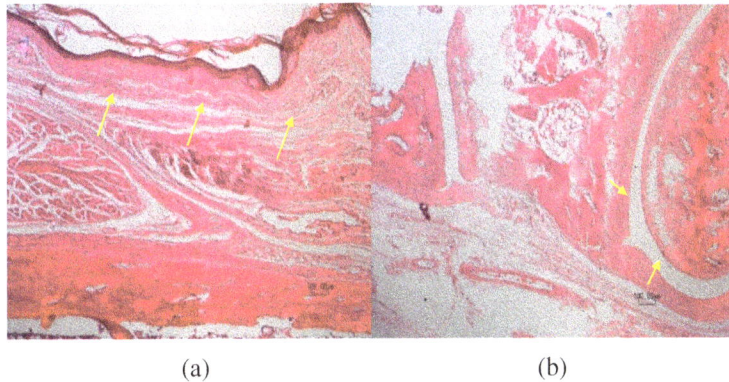

Fig. 8 A section of articular tissue from group (S) or sham. The H&E stained paraffin tissue sections of covering skin tissues (*large arrows*) and articular (*small arrows*) from saline injected group can be seen. The skin (**a**) and articular tissue (**b**) have normal tissue architecture. Scale bar = 100 μm (**a**,**b**)

We further examined the effects of the mixture using the hot-plate test. The present study has demonstrated the analgesic effect of topical mixture of extracts (0.2 g/0.3 ml) significantly increased the response latency time to heat stimulation after 10 days. This could be the possible explanation for its central analgesic activity observed in hotplate test.

We examined our hypothesis also by using the open field test to exclude false positives in nociceptive tests. The open field test is commonly used for pharmacological selection of drugs that act on the locomotor activities [19]. Rats treated with the mixture of extracts displayed significantly better locomotor recovery at the late stages of the treatment when compared to group (N) after 7 days of MIA injection.

We utilized the differential in weight bearing between the left (osteoarthritic) and right (contralateral control) limbs as an indication of joint discomfort by analysis the rat paw prints. The number and intensity of pixel values of left compared to contralateral paw decreased after 3 days of injection of MIA, same as in group (P).

The acute inflammatory response in the MIA model lasts approximately during the first weak, but afterward inflammation plays a minor role in pain and it is more likely caused by biomechanical forces affecting articular cartilage and subchondral bone [34].

The study showed that topical usage of the mixture of the extracts was useful in the treatment of the inflammation induced by MIA. The effect of reducing inflammation was initiated after 3 days. It showed that the formulation has an effect on acute inflammatory response same as diclofenac gel.

Gross morphological observations and histological evaluation of the knee joints were performed to evaluate the protective effect of the mixture of extracts on cartilage and articular tissue structures. The results of the pathological findings and scoring of the lesions showed that topical usage of the selected formula made

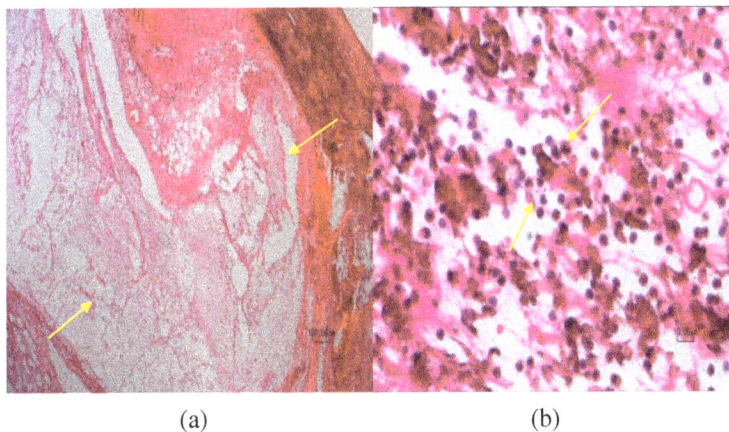

Fig. 9 Pathological findings one day after MIA injection. Severe fibrinopurulent exudates (*arrows*) can be seen within articular and adjacent tissues (**a**&**b**). Scale bar =100 μm (**a**), Scale bar =10 μm (**b**)

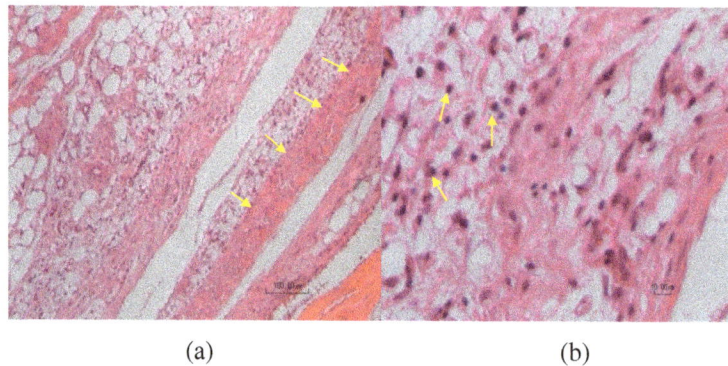

Fig. 10 A section of articular tissue from group (P). A very mild reaction including a few scattered lymphoid cells (*arrows*) can be seen. The same tissue reaction was seen in group (T). Scale bar =100 μm (left handed Fig.) and Scale bar =10 μm (right handed Fig.)

significant changes on the knee of the rats histologically. Compared to vehicle group, in which granulation, tissue formation, tendinal adhesion and mixed inflammatory cell infiltration were seen fourteen days after MIA administration, test and diclofenac groups showed only very mild reactions characterized by negligible edema and a few scattered inflammatory lymphoid cells.

According to the pharmacological responses of each herb extract, it could be concluded that the main effect of the formulation related to *L.inermis* extract efficacy.

Although because of the different active compounds in the extracts, the mechanism of action is unknown but the comparable effect on the inhibition of inflammation and pain compared to diclofenac makes the suggestion that they work through the same pathways.

In conclusion, the present study provided clues for further studies on pharmacological methods to analyze the anti-inflammatory and analgesic activities of topical drugs. The results demonstrated that topical preparation of *L.inermis* and *R.communis* was not only be able to mitigate pain and inflammation but also inhibit MIA-induced histological changes on the knee of the rats. Therefore, this formula could be a good candidate for further studies as a new efficient treatment in patients with osteoarthritis.

Conclusion

This study demonstrated that based on the different anti-inflammatory and analgesic evaluations, the pain and inflammation induced by intra-articular injection of MIA in rats were reduced with topical application of a mixture of *Lawsonia inermis* and *Ricinus communis* extracts. Further clinical studies are required to evaluate the safety and efficacy issues of the extracts mixture.

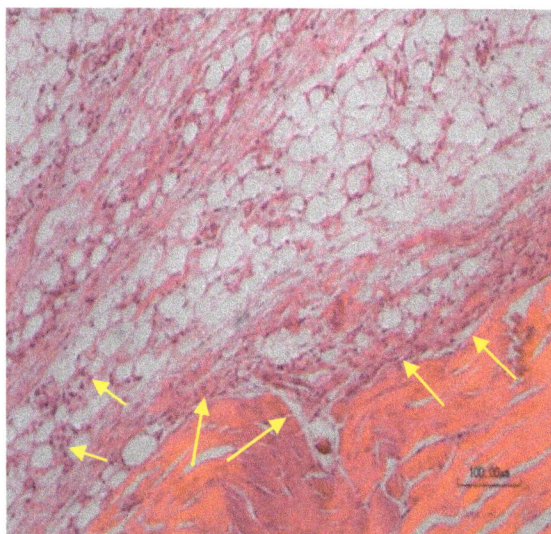

Fig. 11 A section of articular tissue from group (N). 14 days after MIA injection, a mixed inflammatory cell infiltration (*small arrows*) and tendinal adhesion to the adjacent tissue (*large arrows*) are evident. Scale bar =100 μm

Competing interests
The authors declare that they have no competing interests.

Authors' contributions
AZ, MF, MG and SS conceived and designed the experiments. AZ performed experimental procedures. MG produced all histological figures and datas. AZ, MF analyzed the data. MF, MG, AZ contributed materials/analysis tools. AZ, MF, SS and MG wrote the paper. All authors read and approved the final version of the manuscript.

Acknowledgements
This study was the result of a PhD thesis of Atousa Ziaei (no:141) and financial support was provided by a grant (N-128) from Department of Traditional Pharmacy, School of Traditional Medicine, Shahid Beheshti University of Medical Sciences, Tehran, Iran. The authors wish to thank the

Department of Pathology, Faculty of Veterinary Medicine, University of Tehran, for performing the histological tests and their technical assistance.

Author details
[1]Traditional Medicine and Material Medical Research Center; Department of Traditional Pharmacy, School of Traditional Medicine, Shahid Beheshti University of Medical Sciences, Tehran, Iran. [2]Department of Pathology, Faculty of Veterinary Medicine, University of Tehran, Tehran, Iran. [3]Department of Pharmacology and Toxicology, School of Pharmacy, Shahid Beheshti University of Medical Sciences, Tehran, Iran.

References

1. Kennedy DO, Wightman EL. Herbal extracts and phytochemicals: plant secondary metabolites and the enhancement of human brain function. Adv Nutr. 2011;2:32–50. doi:10.3945/an.110.000117.
2. Soares-Bezerra RJ, Calheiros AS, Da Silva Ferreira NC, Da Silva FV, Alves LA. Natural products as a source for new anti-inflammatory and analgesic compounds through the inhibition of purinergic p2x receptors. Pharmaceuticals. 2013;6:650–8.
3. Aghili Khorasani MH. Makhzanol Advieh. 1th ed. Research Institute for Islamic and Complementary Medicine, Iran University of Medical Sciences. Tehran, Iran: Bavardaran Press; 2001. p. 243–55.
4. Aghili Khorasani MH. Gharabadin Kabir. 2nd ed. Tehran: Tehran medical university; 2005. p. 899–901.
5. Tonkaboni MM (1699). Tohfeh al-momenin. In: Rahimi R, Ardekani MS. Farjadmand F, editors. Tehran: Shahid beheshti university of medical sciences; 2007. p.166
6. Guzman RE, Evans MG, Bove S, Morenko B, Kilgore K. Mono-iodoacetate-induced histologic changes in subchondral bone and articular cartilage of rat femorotibial joints: An animal model of osteoarthritis. Toxicol Pathol. 2003;31:619–24.
7. Neugebauer V, Han JS, Adwanikar H. Techniques for assessing knee joint pain in arthritis. Mol Pain. 2007;3:30–42.
8. Alia B, Bashir A. Anti-inflammatory, antipyretic and analgesic effects of Lawsonia inermis L. (henna) in rats. Pharmacol. 1995;51:356–63.
9. Nithya V. Anti-inflammatory activity of Lawsonia ulba Linn., in wistar albino rats. Asian J Sci Tech. 2011;4:001–3.
10. Chaudhary G, Goyal S, Poonia P. Lawsonia inermis Linnaeus: a phytopharmacological review. Int J Pharm Sci Drug Res. 2010;2:91–8.
11. Darmanin S, Wismayer PS, Camilleri Podesta MT, Micallef MJ, Buhagiar JA. An extract from Ricinus communis L. Leaves possesses cytotoxic properties and induces apoptosis in sk-mel-28 human melanoma cells. Nat Prod Res. 2009;23:561–71.
12. Nemudzivhadi V, Masoko P. In vitro assessment of cytotoxicity, antioxidant, and anti-inflammatory activities of Ricinus communis (Euphorbiaceae) leaf extracts. Evid Based Complement Alternat Med. 2014;2014:625961. doi:10.1155/2014/625961.
13. Sengupta S, Velpandian T, Kabir SR, Gupta SK. Analgesic efficacy and pharmacokinetics of topical nimesulide gel in healthy human volunteers: double-blind comparison with piroxicam, diclofenac and placebo. Eur J Clin Pharmacol. 1998;54:541–7.
14. Xu Q, Ming Z, Dart AM, Du XJ. Optimizing dosage of ketamine and xylazine in murine echo cardiography. Clin Exp Pharmacol Physiol. 2007;34:499–507.
15. Horváth A, Tékus V, Boros M, Pozsgai G, Botz B, Borbély E, Szolcsányi J. Transient receptor potential ankyrin 1 (TRPA1) receptor is involved in chronic arthritis: in vivo study using TRPA1-deficient mice. Arthritis Res Ther. 2016;18:6. doi:10.1186/s13075-015-0904-y.
16. Lee Y, Pai M, Brederson JD, Wilcox D, Hsieh G, Jarvis MF, Bitner RS. Monosodium iodoacetate-induced joint pain is associated with increased phosphorylation of mitogen activated protein kinases in the rat spinal cord. Mol Pain. 2011;7:39. doi:10.1186/1744-8069-7-39.
17. Bove SE, Calcaterra SL, Brooker RM, Huber CM, Guzman RE. Weight bearing as a measure of disease progression and efficacy of anti-inflammatory compounds in a model of monosodium iodoacetate-induced osteoarthritis. Osteoarthr Cartilage. 2003;11:821–30.
18. Schuelert N, McDougall JJ. Grading of monosodium iodoacetate-induced osteo- arthritis reveals a concentration-dependent sensitization of nociceptors in the knee joint of the rat. Neurosci Lett. 2009;465:184–8. doi:10.1016/j.neulet.2009.08.063.
19. Rainsford KD, Velo GP, editors. Side-effects of anti-inflammatory drugs, part two studies in major organ systems. Lancaster: MTP press limited; 1987. p. 114.
20. Beyreuther B, Callizot N, Stohr T. Antinociceptive efficacy of lacosamide in the monosodium iodoacetate rat model for osteoarthritis pain. Arthritis Res Ther. 2007;9:R14.
21. Archer J. Tests for emotionality in rats and mice: a review. Anim Behav. 1973;21:205–35. doi:10.1016/S0003-3472(73)80065-X.
22. Lacroix L, Broersen L, Weiner I, Feldon J. The effects of excitotoxic lesion of the medial prefrontal cortex on latent inhibition, prepulse inhibition, food hoarding, elevated plus maze, active avoidance and locomotor activity in the rat. Neurosci. 1998;84:431–42.
23. Dijkstra JR, Meek MF, Robinson PH, Gramsberge A. Methods to evaluate functional nerve recovery in adult rats: Walking track analysis, video analysis and the withdrawal reflex. J Neurosci Meth. 2000;96:89–96.
24. Hasler N, Klette R, Agnew W. In: Pariman D, North H, Mcneill S, editors. Footprint recognition of rodents and insects. New Zealand: Landcare Reasearch Ltd; 2004. p. 167–73.
25. South SM, Smith MT. Apparent insensitivity of the hotplate latency test for detection of antinociception following intraperitoneal, intravenous or intracerebroventricular M6G administration to rats. J Pharmacol Exp Ther. 2002;286:1326–32.
26. Hajarolasvadi N, Zamani MJ, Sarkhail P, Khorasani R, Mohajer M, Amin G, Shafiee A, Sharifzadeh M, Abdollahi M. Comparison of antinociceptive effects of total, water, ethyl acetate, Ether and N-Butanol extracts of Phlomis anisodonta boiss and indomethacin in mice. Int J Pharmacol. 2006;2:209–12.
27. Fereidoni M, Ahmadiani A, Semnanian S, Javan M. An accurate and simple method for measurement of paw edema. J Pharmacol Toxicol Methods. 2000;43:11–4.
28. Luna LG. Manual of histologic staining methods of the armed forces institute of pathology. 3rd ed. New York: The Blakiston Division, Mc Graw Hill Book Company; 1960. p. 8–9. 38–39.
29. Woong Park C, Wan Ma K, Woo Jang S, Son M, Joo KM. Comparison of Piroxicam Pharmacokinetics and anti-inflammatory effect in rats after Intra-articular and intramuscular administration. Biomol Ther (Seoul). 2014; 22:260–6. doi:10.4062/biomolther.2014.037.
30. B.McMahon S, Koltzenburg M, Tracey I, Turk D. Wall & Melzack's textbook of Pain. Sixth ed. Philadelphia, PA, USA: Elsevier/Churchill Livingstone; 2013.
31. Makhija IK, Dhananjaya DR, Kumar VS, Devkar R, Khamar D, Manglani N, Chandrakar S. Lawsonia inermis-from traditional use to scientific assessment. Afr J Pharm Sci Pharm. 2011;2:145–65.
32. Rashid MH, Theberge Y, Elmes SJ, Perkins MN, McIntosh F. Pharmacological validation of early and late phase of rat mono-iodoacetate model using the Tekscan system. Eur J Pain. 2013;17:210–22. doi:10.1002/j.1532-2149.2012.00176.x.
33. Eidman DS, Benedito MA, Leite JR. Daily changes in pentylenetetrazol-induced convulsions and open-field behavior in rats. Physiol Behav. 1990;47:853–6.
34. Kumari RR, More AS, Gupta G, Lingaraju MC, Balaganur V, Kumar P. Effect of alcoholic extract of Entada pursaetha DC on monosodium iodoacetate-induced osteoarthritis pain in rats. Indian J Med Res. 2015;141:454–62. doi:10.4103/0971-5916.159296.

16

Cost analysis of pharmaceutical care provided to HIV-infected patients: an ambispective controlled study

Renata Cavalcanti Carnevale[1], Caroline de Godoi Rezende Costa Molino[1], Marília Berlofa Visacri[1*], Priscila Gava Mazzola[1] and Patricia Moriel[1,2]

Abstract

Background: Studies have shown that pharmaceutical care can result in favorable clinical outcomes in human immunodeficiency virus (HIV)-infected patients, however, few studies have assessed the economic impact. The objective of this study was to evaluate the clinical and economic impact of pharmaceutical care of HIV-infected patients.

Methods: A controlled ambispective study was conducted in Brazil from January 2009 to June 2012. Patients were allocated to either intervention or control group. The control group was followed according to standard care while the intervention group was also followed by a pharmacist at each physician appointment for one year. Effectiveness outcomes included CD4+ count, viral load, absence of co-infections and optimal immune response, and economic outcomes included expenses of physician and pharmaceutical appointments, laboratory tests, procedures, and hospitalizations, at six months and one year.

Results: Intervention and control groups included 51 patients each. We observed significant decreases in total pharmacotherapy problems during the study. At six months, the intervention group contained higher percentages of patients without co-infections and of patients with CD4+ >500 cells/mm^3. None of the differences between intervention and control group considering clinical outcomes and costs were statistically significant. However, at one year, the intervention group showed higher percentage of better clinical outcomes and generated lower spending (not to procedures). An additional health care system daily investment of US$1.45, 1.09, 2.13, 4.35, 1.09, and 0.87 would be required for each additional outcome of viral load <50 copies/ml, absence of co-infection, CD4+ >200, 350, and 500 cells/mm^3, and optimal immune response, respectively.

Conclusion: This work demonstrated that pharmaceutical care of HIV-infected patients, for a one-year period, was able to decrease the number of pharmacotherapy problems. However, the clinical outcomes and the costs did not have statistical difference but showed higher percentage of better clinical outcomes and lower costs for some items.

Keywords: Pharmacoeconomics, Pharmaceutical care, HIV-infected patients

* Correspondence: mariberlofa@gmail.com
[1]Department of Clinical Pathology, Faculty of Medical Sciences (FCM), University of Campinas (UNICAMP), Alexander Fleming, 105, 13083-881 Campinas, SP, Brazil
Full list of author information is available at the end of the article

Introduction

Since 1996, Brazil has had a public health system program that provides free antiretroviral therapy, laboratory tests, and procedures to HIV-infected patients. This program has been internationally recognized as a major initiative against HIV [1]. However, this program alone does not guarantee safety and effectiveness of treatment because HIV treatment requires long-term therapy. Treatment of HIV includes a large number of drugs and drug interactions, and requires careful monitoring of therapy, with the goal of decreasing viral resistance and drug-related problems [1-3].

Studies have investigated the effects of pharmaceutical care on the rational use of drugs in HIV-infected patients [4-6]. March et al. demonstrated that HIV-infected patients followed by a clinical pharmacist show significant improvements in CD4+ levels and viral load and a decrease in toxic effects related to treatment [7]. This reduction in toxicity improves the quality of life and treatment adherence of the patients [8]. In addition, a systematic analysis (including data from January 1980 to June 2011) revealed that providing pharmaceutical care to HIV-infected patients was associated with statistically significant improvements in treatment adherence and had a positive impact on viral suppression [9].

Despite the variety of pharmaceutical care studies conducted with HIV-infected patients, remarkably few include an economic analysis. There is a need to go beyond the investigation of clinical outcomes generated by pharmaceutical care. Studies that include the economic impact of pharmaceutical care are necessary to justify the implementation or expansion of pharmaceutical care services [10].

In addition to the lack of economic studies on pharmaceutical care conducted with HIV-infected patients, another limitation is that, even though the studies available demonstrate that pharmaceutical care practice can contribute to the reductions of costs, they focus only on the costs associated with drugs, physician appointments, and hospitalizations. The available literature does not present studies regarding the impact of pharmaceutical care on the costs associated with laboratory tests and procedures [9,11-13]. Moreover, the majority of pharmacoeconomic studies present many methodological limitations, such as the lack of a control group and non-inclusion of costs associated with pharmacist appointments [14]. Thus, it has become imperative to conduct well-designed studies in the area of pharmaceutical care in order to obtain a clearer comprehension of its economic impact [14]. Well-designed studies investigating economic impact should be encouraged because they enable the rationalization of resources in health care, where the available resources are limited [15].

This study was designed to perform a pharmacoeconomic analysis of the impact of pharmaceutical care on HIV-infected patients over a one-year period by measuring both clinical and health care system economic outcomes.

Methods

This was a one-year, ambispective, controlled study, with a systematic sample by quota controls, paired according to random characteristics. A retrospective chart review and a prospective pharmaceutical care follow-up were conducted. The study was conducted at a hospital in the state of São Paulo, Brazil. The Hospital Ethics Committee approved the research, and informed consent was obtained from all patients.

The inclusion criteria for the study were as follows: outpatients diagnosed with HIV/AIDS (Human Immunodeficiency Virus/Acquired Immunodeficiency Syndrome), aged between 18 and 60 years, having body mass index (BMI) lower than 30 kg/m^2, and receiving antiretroviral therapy (ART). Obese patients were not included because they present higher incidences of hyperlipidemia, hypertension, and insulin resistance, and because some HIV/AIDS medications such as protease inhibitors can cause weight gain and fat accumulation, it would not be possible to determine whether the weight gain was related to the medication or to the background disease in such patients [16-19]. Patients who were unable to return for later appointments/exams, who refused to participate, who have psychiatric disease (that unable them to follow the medical appointments schedule and the pharmacist interventions), and those who were pregnant were excluded. Patients were enrolled in the study from January 2009 to June 2011 and were assigned in a 1:1 ratio to either intervention or control group by the clinical pharmacy team. Control group patients were matched to intervention group patients according to gender and baseline CD4+ count.

For one year, the intervention group was followed by the clinical pharmacy staff, composed of two pharmacists trained by the hospital clinical pharmacy team regarding HIV/AIDS and pharmaceutical care, after routine medical appointments at the hospital, using a method developed and adapted to the reality of the hospital, based on the Pharmacist's Workup of Drug Therapy (PWDT) method [20]. The control group was not followed by the clinical pharmacy team, and its data were collected through review of medical charts encompassing the same period.

Initial and final pharmacotherapy problems were accounted for and classified as necessity, effectiveness, safety, or therapy compliance pharmacotherapy problems only for the intervention group [21]. The clinical pharmacy team performed written and verbal pharmacist interventions with the intervention group, which were accounted for and classified as pharmacist-patient or pharmacist-physician interventions and as resolutive pharmacotherapy problems, preventive pharmacotherapy problems, quality of life, or referral to other medical specialties interventions. The classifications used for pharmacotherapy problems and pharmacist interventions are in accordance with those used in another publication by the authors [22].

The five effectiveness outcomes were as follows: CD4+ count higher than 200 cells/mm^3, 350 cells/mm^3, and 500 cells/mm^3; viral load lower than 50 copies/ml; and absence of co-infections. The co-infections considered by the study were as follows: bacterial co-infections (urinary infection, shigellosis, infected sebaceous cysts, cellulitis, pneumonia, and hordeolums), viral co-infections (cytomegalovirus, influenza, *Herpes zoster*, *Herpes simplex*, human papillomavirus, viral conjunctivitis, and warts), parasitic co-infection (microsporidiosis, isosporiasis, coccidiosis, and neurocryptococcosis), and fungal co-infections (oral moniliasis, onychomycosis, and tinea pedis). Effectiveness outcomes were measured at six months and one year of study and were obtained through medical chart review for both groups. Additionally, using a decision tree model, we established the number of patients from both groups that achieved, after one year of study, an optimal immune response as characterized by viral load <50 copies/ml, absence of co-infection, and CD4+>500 cells/mm^3.

For cost analysis, we identified the number of appointments (medical/nursing/nutrition/physical therapy/speech therapy/dental), laboratory tests, procedures, and hospitalizations per patient in the first six months, the last six months, and in one year, for both groups, through review of their medical charts. For the intervention group, we also included the cost of the pharmacist appointment. The DATASUS database [23] provided the monetary values for all these items. Values were quoted in US dollars ($).

Cost analysis was performed for the one-year period, considering both the effectiveness and the costs of appointments, laboratory tests, procedures, hospitalizations, total cost, and total cost without procedures.

Statistical analysis of the results was performed by SAS System for Windows (Statistical Analysis System, version 9.2). For baseline characteristics analysis, chi-square, Fisher's exact, and Mann–Whitney tests were performed. For co-infection, CD4+ and viral load analysis and generalized estimating tests were performed. For costs analysis, ANOVA for repeated measures, with a transformation by positions, was performed. The significance level was set at 5% (P ≤0.050).

Results

The study screened 140 HIV-infected patients being treated at the hospital on an outpatient basis. Thirty-eight patients were excluded: two were pregnant; nine interrupted the treatment at the hospital; eight were transferred from the hospital; and nineteen had not returned for the second pharmaceutical appointment in the first six months of the study (Figure 1). Finally, 51 patients each were allocated to intervention and control groups. A medical chart review provided the demographic data and initial information for both study groups (Table 1). The two study groups had similar baseline characteristics, indicating homogeneity.

There were a total of 230 pharmaceutical appointments (143 in the initial six months and 87 in the final six months). During these appointments, 219 pharmacist interventions were performed. Among them, 185 (84.5%) were pharmacist-patient interventions and 34 (15.5%) were pharmacist-physician interventions; 116 (53.0%) were preventive interventions, 55 (25.1%) were resolutive interventions, 42 (19.2%) were quality of life interventions, and six (2.7%) were referral to other medical specialties

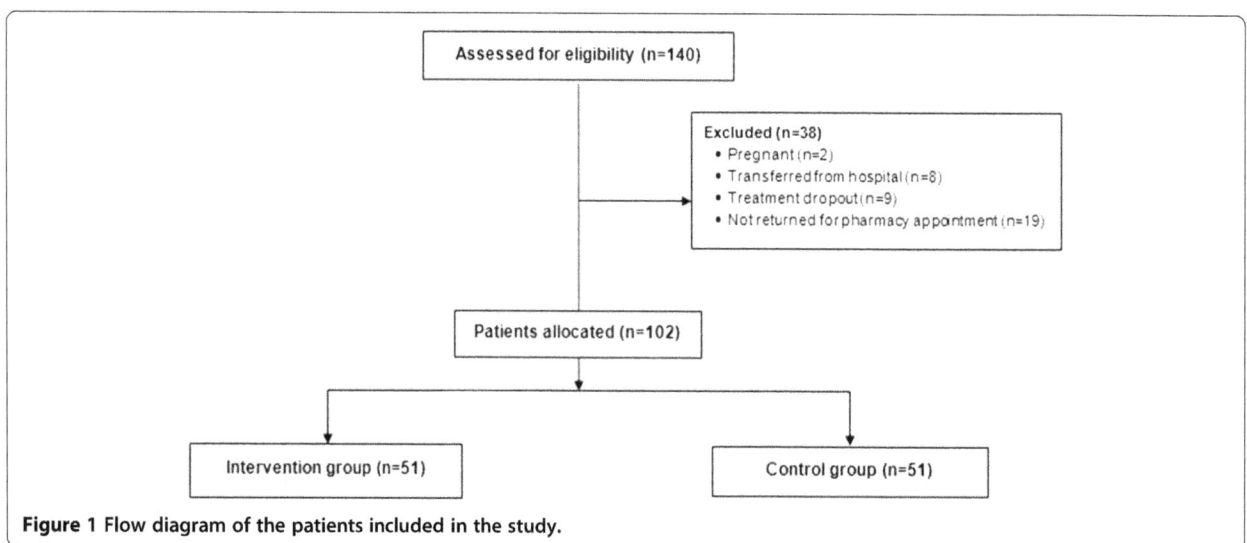

Figure 1 Flow diagram of the patients included in the study.

Table 1 Baseline characteristics of intervention group and control group

Characteristics	Control group N=51	Intervention group N=51	P value
Age (Mean [SD], years)	40.5 [9.2]	41.3 [8.8]	0.580[a]
Men - % (n)	66.7 (34)	66.7 (34)	1.000[b]
Ethnicity - % (n)			0.830[b]
Caucasian	70.6 (36)	68.6 (35)	
Black/ african descent	29.4 (15)	31.4 (16)	
HIV Diagnosis(Mean [SD], years)	7.5 [5.6]	8.3 [6.4]	0.690[a]
HIV Treatment Duration (Mean [SD], years)	5.7 [4.2]	6.5 [5.5]	0.780[a]
Number of tablets/day (Mean [SD])	9.3 [4.4]	10.1 [4.2]	0.250[a]
ART changes during the first 4 weeks of the study - % (n)	9.8 (5)	7.8 (4)	1.000[c]
CD4 + (Mean [SD], cells/mm^3)	304.0 [277.1]	310.4 [302.0]	0.980[a]
CD4 + >200 cells/mm^3 % (n)	56.9 (29)	54.9 (28)	0.840[b]
CD4 + >350 cells/mm^3 % (n)	31.4 (16)	33.3 (17)	0.830[b]
CD4 + >500 cells/mm^3 % (n)	15.7 (8)	17.7 (9)	0.800[b]
Viral load <50 copies/ml % (n)	60.8 (31)	64.8 (33)	0.190[b]
Number of Comorbidities (Mean [SD])	2.5 [1.6]	2.8 [2.1]	0.730[a]
Type of comorbidities % (n)			
Hepatitis C	23.5 (12)	21.6 (11)	0.630[b]
Tobaccoism	15.8 (8)	11.8 (6)	0.570[b]
Neurotoxoplasmosis	9.8 (5)	9.8 (5)	0.510[b]
Hypertriglyceridemia	3.9 (2)	9.8 (5)	0.440[c]
Pulmonary tuberculosis	13.7 (7)	3.9 (2)	0.160[c]
ART regimen % (n)			0.800[b]
TDF+3TC+EFV	17.6 (9)	21.6 (11)	
AZT+3TC+EFV	15.7 (8)	21.6 (11)	
AZT+3TC+LPV/r	9.8 (5)	7.8 (4)	
TDF+3TC+LPV/r	11.8 (6)	11.8 (6)	
Others	45.1 (23)	37.2 (19)	
Substance abuse % (n)			0.418[b]
Alcohol	19.6 (10)	29.4 (15)	
Tobacco	27.4 (14)	33.3 (17)	
Illicit drugs	13.73 (7)	7.8 (4)	

Note: [a]Mann-Whitney test; [b]Chi-square test; [c]Fisher's exact test.
Abbreviations: ART, antiretroviral therapy; AZT, zidovudine; CD4+, lymphocyte T CD4+; EFV, efavirenz; LPV/r, lopinavir/ritonavir; n, absolute number of patients; SD, standard deviation; TDF, tenofovir; 3TC, lamivudine.

interventions. We also observed significant decreases in total pharmacotherapy problems (from 248 to 145; 41.5%, P <0.001), necessity problems (from 55 to 26; 52.7%, P <0.001), and safety problems (from 161 to 96; 40.4%, P <0.001). A decrease in the other pharmacotherapy problems was also detected; however, it was not statistically

significant: effectiveness problems (from 12 to 11; 8.4%, P =1.0000) and compliance problems (from 20 to 12; 40.0%, P =0.760).

Regarding clinical outcomes, in the initial six months, the intervention group contained higher percentages of patients without co-infections and of patients with CD4+ >500 cells/mm^3. At one year, the intervention group showed higher percentage of better clinical outcomes: absence of co-infection, viral load <50 copies/ml, CD4+ >200 cells/mm^3, CD4+ >350 cells/mm^3, and CD4+ >500 cells/mm^3 (Table 2). However, none of these differences was statistically significant. In addition, by using the decision tree model to establish the number of patients from each study group that achieved an optimal immune response (Figure 2), it was possible to infer that pharmaceutical care improves a patient's immune response.

At six months, the intervention group presented with two bacterial, five viral, and two fungal co-infections and, at one year, presented with two bacterial, one viral, two parasitic, and one fungal co-infections. At six months, the control group presented with five bacterial, three viral, two parasitic, and one fungal co-infections, and at one year, presented with one bacterial, five viral, and three parasitic co-infections.

At one year of study, the intervention group spent less per day on appointments, laboratory tests, and hospitalizations, but spent more on procedures and in total than the control group. Moreover, only the intervention group spent on pharmaceutical appointments. Compared with the control group, the intervention group annually generated savings per patient of $3.20 associated with appointments, $23.19 with laboratory tests, and $5.94 with hospitalizations. The intervention group also generated additional annual costs per patient of $50.60 associated with procedures, $12.88 with pharmaceutical appointments, and $31.13 with total costs (Table 3). However, the difference in costs between the groups was not statistically significant. The stark contrast in the costs associated with procedures was caused by two hip surgeries performed on patients from the intervention group, which together added $1,916.09 to the total expenses. This amount corresponds to 48.0% of the total spent on procedures in the first six months of the study ($3,991.04). Excluding the costs of these procedures from the total costs, the results demonstrate that compared with the control group, the intervention group would have spent $19.40 less per patient per year (Table 3).

Cost analysis identified the additional costs associated with procedures and total costs required to achieve each of the clinical outcomes outlined in the study (Table 4). Moreover, we found that, for each $1.00 spent on pharmaceutical care, there was a loss of $1.42 per day. However, when the costs associated with procedures were excluded

Table 2 Co-infection, viral load and CD4+ at baseline, 6 months, and at one year of study

	Control Group N=51			Intervention Group N=51			P value[a]
	Basal % (n)	6 months % (n)	1 year % (n)	Basal % (n)	6 months % (n)	1 year % (n)	
Absence of co-infection	/	72.6 (37)	56.9 (29)	/	76.5 (39)	64.7 (33)	0.092
Viral load <50 copies/ml	60.8 (31)	76.5 (39)	68.6 (35)	64.8 (33)	58.8 (30)	74.5 (38)	0.869
CD4+>200 cells/mm^3	56.9 (29)	68.6 (35)	74.5 (38)	54.9 (28)	70.8 (34)	78.4 (40)	0.793
CD4+>350 cells/mm^3	31.4 (16)	37.3 (19)	49.0 (25)	33.3 (17)	37.5 (18)	51.0 (26)	0.977
CD4+>500 cells/mm^3	15.7 (8)	17.7 (9)	19.6 (10)	17.7 (9)	20.8 (10)	27.5 (14)	0.599

Note: [a]Statistical significance value - Generalized estimating equations (GEE) test.
Abbreviation: CD4+, lymphocyte T CD4+.

from final costs, for each $1.00 spent on pharmaceutical care, there was a benefit of $2.51 per day. No relationship could be identified between the total daily costs generated by the patients and the reductions of pharmacotherapy problems (P =0.292; correlation R =0.15039; Spearman correlation coefficient test), or between the total costs and the number of pharmacist interventions (P =0.706; correlation R = −0.05412; Spearman correlation coefficient test).

Discussion

Pharmaceutical interventions were mostly of the pharmacist-patient type, which prevented therapy compliance errors (i.e., the patients needed clarifications regarding the use of medication, especially regarding dosage, drug interactions, and adherence). This type of intervention can help increase patient adherence to therapy. Hirsch et al. demonstrated in a cohort study with 2,234 patients that patients undergoing pharmaceutical care had greater adherence to antiretroviral therapy than patients not undergoing pharmaceutical care [6].

The decreases observed for all pharmacotherapy problem types are consistent with the literature. Studies have shown that pharmacist interventions can effectively identify, prevent, and solve pharmacotherapeutic problems [24,25]. Problems relating to safety were the most frequently encountered in our study. Other researchers have also identified a high frequency of issues related to inappropriate dosage and safety [5,26-29]. Carcelero et al. demonstrated that the most frequent issues with hospitalized HIV-infected patients are caused by combinations of contraindicated or not recommended drugs and by dosage errors, which happen in approximately one in five patients [5].

During one year of study, compared to the control group, the intervention group showed higher percentage of clinical outcomes, however there was no statistical difference. The better clinical response is associated with slower disease progression and a lower risk of complications, opportunistic infections, and co-infections [1,30-32]. We speculate that owing to these better clinical outcomes, the intervention group needed less hospitalization, laboratory tests, and medical appointments than the control group did.

Even though the difference in costs between the groups was not statistically significant, we can expect to see an overall, long-term cost analysis for the intervention group due its better clinical outcomes than the control group.

The lower costs associated with appointments and hospitalizations generated by the intervention group, compared with those of the control group, are consistent with the literature. Horberg et al. [13] and McPherson-Baker et al. [33] showed that the pharmacist's presence may decrease the number of appointments and, therefore, the costs for HIV-infected patients. A systematic review that included 32 articles pertaining to the impact of pharmaceutical care on HIV-infected patients showed that pharmaceutical care is associated with cost savings because it decreases the number of physician appointments, hospitalizations, and emergency visits [9]. A study in China found that total hospitalization costs in a group undergoing pharmaceutical care were significantly lower than those in a control group ($1,442.3 [684.9] vs. $1,729.6 [773.7], P <0.001) [34]. Furthermore, a Taiwanese study showed that the replacement of intravenous levofloxacin with its oral form, performed by a pharmacist, decreased hospital stays from 27.2 to 16.1 days (P =0.001), thereby lowering hospital costs [35]. Nevertheless, we found no studies in the literature that described the impact that pharmaceutical care has on the costs associated with laboratory tests and procedures.

In this study, an economic analysis that correlates the effectiveness and the costs of pharmacotherapy demonstrated that pharmaceutical care is dominant (less expensive and more effective), when we consider the effectiveness outcomes and the costs associated with appointments, laboratory tests, and hospitalizations. However, the intervention group generated higher costs associated with procedures and total costs than those of the control group. Furthermore, this study demonstrates

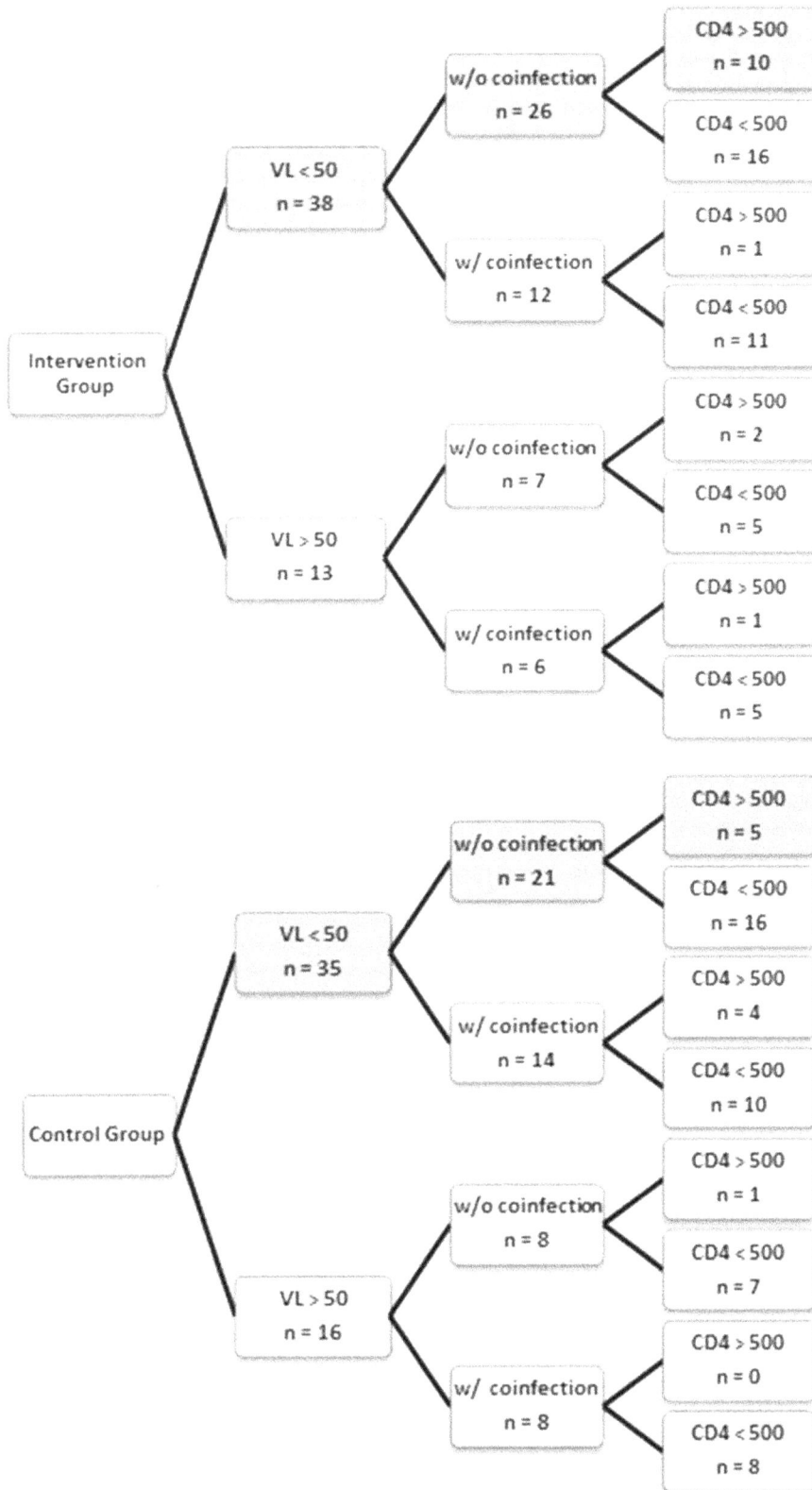

Figure 2 Optimal response immune for control and intervention groups. Abbreviation: CD4, CD4+ lymphocites; VL, viral load; w/o, without; w/, with.

Table 3 Study length of time and total daily costs (US$) for control and intervention groups

	Control Group N=51			Intervention Group N=51		
Study period	**6 m (i)**	**6 m (f)**	**Final**	**6 m (i)**	**6 m (f)**	**Final**
Length of time (mean [SD], days)	180.2[41.8]	190.5[6.4]	370.7[41.3]	196.8[29.3]	190.2[56.4]	387.0[39.8][a]
Appointments						
Total cost (US$) /day	8.65	6.49	**7.53**	8.01	6.12	**7.08**
Individual mean [SD] (US$)	0.17[0.08]	0.13[0.09]	**0.15[0.07]**	0.16[0.09]	0.12[0.08]	**0.14[0.07]**
Laboratory tests						
Total cost (US$) /day	38.07	25.35	**31.48**	33.33	22.96	**28.24**
Individual mean [SD] (US$)	0.75[0.74]	0.50[0.46]	**0.62[0.43]**	0.65[0.61]	0.45[0.43]	**0.55[0.44]**
Procedures						
Total cost (US$) /day	3.75	4.81	**4.29**	20.28	2.11	**11.36**
Individual mean [SD] (US$)	0.07[0.22]	0.09[0.21]	**0.08[0.17]**	0.40[1.11]	0.04[0.09]	**0.22[0.57]**
Hospitalization						
Total cost (US$) /day	2.62	2.53	**2.57**	2.30	1.17	**1.74**
Individual mean [SD] (US$)	0.05[0.30]	0.05[0.18]	**0.05[0.17]**	0.05[0.13]	0.02[0.10]	**0.03[0.09]**
Pharmacist						
Total cost (US$) /day	0.0	0.0	**0.0**	2.20	1.39	**1.80**
Individual mean [SD] (US$)	NA	NA	**NA**	0.05[0.02]	0.03[0.02]	**0.04[0.02]**
Total						
Final cost/day (US$)	53.09	39.18	**45.88**	66.13	33.74	**50.23**
Individual mean [SD] (US$)	1.04[0.99]	0.77[0.70]	**0.90[0.60]**	1.30[1.33]	0.66[0.55]	**1.00[0.81]**
Total excluding procedures						
Final cost/day (US$)	49.34	34.36	**41.58**	45.84	31.63	**38.87**
Individual mean [SD] (US$)	0.97[0.94]	0.67[0.63]	**0.82[0.56]**	0.90[0.71]	0.62[0.05]	**0.77[0.53]**

Note: [a] ANOVA results for repeated measures with a transformation by positions (P=0.057).
Abbreviations: 6m (i), initial 6 months; 6m (f), final 6 months; SD, Standard deviation.
Obs. The cost is the sum of the daily costs for all patients.

the importance of considering the costs associated with procedures. Here, if costs of procedures were disregarded when calculating the daily costs, the total costs of the intervention group would have been lower than those of the control group.

Table 4 Incremental Cost Effectiveness Ratio analysis per day for procedures and total costs (US$)

For each additional outcome of:	ICER (US $/day)	ICER (US$/day)
	Procedures	Total Cost (with procedures)
Viral load <50 copies/ml	2.36	1.45
Absence of co-infection	1.77	1.09
CD4+>200 cells/mm^3	3.53	2.18
CD4+>350 cells/mm^3	7.07	4.35
CD4+>500 cells/mm^3	1.77	1.09
Optimal immune response	1.41	0.87

Abbreviation: ICER, Incremental Cost Effectiveness Ratio.

Cost analysis identified a negative relationship when considering total cost, which contradicts the literature. According to Brennan et al., a $1.00 investment in pharmaceutical care showed a $3.00 return [36]. A meta-analysis demonstrated that 85% of the studies describe positive economic impacts of pharmaceutical care and concluded that the median benefit:cost ratio was 4.68:1 [10]. However, it should be noted that costs associated with laboratory tests and procedures were not included in these studies. In our study, by disregarding the procedures cost, the relationship becomes positive (2.51:1). Inclusion of costs associated with laboratory tests and procedures explains why this study showed different results than the results from the literature, and these differences clarify the need for well-designed studies that include the costs associated with procedures and laboratory tests, for a better understanding of the relationships among pharmaceutical care, HIV-infected patients, and the economy.

Limitations

This study has some limitations. There was no randomization of patients; the pharmacy staff was not blinded; pharmacotherapy problems were not verified for the control group (it was considered unethical to identify pharmacotherapy problems without providing any intervention); and the biggest limitation was our inability to retrieve the costs associated with the use of drugs, due to lack of information in the patient's medical charts. Several studies have analyzed the costs associated with the use of drugs [9,11-13,37] because they make a significant contribution to health care costs, especially in the context of hospital care, which represents 15%–25% of total health care costs. In a study conducted at the Maine Medical Center to guide the use of antibiotics, the pharmacist performed 74 interventions, which reduced the costs associated with antibiotics use, especially by replacing parenteral with oral formulations, generating savings of approximately $400.00 per patient and decreasing the length of hospital stay [38]. Therefore, with more comprehensive patient data, important additional savings regarding the use of drugs to treat co-infections could have been verified, since the intervention group had fewer co-infections than the control group did. For example, tuberculosis is common co-infection among HIV-infected patients and its treatment consists of a combination of rifampicin, isoniazid, and pyrazinamide [32], generating a cost of $316.56 per patient [39].

Conclusion

Our study presents important information about the impact that pharmaceutical care of HIV-infected patients can have on costs associated with procedure and laboratory tests. This information could not be found elsewhere in the literature, which indicates the need for well-designed and more complete studies.

This work demonstrated that pharmaceutical care of HIV-infected patients, for a one-year period, was able to decrease the number of pharmacotherapy problems. In addition, the intervention group presented higher percentage of better clinical outcomes and lower costs associated with appointments, laboratory tests, and hospitalizations than control group, however, there was no statistical difference; and, conversely, higher total costs and costs associated with procedures than those of the control group (no statistical significance). Additional pharmacoeconomic studies focused on pharmaceutical care are necessary to achieve a more comprehensive and reliable analysis.

Competing interests
The authors declare that they have no competing interests.

Authors' contributions
RCC, CGRCM, PGM and PM were responsible for concept and design. RCC and CGRCM collected data. RCC, CGRCM, PGM and PM interpreted data. RCC,

MBV and PM were involved in the writing of manuscript. MBV and PM revised the manuscript. All authors read and approved the final manuscript.

Acknowledgments
The researchers would like to thank the hospital medical staff for their support and collaboration during the research, and Coordination for the Improvement of Higher Level Personnel (CAPES) and State of São Paulo Research Foundation (FAPESP) for financial support.

Author details
[1]Department of Clinical Pathology, Faculty of Medical Sciences (FCM), University of Campinas (UNICAMP), Alexander Fleming, 105, 13083-881 Campinas, SP, Brazil. [2]Faculty of Pharmaceutical Sciences (FCF), University of Campinas (UNICAMP), Sérgio Buarque de Holanda, 25, 13083-859 Campinas, SP, Brazil.

References
1. Brazil, Ministry of Health, Secretária de Vigilância em Saúde, Programa Nacional de DST e Aids: Recomendações para Terapia Anti–retroviral em Adultos Infectados pelo HIV 2008 [http://www.ensp.fiocruz.br/portal-ensp/judicializacao/pdfs/491.pdf]
2. Dipiro J, Talbert R, Yees G, Matzke G, Wells B, Posey L: Pharmacotherapy: A Pathophysiologic Approach. 6th edition. Rio de Janeiro: Mcgraw Hill Companie; 2007.
3. Okie S: Fighting HIV-Lessons from Brazil. N Engl J Med 2006, 354:1977–1981.
4. Ma A, Chen DM, Chau FM, Saberi P: Improving adherence and clinical outcomes through an HIV pharmacist's interventions. AIDS Care 2010, 22:1189–1194.
5. Carcelero E, Tuset M, Martin M, De Lazzari E, Codina C, Miró J, Gatell J: Evaluation of antiretroviral-related errors and interventions by the clinical pharmacist in hospitalized HIV-infected patients. HIV Med 2011, 12:494–499.
6. Hirsch J, Gonzales M, Rosenquist A, Miller T, Gilmer T, Best B: Antiretroviral therapy adherence, medication use, and health care costs during 3 years of a community pharmacy medication therapy management program for Medi-Cal beneficiaries with HIV/AIDS. J Manag Care Pharm 2011, 17:213–223.
7. March K, Mak MM, Louie SG: Effects of pharmacists' interventions on patient outcomes in an HIV primary care clinic. Am J Heal Syst Pharm 2007, 64:2574–2578.
8. Mocroft A, Youle M, Moore A, Sabin CA, Madge S, Lepri AC, Tyrer M, Chaloner C, Wilson D, Loveday C, Johnson MA, Phillips AN: Reasons for modification and discontinuation of antiretrovirals: results from a single treatment centre. AIDS 2001, 15:185–194.
9. Saberi P, Dong BJ, Johnson MO, Greenblatt RM, Cocohoba JM: The impact of HIV clinical pharmacists on HIV treatment outcomes: a systematic review. Patient Prefer Adherence 2012, 6:297–322.
10. Schumock GT, Butler MG, Meek PD, Vermeulen LC, Arondekar BV, Bauman JL: Evidence of the economic benefit of clinical pharmacy services: 1996–2000. Pharmacotherapy 2003, 23:113–132.
11. Bozek PS, Perdue BE, Bar-Din M, Weidle PJ: Effect of pharmacist interventions on medication use and cost in hospitalized patients with or without HIV infection. Am J Health Syst Pharm 1998, 55:1151–1155.
12. Engles-Horton LL, Skowronski C, Mostashari F, Altice FL: Clinical guidelines and pharmacist intervention program for HIV-infected patients requiring granulocyte colony-stimulating factor therapy. Pharmacotherapy 1999, 19:356–362.
13. Horberg M, Hurley L, Silverberg M, Kinsman C, Quesenberry C: Effect of clinical pharmacists on utilization of and clinical response to antiretroviral therapy. J Acquir Immune Defic Syndr 2007, 44:531–539.
14. De Rijdt T, Willems L, Simoens S: Economic effects of clinical pharmacy interventions: a literature review. Am J Health Syst Pharm 2008, 65:1161–1172.
15. Areda CA, Bonizio RC, Freitas O: Pharmacoeconomy : an indispensable tool for the rationalization of health costs. Braz J Pharm Sci 2011, 47:231–240.

16. Bavinger C, Bendavid E, Niehaus K, Olshen RA, Olkin I, Sundaram V, Wein N, Holodniy M, Hou N, Owens DK, Desai M: Risk of cardiovascular disease from antiretroviral therapy for HIV : a systematic review. *PLoS One* 2013, 8:e59551.

17. Dube MP: Disorders of glucose metabolism in patients infected with human immunodeficiency virus. *Clin Infect Dis* 2000, 31:1467–1475.

18. Friis-Møller N, Sabin CA, Data Collection on Adverse Events of Anti-HIV Drugs (DAD) Study Group, Weber R, D'Arminio Monforte A, El-Sadr WM, Reiss P, Thiébaut R, Morfeldt L, De Wit S, Pradier C, Calvo G, Law MG, Kirk O, Phillips AN, Lundgren JD: Combination antiretroviral therapy and the risk of myocardial infarction. *N Engl J Med* 2003, 349:1993–2003.

19. Crum-Cianflone N, Roediger MP, Eberly L, Headd M, Marconi V, Ganesan A, Weintrob A, Barthel RV, Fraser S, Infectious Disease Clinical Research Program HIV Working Group, Agan BK: Increasing rates of obesity among HIV-infected persons during the HIV epidemic. *PLoS One* 2010, 5:e10106.

20. Strand LM, Cipolle RJ, Morley PC: Documenting the clinical pharmacists activities: back to basics. *Drug Intell Clin Pharm* 1988, 22:63–67.

21. University of Minnesota College of Pharmacy. Pharmacy workup notes [http://www.pharmacy.umn.edu/medmanagenotes/]

22. Molino CGRC, Carnevale RC, Rodrigues AT, Visacri MB, Moriel P, Mazzola PG: Impact of pharmacist interventions on drug-related problems and laboratory markers in outpatients with human immunodeficiency virus infection. *Ther Clin Risk Manag* 2014, 10:631–639.

23. DATASUS: SGTAP - Sistema de Gerenciamento da Tabela de Procedimentos, Medicamentos e OPM do SUS [http://sigtap.datasus.gov.br/tabela-unificada/app/sec/inicio.jsp].

24. Ruiz I, Olry A, López MA, Prada JL, Causse M: Prospective, randomized, two-arm controlled study to evaluate two interventions to improve adherence to antiretroviral therapy in Spain. *Enferm Infecc Microbiol Clin* 2010, 28:409–415.

25. Martin S, Wolters P, Calabrese S, Toledo-Tamula MA, Wood LV, Roby G, Elliott-DeSorbo DK: The antiretroviral regimen complexity index. A novel method of quantifying regimen complexity. *J Acquir Immune Defic Syndr* 2007, 45:535–544.

26. Mok S, Minson Q: Drug-related problems in hospitalized patients with HIV infection. *Am J Health Syst Pharm* 2008, 65:55–59.

27. Rastegar D, Knight A, Monolakis J: Antiretroviral medication errors among hospitalized patients with HIV infection. *Clin Infect Dis* 2006, 43:933–938.

28. Pastakia S, Corbett A, Raasch R, Napravnik S, Correll T: Frequency of HIV-related medication errors and associated risk factors in hospitalized patients. *Ann Pharmacother* 2008, 42:491–497.

29. Misson J, Clark W, Kendall M: Therapeutic advances: protease inhibitors for the treatment of HIV-1 infection. *J Clin Pharm Ther* 1997, 22:109–117.

30. Osterberg L, Blaschke T: Adherence to medication. *N Engl J Med* 2005, 353:487–497.

31. Langford SE, Ananworanich J, Cooper DA: Predictors of disease progression in HIV infection : a review. *Aids Res Ther* 2007, 4:1–14.

32. Brazil, Ministry of Health, Secretaria de Vigilancia em Saúde, Departamento de DST Aids e Hepatites Virais: Boletim Epidemiológico - AIDS e DST. 2012 [http://www.aids.gov.br/sites/default/files/anexos/publicacao/2011/50652/boletim_aids_2011_final_m_pdf_26659.pdf]

33. McPherson-Baker S, Malow RM, Penedo F, Jones DL, Schneiderman N, Klimas NG: Enhancing adherence to combination antiretroviral therapy in non-adherent HIV-positive men. *AIDS Care* 2000, 12:399–404.

34. Shen J, Sun Q, Zhou X, Wei Y, Qi Y, Zhu J, Yan T: Pharmacist interventions on antibiotic use in inpatients with respiratory tract infections in a Chinese hospital. *Int J Clin Pharm* 2011, 33(6):929–933.

35. Yen Y-H, Chen H-Y, Wuan-Jin L, Lin Y-M, Shen WC, Cheng K-J: Clinical and economic impact of a pharmacist-managed i.v.-to-p.o. conversion service for levofloxacin in Taiwan. *Int J Clin Pharmacol Ther* 2012, 50:136–141.

36. Brennan TA, Dollear TJ, Hu M, Matlin OS, Shrank WH, Choudhry NK, Grambley W: An integrated pharmacy-based program improved medication prescription and adherence rates in diabetes patients. *Health Aff (Millwood)* 2012, 31:120–129.

37. Lee AJ, Boro MS, Knapp KK, Meier JL, Korman NE: Clinical and economic outcomes of pharmacist recommendations in a Veterans Affairs medical center. *Am J Health Syst Pharm* 2002, 59:2070–2077.

38. Janknegt R, Meer JWM van der: Sequential therapy with intravenous and oral cephalosporins. *J Antimicrob Chemother* 1994, 33:169–177.

39. Brazilian Health Surveillance Agency (ANVISA): Preços máximos de medicamentos por princípio ativo para compras públicas – monodrogas/ preços fábrica (PF) e preço máximo de venda ao governo (PMVG) [http://portal.anvisa.gov.br/wps/wcm/connect/de29e2004baf729293c5dbbc0f9d5b29/LISTA_CONFORMIDADE_GOV_2012-06-19.pdf?MOD=AJPERES. Accessed July 12, 2014].

17

Carboxylate derivatives of tributyltin (IV) complexes as anticancer and antileishmanial agents

Durdana Waseem[1], Arshad Farooq Butt[2], Ihsan-ul Haq[1], Moazzam Hussain Bhatti[2] and Gul Majid Khan[1*]

Abstract

Background: Tributyltin (IV) compounds are promising candidates for drug development. In the current study, we evaluated in-vitro and *in-silico* profile of carboxylate derivatives of tributyltin (IV) complexes.

Methods: ADMET and drug-likeliness properties were predicted using MetaPrint2D React, preADMET, SwissADME and Molsoft tools. SwissTargetPrediction predicted molecular targets for compounds. In-vitro bioactivity was evaluated by quantifying cytotoxicity against HepG2, THP-1 cell lines, isolated lymphocytes and *leishmania* promastigotes as well as measuring protein kinase (PK) inhibition activity.

Results: Results indicate partial compliance of compounds with drug-likeliness rules. Ch-409 complies with WDI and Lipinski rules. ADMET profile prediction shows strong plasma protein binding except for Ch-409, low to high GI absorption and BBB penetration (C_{brain}/C_{blood} = 0.942–11; caco-2 cells permeability 20.13–26.75 nm/sec), potential efflux by P-glycoprotein, metabolism by CYP3A4, medium inhibition of hERG, mutagenicity and capacity to be detoxified by glutathionation and glucuronidation. Molecular targets include proteases, enzymes, membrane receptors, transporters and ion channels where Ch-409 targets membrane receptors only. Compounds are significantly ($p < 0.05$) cytotoxic against HepG2 cell line and *leishmania* as compared with normal isolated lymphocytes. Ch-459 indicates highest toxicity against *leishmania* (mortality 97.9 ± 3.99%; LC50 0.323 ± 0.002 µg/mL) whereas Ch-409 possesses maximum cytotoxicity against HepG2 cell line (IC50 0.08 ± 0.001 µg/mL) as well as 97.5 ± 1.98% (LC50 0.954 ± 0.158 µg/mL) mortality of *leishmania* promastigotes. It was observed that antileishmanial effect was reduced by 16.38%–34.38% and 15–38.2% in the presence of NaN_3 and mannitol respectively. PK inhibition and reactive oxygen species production are possible mechanisms for cytotoxicity.

Conclusions: Selected carboxylate derivatives of tributyltin (IV) complexes possess significant antileishmanial and cytotoxic potential. These are promising compounds for the development of antileishmanial and anticancer drugs.

Keywords: Organotin (IV), Anticancer, Antileishmanial, ADMET, Protein kinase inhibition

Background

Cancer and leishmaniasis are major threats to humans causing significant morbidity and mortality worldwide. Leishmaniasis is caused by transmission of *leishmania* parasite through sand fly in both endemic and non-endemic areas [1]. Lack of effective measures to control both parasite and sand fly are major factors for the spread of disease. Current therapies are inadequate to manage cancer and leishmaniasis due to diversity of molecular disruptions and development of resistance respectively. Cancer evolves by deregulating endogenous functions of molecular proteins, which in turn can be targeted to impede cancer progression. Anticancer drugs are developed and investigated against angiogenesis, extracellular matrix proteins and a variety of signal transduction pathways, including mitogen-activated protein kinase (MAPK), Janus-activated kinase, transforming growth factor-beta, p53, Ras, Wnt and Akt signaling [2, 3]. Treatment strategies against leishmaniasis involve killing parasite by DNA fragmentation, formatting aqueous pores

* Correspondence: gmkhan@qau.edu.pk
[1]Department of Pharmacy, Quaid-i-Azam University, Islamabad 45320, Pakistan
Full list of author information is available at the end of the article

in promastigotes cell membrane, oxidative mitochondrial damage, decreasing mitochondrial membrane potential, affecting peptidases that constitute *leishmania* genome and disrupting kinases responsible for *leishmania* division and differentiation [4]. Glycogen synthase kinase that control leishmania cell cycle, is a new potential target for antileishmanial drugs [5].

Regression of cancer and leishmaniasis is a challenge that can be accomplished by developing efficacious and cost-effective drugs. Among multiple synthetic drugs, organometallic compounds are prospective candidates for anticancer and antileishmanial drug discovery [6, 7]. Organometallics including pentavalent antimonials [8] and platin derivatives [9] have been used for over three decades for the management of leishmaniasis and cancer respectively [10]. Sodium stibogluconate and meglumine antimoniate are first line drugs against all forms of leishmaniasis [11]. On the other hand, carboplatin, oxaliplatin and cisplatin are commonly employed metal based drugs against ovarian, breast, head/neck, bladder, lung and colorectal cancers [12]. Efficacy of these compounds is compromised due to substantial risk of toxicities and emergence of resistance [8, 12]. Clinical limitations and inadequate control of subject diseases demand to investigate new drugs. It is general consensus that there are other metals in periodic table with therapeutic potential. Structural diversity and redox and catalytic properties of organometallics make them promising drug candidates. Among these, organotin (IV) compounds have caught the attention of researchers for their prospective biocidal activities. Carboxylate derivatives of organotin (IV) compounds have been previously investigated for their anticancer and antileishmanial profile [10]. Novel tin based compounds have been characterized with proven antibacterial, antifungal and antitumor activities [13, 14]. Considering the growing importance of organotin (IV) compounds in medicine, the present study was designed to evaluate the cytotoxic potential of tributyltin (IV) compounds against cancer cells and *leishmania*. The rationale was to appraise metal based drugs that can be effective and efficacious in managing rapidly spreading cancers and leishmaniasis. We assessed *in-silico* drug-likeness, ADMET profile and in-vitro anticancer and antileishmanial activities of new carboxylate derivatives of tributyltin (IV) ligand.

Methods
Chemicals, cell lines and strains
Standards including surfactin, amphotericin B and vincristine were procured from Sigma-Aldrich (Steinheim, Germany). Doxorubicin was purchased from Merck (Darmstadt, Germany). Medium ISP4 for protein kinase (PK) assay was prepared in the laboratory. Unless stated otherwise, all other chemicals were purchased from

Sigma-Aldrich (Germany). Human leukemia (THP-1) (ATCC # TIB-202) and human hepatoma (HepG2) (RBRC-RCB1648) cell lines were used for cytotoxicity assays. *Streptomyces* 85E and *Leishmania tropica* kwh 23 were used for protein kinase inhibition and antileishmanial assays respectively.

Compounds
Carboxylate derivatives of tributyltin (IV) backbone were selected from library of synthetic compounds present at our laboratory (Fig. 1). These compounds were selected based on structural similarity to compounds previously reported to possess cytotoxic profile [10]. These included bis(tributylstannyl) 2,2'-(1,4-phenylenebis(oxy))-diacetate (Ch-409), ethyl (Z)-4-(4-oxo-4-((tributylstannyl)oxy)but-2-enamido)benzoate (Ch-431), tributylstannyl (Z)-4-(cyclohexylamino)-4-oxobut-2-enoate (Ch-442), tributylstannyl 4-(4-oxo-4-((tributylstannyl)oxy)butanamido)benzoate (Ch-448), tributylstannyl 2-(naphthalene-1-ylcarbamoyl)benzoate (Ch-450), tributylstannyl (Z)-4-oxo-4-(phenylamino)but-2-enoate (Ch-458) and tributylstannyl (Z)-4-((2,3-dimethylphenyl)amino)-4-oxobut-2-enoate (Ch-459). Synthesis and characterization data on these compounds are submitted for publication elsewhere.

In-silico screening
Drug-likeliness prediction
PreADMET and Molsoft tools were utilized to determine the drug-likeness of tributyltin (IV) compounds and some marketed drugs [15]. PreADMET calculates drug-likeness of compounds based on Lipinski rule, lead-like rule, CMC-like rule, MDDR-like rules and World Drug Index (WDI) rule. 2D structural models were drawn in ChemBioDraw Ultra version 12.0 (Cambridge Software) and SMILES of each compound were translated into molfile by online SMILES translator and structure file generator (National Cancer Institute) [16]. Molfile data was added into the database to predict drug-likeness properties. Drug-likeness score was calculated from Molsoft using SMILES as input.

ADMET profile prediction
ADMET profile of tributyltin (IV) compounds was predicted using PreADMET and SwissADME tools [17]. Molfiles created for each compound were added into the database and searched for ADMET properties. Degree of plasma protein binding (PPB) is categorized in preADMET as strongly bound if %PPB > 90% and weakly bound if %PPB < 90%. Blood brain barrier (BBB) penetration is presented as concentration ratio of steady-state of radiolabeled compounds in brain (C_{brain}) and peripheral blood (C_{blood}). Compounds are classified into high, middle and low absorbing into CNS with

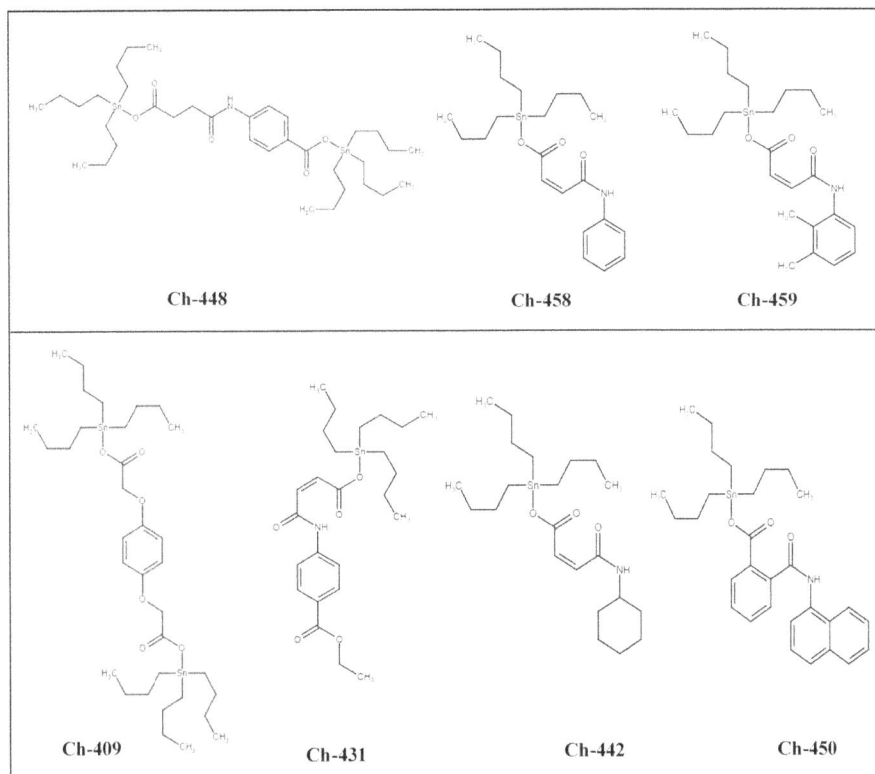

Fig. 1 Structures of tributyltin (IV) compounds

C_{brain}/C_{blood} values of >2, 2-0.1 and <0.1 respectively. For assessing intestinal absorption, Caco-2 cell model categorizes compounds as low, middle and highly permeable corresponding to values <4 nm/sec, 4–70 nm/sec and >70 nm/sec respectively. SwissADME predicts BBB penetration and GI absorption by BOILED-Egg method [18]. It also classified compounds as targets of p-glycoprotein (p-gp) efflux, inhibitors of cytochrome P450 enzymes CYP2C9, CYP2C19, CYP2D6 and CYP3A4 and substrates for metabolism by CYP2D6 and CYP3A4. PreADMET anticipated toxicity of compound on models of Ames test with or without metabolic activation by S9 (rat liver homogenate) against strains of *Salmonella typhimurium* TA100 and TA1535 and rodent carcinogenicity constructed on National Toxicology Program and FDA US data on in-vivo 2 year carcinogenicity tests of mice and rats. Results are produced are positive or negative mutagenicity or carcinogenicity.

Metabolism of compounds via phase I and phase II reactions was predicted using MetaPrint2D React [19, 20] subjected to similarity to known sites of metabolism. It calculates normalized occurrence ration (NOR) indicating relative likelihood of metabolism, which occurs at a specific site in the molecule.

Molecular target prediction

Molecular targets were predicted by SwissTargetPrediction online tool [21]. Query molecules were drawn in 2D using the javascript-based molecular editor of ChemAxon and submitted to the database. SwissTargetPrediction envisages molecular targets based on chemical similarity (2D) and/or structural similarity (3D) among bioactive molecules. A threshold for 3D and 2D similarity values has been set to 0.75 and 0.45 respectively. Compounds having values beyond these thresholds are not listed.

In-vitro screening
Cytotoxicity against THP-1 cell line

Cytotoxicity of tributyltin (IV) compounds against THP-1 cell line was determined by 3-(4,5-dimethylthiazol-2-yl)-2,5-diphenyl tetrazolium bromide (MTT) assay [22]. THP-1 cells were cultured in complete growth medium comprising RPMI-1640 (pH 7.4) supplemented with 2.2 g/L $NaHCO_3$ and 10% v/v heat inactivated fetal bovine serum (HIFBS). An aliquot of 20 μL of samples in 1% DMSO in PBS and 180 μL of THP-1 cells were mixed in 96-well plate. Cells were added at an assay density of 1×10^4 cells/mL whereas sample/standard was added to achieve the final concentration of 20 μg/mL.

The plate was incubated at 37 °C for 72 h in humidified 5% carbon dioxide incubator (Panasonic, Japan MCO-18 AC-PE). Vincristine and 1% DMSO in PBS were used as positive and negative controls respectively. After incubation, 20 μL of pre-filter sterilized MTT solution (4 mg/mL in distilled water) was added in plates and incubated for 4 h at 37 °C in CO_2 incubator. Later, colored formazan crystals were separated by removing supernatant and dissolved in 100 μL of DMSO. Reaction was allowed to stand for 1 h to ensure complete dissolution and absorbance was measured at 540 nm using microplate reader (Biotech USA, Elx 800).

Cytotoxicity assays against HepG2 cell line
Cytotoxicity was further evaluated against HepG2 cell line by sulforhodamine B (SRB) colorimetric assay [22]. Dulbecco's Modified Eagle Medium (DMEM) supplemented with 10% FBS, 100 μg/mL streptomycin sulfate, 100 IU/mL penicillin G sodium and 0.25 μg/mL amphotericin B was used to culture HepG2 cells in CO_2 (5%) incubator (Panasonic, Japan MCO-18 AC-PE) at 37 °C. An aliquot of 20 μL (1% DMSO in PBS) of samples was added to 180 μL of cell culture at an assay density of 1×10^5 cells/mL in 96-well plate. The plate was incubated at 37 °C for 72 h in CO_2 incubator. Final concentration of compounds/standard was 20 μg/mL. Doxorubicin and 1% v/v DMSO in PBS ere used as positive and negative controls respectively. An equivalent number of cells in twelve wells of 96-well plate were incubated for 1 h at 37 °C and labeled as day zero control. Later, cells were fixed by adding 50 μL of cold 20% w/v TCA for 1 h at 4 °C. These were washed with tap water, air dried and stained with 50 μL of 0.057% w/v SRB in 1% v/v acetic acid for 30 min at room temperature. Cells were again washed with 1% v/v acetic acid, dried overnight and 200 μL of 10 mM Tris base (pH 10) was used to solubilize the bound dye for 1 h. Absorbance was measured at 515 nm using a microplate reader. Percentage of growth inhibition was calculated as: % inhibition = $100 - [(A_s - A_o) / (A_n - A_o) \times 100]$, where, A_o, A_s and A_n are absorbance of day zero control, samples and negative control respectively. IC50 values were determined using 3-fold dilutions of the samples.

Cytotoxicity against isolated lymphocytes
Lymphocytes were isolated using previously described protocol with some modifications [23, 24]. Informed consent was obtained from volunteers and procedure was conducted according to international ethical guidelines after gaining approval from the ethical committee of the Quaid-i-Azam University. A volume of 3 mL of blood was obtained from a healthy donor by venipuncture and diluted (1:1) with PBS. It was layered over 2 mL Histopaque-1077 and centrifuged at 800 × g

for 20 min. The buffy coat was aspirated into 5 mL of PBS and centrifuged at 350 rpm for 4 min to pellet the lymphocytes. The pellet was suspended in 1 mL of RPMI-1640 and cell density was adjusted to get 1×10^5 cells/mL. For cytotoxicity determination, 20 μL of samples (20 μg/mL) or vincristine or 1% DMSO in PBS and 180 μL of lymphocyte suspension were incubated in 96-well plate at 37 °C for 24 h in humidified 5% carbon dioxide incubator (Panasonic, Japan MCO-18 AC-PE). Phytohaemagglutinin (PHA) was added in medium to stimulate lymphocyte growth. Afterwards, MTT assay was done as described above. IC50 values were determined using 3-fold dilutions of the samples.

Antileishmanial activity
Antileishmanial activity against the promastigotes of Leishmania tropica kwh 23 was evaluated by a quantitative colorimetric assay using 3-(4,5-dimethylthiazol-2-yl)-2, 5-diphenyl tetrazolium bromide (MTT) with minor modifications [25, 26]. Leishmania tropica parasites were cultured in Medium 199 supplemented with 10% FBS, 100 μg/mL streptomycin sulfate and 100 IU/mL penicillin G at 24 °C. A volume of 20 μL of extracts (100 μg/mL; DMSO ≤ 1% in PBS) and amphotericin B (0.33–0.004 μg/mL) were incubated with 180 μL of promastigotes at seeding density 2×10^6 cells/mL in 96-well flat bottom plate at 25 °C for 72 h. Negative control wells contained 1% DMSO in PBS. All samples were run in triplicate. Afterwards, plates were incubated for 4 h at 24 °C with 20 μL of MTT (4 mg/mL in distilled water) to determine the cell viability. Supernatant from each well was carefully removed leaving behind formazan crystals. Colored formazan crystals were dissolved in 100 μL of DMSO by setting those aside for 1 h to ensure complete dissolution. Cell viability was estimated by measuring absorbance at 540 nm using microplate reader and percentage growth inhibition was calculated.

Determining photosensitizing effect against leishmania
Photosensitizing effect of tributyltin (IV) compounds was determined in three parallel groups [27]. Samples and controls were exposed for 15 min to sunlight (168 W/m^2 of sun intensity) or sunlight with IR filter or dark conditions. The relative intensity of sunlight was measured by a CCD spectrometer (Ocean Optics, model HR4000). Later, plates were incubated at 25 °C for 72 h and cell viability was determined by MTT assay as given above. In this assay, samples were tested at concentrations showing less than 55% inhibition in primary antileishmanial assay to exclude false positive.

Determining ROS mediated antileishmanial activity
Leishmania tropica kwh 23 promastigotes were treated in three groups [27]. First group was exposed to samples

along with 0.1 mM sodium azide (NaN$_3$), second group to samples with 1 mM mannitol and third group comprised of all controls. In third group, promastigotes were treated in different wells with samples only (sample control), 1% DMSO in PBS only (negative control-I), amphotericin B only (positive control), 0.1 mM NaN$_3$ only (negative control-II) and 1 mM mannitol only (negative control-III). Plates were incubated followed by MTT assay described above.

Protein kinase inhibition assay

Protein kinase inhibitory activity of the tributyltin (IV) compounds was measured against *Streptomyces* 85E strain using previously described protocol [28]. Culture of *Streptomyces* 85E was refreshed in tryptic soy broth and 100 μL of this was swabbed on sterile ISP4 medium under aseptic conditions. Sterile filter paper discs (6 mm) impregnated with 5 μL of samples (10 mg/mL in DMSO) or surfactin (2 mg/mL in DMSO; positive control) or DMSO (negative control) were placed on *Streptomyces* swabbed petri plate and incubated for 72-96 h at 30 °C. Diameter (mm) of zone of inhibition (ZOI) around all samples and controls was measured as clear zone (CZ) and bald zone (BZ). Clear zone represents *Streptomyces* growth inhibition whereas bald zone shows inhibition of hyphae and spore formation. BZ is indicative of PK inhibition.

Statistical analysis

Data is presented as Mean ± SD of respective parameters in triplicate analysis. One Way Analysis of Variance (ANOVA) was applied to measure significance of results. $p < 0.05$ was considered statistically significant. Analysis was done using GraphPad Prism 5.0 software.

Results and discussion
Drug-likeliness prediction

Drug-likeliness prediction is important to optimize pharmaceutical and pharmacokinetic properties of compounds [29]. Tributyltin (IV) carboxylate compounds partially comply with selected rules of drug-likeliness. Ch-409 was in 90% cutoff range of WDI rule and complies with all conditions of Lipinski rule. Ch-458, 431, 448, 459 and 442 are mid-structures whereas Ch-450 is drug-like according to MDDR-like rule (Fig. 2). In practice, we have drugs in market that do not completely comply with drug-likeliness rules but are used due to their high beneficial effects for humans to treat cancer. For example, vincristine, which violates CMC-like, lead-like and Lipinski rules and complies with MDDR-like rule. Besides, cisplatin does not completely comply with any of the above rules. Drug-likeliness scores computed from Molsoft tool also indicate these compounds as moderately drug-like. Higher the score, greater the drug-likeliness conforming to available drugs [30]. Tributyltin (IV) compounds scores are -1.11, 0.42,−0.23, 0.15, 0.40,−0.49 and 0.27 for Ch-409, Ch-431, Ch-442, Ch-448, Ch-450, Ch-458 and Ch-459 respectively. On the other hand, cisplatin, vincristine, doxorubicin, amphotericin B, dactinomycin and sorafenib have drug-likeliness scores of -1.12, 1.38, 1.02, 0.9,−1.00 and 0.51 respectively. Thus, our compounds have comparable drug-likeliness profile with marketed drugs and are good drug candidates.

ADMET prediction

ADME analysis done by PreADMET predicts that tributyltin (IV) carboxylate compounds have middle to high BBB permeability based on C$_{brain}$/C$_{blood}$ ratio of 0.942–11 whereas SwissADME predicts no BBB crossing since these compounds are also substrates for p-glycoprotein efflux (Table 1). P-gp is present on the apical surface of endothelial cells of blood brain barrier and impedes the entry of various drugs [31]. All compounds strongly bind with plasma protein except Ch-409 and have low to high GI absorption (caco-2 cells permeability 20.13–26.75 nm/sec). These compounds can be formulated into oral dosage form. Ch-409 is inhibitor of CYP2C19; Ch-450 and Ch-409 are inhibitors of CYP2C9; Ch-458, Ch-431, Ch-450, Ch-448, Ch-459 and Ch-442 are of CYP2D6 and Ch-450, Ch-409 and Ch-448 inhibit

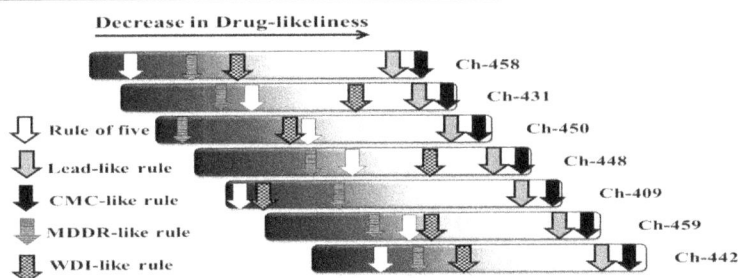

Fig. 2 Drug-likeliness profile of tributyltin (IV) compounds: The color from black to white indicates decrease in compliance with drug-likeliness rules. Placement of arrows on compliance bar shows the extent to which a compound conform to respective rule depending upon number of the conditions fulfilled for each rule. It is predicted from PreADMET

Table 1 ADME prediction of tributyltin (IV) compounds

Samples	PPB (%)	ADME Profile								Toxicity Profile					
		BBB Permeability		Swiss Pred[a]	Lipophilicity Consensus Log $P_{o/w}$[a]	Water Sol[a]	GI Abs[a]	Caco-2 Cells (nm/sec)	P-gp Substrate[a]	Ames Test					hERG Inhibition
		PreADMET (C_{brain}/C_{blood})	Pred							Pred	TA100		TA1535		
											+S9	-S9	+S9	-S9	
Ch-458	100	0.965	Middle	No	4.36	Poor	High	21.34	Yes	M	-ve	+ve	+ve	+ve	Medium
Ch-431	100	2.97	High	No	4.54	Poor	High	21.43	Yes	M	-ve	-ve	-ve	+ve	Medium
Ch-450	100	1.05	Middle	No	6.20	Insol	Low	26.75	Yes	M	-ve	-ve	+ve	+ve	Medium
Ch-448	100	0.971	Middle	No	7.58	Insol	Low	21.68	Yes	M	-ve	-ve	-ve	+ve	Medium
Ch-409	-ve	1.49	Middle	No	7.57	Insol	Low	22.28	Yes	M	-ve	+ve	-ve	-ve	Medium
Ch-459	100	0.942	Middle	No	4.93	Poor	High	22.03	Yes	M	-ve	-ve	-ve	+ve	Medium
Ch-442	100	1.14	Middle	No	4.35	Poor	High	21.34	No	M	-ve	-ve	+ve	+ve	Medium

[a]Data predicted from Swiss ADME tool. Sol = solubility; abs = absorption; Insol = insoluble; M = mutagen; -ve means no toxicity in Ames test; +ve means toxicity predicted in Ames test; Pred = prediction

CYP3A4. No compound is substrate of CYP2D6 whereas all others except Ch-409, Ch-458 and Ch-442 are strong substrates for metabolism by CYP3A4. Our compounds were found mutagenic in Ames test either by point or frame-shift mutations (Table 1). Metabolic activation predicts mutagenicity of metabolites of Ch-458, Ch-450 and Ch-442. Carcinogenicity prediction was "out of range" in the database expect for Ch-409, which was not carcinogenic in rat model. Human ether a go-go-related (hERG) gene encodes cardiac potassium channels that mediate repolarization phase. Inhibition of these prolong QTc interval along with the risk of cardiac arrhythmias [32]. Our compounds show medium risk of hERG inhibition. Since, compounds show very high PPB and very low IC/LC50 values in in-vitro analysis; therefore, it is necessary to assess the concentration at which hERG inhibition risk is predominant.

Metabolic sites predicted by MetaPrint2D React are highlighted as red ($0.66 \leq$ NOR ≤ 1.00), orange ($0.33 \leq$ NOR < 0.66), green ($0.15 \leq$ NOR < 0.33), white ($0.00 \leq$ NOR < 0.15) and grey (little/no data) corresponding to NOR where high NOR means most frequently reported site in metabolism database (Fig. 3). It was found that besides dealkylation, hydroxylation and oxidation, all compounds are possibly metabolized by multiple phase I and phase II reactions. Ch-409 can undergo acetylcysteination and glutathionation; Ch-431 is metabolized by demethylation and glucuronidation; Ch-448 by glucuronidation; Ch-450 go through epoxidation, glutathionation, sulfonation, oxidative deamination and methoxylation whereas

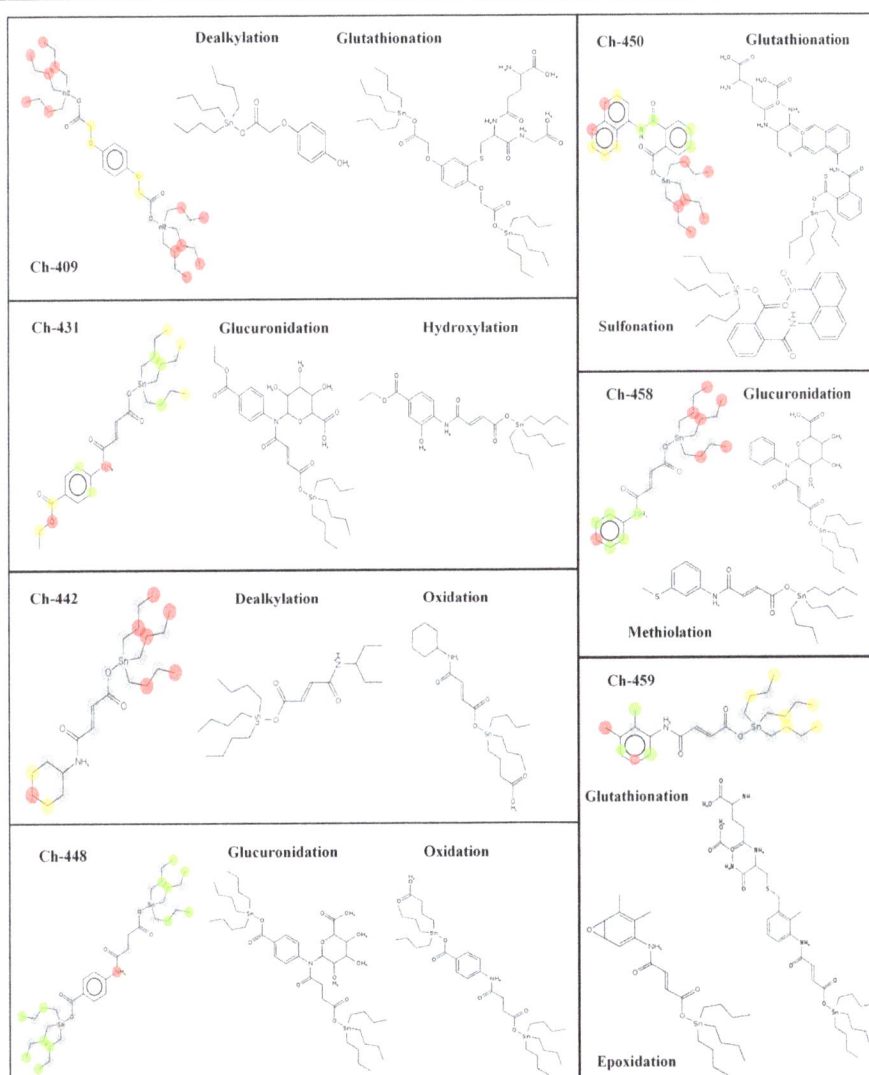

Fig. 3 Predicted metabolic sites and metabolites of tributyltin (IV) compounds. Structures with colored circles indicate the metabolic sites predicted by MetaPrint2D React. Color codes are given based on normalized occurrence ratio. Red = $0.66 \leq$ NOR ≤ 1.00; orange = $0.33 \leq$ NOR < 0.66; green = $0.15 \leq$ NOR < 0.33; white = $0.00 \leq$ NOR < 0.15 and grey = little/no data. Two possible metabolites for each compound are given with NOR ≥ 0.33

epoxidation, glucuronidation, methiolation, methoxylation are predicted for Ch-458 and epoxidation, glutathionation and methoxylation for Ch-459 (Fig. 3). Glucuronidation and glutathione metabolism of compounds make these hydrophilic and ionized at physiological pH. This also reduces their affinity with cellular target [33]. It is proposed that metabolism at multiple sites will excrete the compounds out of the body with less side effects of metabolites.

Molecular target prediction

Molecular target prediction by SwissTargetPrediction tool provided possible interaction sites for tributyltin (IV) compounds. These include proteases, enzymes, transcription factor, receptors, ion channels and other proteins (Fig. 4). Although the probabilities of interaction with targets was low (range: 0.01–0.1) based on ChEMBL database; however, in-vitro analysis depicts good bioactivity profile of these compounds. This means that they interact strongly with cellular proteins and modify their functions to kill cancer cells and *leishmania* parasite. It was predicted that Ch-409 can bind with membrane receptors such as opioid (mu, kappa, delta) and nociceptin receptors. On the contrary, Ch-431 dominantly aims enzymes (47%) acetylcholinesterase, inosine-5'-monophosphate dehydrogenase 2 and tyrosyl-DNA phosphodiesterase 1; transcription factor (7%) hypoxia-inducible factor 1-alpha and other proteins (33%) including microtubule-associated protein tau and muscleblind-like protein 1, 2 and 3. Ch-442 was predicted to interact with serine proteases (60%) cathepsin G, granzyme B and H, chymotrypsin-C and chymotrypsin-like elastase family member 2A and enzymes (40%) peptidyl-prolyl cis-trans isomerase FKBP1A and B and peptidyl-prolyl cis-trans isomerase FKBP4 and 5. Ch-448 can regulate transporters (47%), for examples, excitatory amino acid transporters 1, 2, 3, 4 and 5. Other proteins include tyrosyl-DNA phosphodiesterase 1, FAD-linked sulfhydryl oxidase ALR;

muscleblind-like proteins and membrane metalloendopeptidase-like 1 (soluble form). Ch-450 targets 67% proteases (alpha-trypsin chain 1, trypsin 2 and 3, activation peptide fragment 1, urokinase-type plasminogen activator long chain A, tissue-type plasminogen activator, hepatocyte growth factor activator long chain, apolipoprotein-a), 7% other enzymes (enzyme FAD-linked sulfhydryl oxidase ALR), 13% transcription factors (oxysterols receptor LXR-alpha and beta) and 13% unclassified proteins (plectin, microtubule-associated protein tau). Ch-458 can dominantly control serine proteases (73%) including chymase, chymotrypsin-C, cathepsin G, Granzyme B and H, chymotrypsin-like elastase family member 1, 2A, 2B, 3A and 3B and neutrophil elastase as well as acetylcholinesterase, poly [ADP-ribose] polymerase 14 and microtubule-associated protein tau. Besides enzymes (74%; telomerase reverse transcriptase, cathepsin G, monoglyceride lipase), Ch-459 can also interact with ion channels (13%) like ATP-sensitive inward rectifier potassium channels 11, 1 and 8. It has been previously reported that some of these proteins are positive and negative regulators of cancer. For examples, microtubule-associated protein tau is associated with paclitaxel resistance in breast and gastric cancer patients [34, 35] and upregulated hepatocyte growth factor activator and trypsin like proteases in cancer tissues are involved with carcinogenesis and metastasis [36]. In contrast, muscleblind-like protein 1 is implicated in suppression of breast cancer metastatic colonization [37]; granzymes play key role in antitumor immunity [38] and FKBP1A is a target for anticancer drug rapamycin [39]. Predicted interaction of our compounds with previously reported proteins in cancer provides evidence for their beneficial role.

Cytotoxicity of tributyltin (IV) compounds

Cytotoxicity of tributyltin (IV) compounds was quantified against HepG2, THP-1 cell lines and isolated

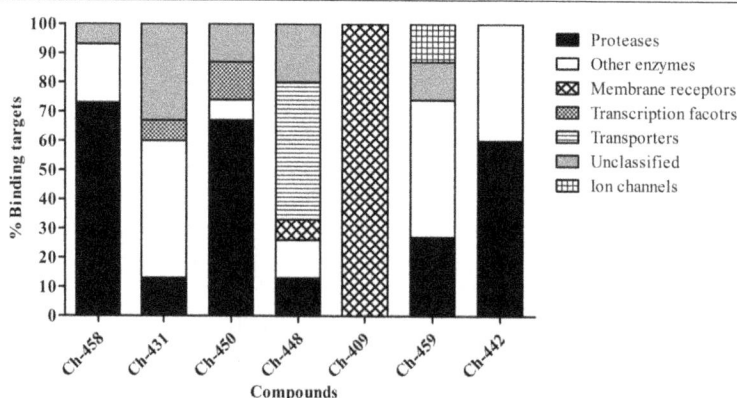

Fig. 4 Predicted molecular targets for tributyltin (IV) compounds. Molecular target prediction is done by SwissTargetPrediction tool. Each bar represents the targets for each compound based on structural homology and binding potential of similar compounds in database. Unclassified shows the proteins that are not classified into any group

lymphocytes at 20 μg/mL to compare effect at same concentration (Table 2). All compounds showed significantly higher ($p < 0.05$) cytotoxicity against HepG2 cell line except Ch-442. Ch-450 and Ch-459 exhibited significant cytotoxicity against THP-1 cells whereas activity of other compounds was lower than 50% at same concentration. On the contrary, Ch-409, Ch-459 and Ch-442 were toxic against normal isolated lymphocytes. However, IC50 values of these compounds for HepG2 cells were 10–100 times lower than those for isolated lymphocytes (Table 2). There was no significant cytotoxicity of other compounds against normal cells. This partially selective response against cancer cell lines is beneficial in targeting cancer cells whereas limiting damage to normal cells. Results are comparable with standard doxorubicin against HepG2 cells while lower in case of vincristine against THP-1 cells and lymphocytes. It can be seen that vincristine is significantly toxic against normal lymphocytes. Our compounds showed cytotoxicity against HepG2 cell line comparable to previously reported data on oxaliplatin and cisplatin [40]. On the contrary, lymphocyte cytotoxicity was more pronounced in carboplatin and cisplatin [23].

It was reported that carboxylate derivatives of organotin such as phenylacetate, benzoate and cinnamates were found effective against tumor cell lines. Some of the di-n-butyltin compounds were proved more potent than cisplatin [41]. In line with this, our results are comparable with previous study where different organotin (IV) carboxylate compounds revealed significant anticancer activity against kidney fibroblast (BHK-21) and lung carcinoma (H-157) cell lines [10]. This indicates prospective of tributyltin (IV) carboxylate compounds as potential candidates for anticancer drug development. Further screening of compounds used in present study is recommended against a range of cancer and normal cell lines to evaluate their efficacy and selectivity. Several reports presented that there is no well-defined mechanism by which organotin compounds can interact with cancer cells. Their intercalation with phosphodiester backbone of DNA is reported, altering intracellular breakdown of phospholipids of endoplasmic reticulum [42, 43]. Organotin compounds may also bind with membrane proteins, cellular kinases, ATPase or glycoproteins [44]. We have found these compounds as protein kinase inhibitors, which can be one of the mechanisms for cytotoxicity. However, detailed mechanism of action of these compounds is to be elucidated.

Antileishmanial activity
Tributyltin (IV) compounds demonstrated highly significant ($p < 0.05$) antileishmanial activity with >90% lethality and very low LC50s ranging from 0.954 ± 0.158 μg/mL to 0.078 ± 0.002 μg/mL (Table 3). Lowest LC50 was observed by Ch-431 that appears equipotent to the standard amphotericin B. It has been reported that sodium stibogluconate showed IC50s of 64 μg/mL and 22 μg/mL against axenic log-phase promastigotes and cellular meta-cyclic promastigotes respectively [45]. Our compounds appear to be more potent than sodium stibogluconate. Compounds were further tested for their photocatalytic activity by exposing to sunlight, sunlight with IR filter and dark conditions. There was 0–32% toxicity against *leishmania* when exposed to light and dark conditions without samples. Compounds showed no significant photosensitizing effect after normalizing the data indicating that their activity is independent of light conditions. Samples were further tested in the presence of ROS scavengers NaN_3 and mannitol, which scavenge singlet oxygen [46] and hydroxyl radicals [47] respectively. ROS are important molecules in controlling *leishmania* infection that are generated by macrophages during phagocytosis of parasite [48]. It was observed that antileishmanial activity of compounds was reduced by 16.38%–34.38% in the presence of NaN_3 whereas it was reduced by 15–38.2% in the presence of mannitol as compared with 16% and 10% decline for amphotericin B in the presence of NaN_3 and mannitol respectively. Ch-442 showed selective toxicity against *leishmania* with 95.8 ± 1.16% lethality as compared with 12.8 ± 0.37% and 44.6 ± 0.18% cytotoxicity against HepG2 and THP-1 cells respectively. Moreover, antileishmanial L50 (0.088 ± 0.009 μg/mL) is approximately 15 times lower than IC50 (14.9 ± 0.25 μg/mL) against isolated lymphocytes. Activity of Ch-442 was reduced by 22% and 38.2% in the presence of NaN_3 and mannitol respectively. These results indicate that ROS production by compounds is one of the mechanisms for antileishmanial effect.

Structure-activity relationship
Tributylstannyl carboxylate is the primary moiety responsible for cytotoxicity of these compounds. We compared all compounds with Ch-458, which has double bond at position 2, phenylamino ring and one tributylstannyl group with an IC50 of 1.58 μg/mL against HepG2 cells. Replacing the oxo-phenylaminobutanoic acid ligand with phenylenebis(oxy) diacetic acid has enhanced the potency of Ch-409 by 19-fold providing maximum cytotoxicity with lowest IC50 value. Dimethyl substitution at phenylamino ring in Ch-459 augmented its potency by 2.54-fold compared to Ch-458. On the contrary, substitutions of naphthalene-1-ylcarbamoyl, ethoxycarbonyl at position 4 on phenylamino group and missing double bond at position 2 reduced potency of compounds Ch-450, Ch-431 and Ch-448 by 1.77, 3.46 and 2.18-folds respectively. However, presence of cyclohexyl ring instead of phenyl may have hindered binding

Table 2 Cytotoxicity and PK inhibition activity of tributyltin (IV) compounds

Samples	Cytotoxicity					Protein kinase inhibition assay				
	HepG2 (20 µg/mL)	IC50 (µg/mL)	THP-1 (20 µg/mL)	Isolated lymphocytes (20 µg/mL)	IC50 (µg/mL)	ZOI (mm) at 50 µg/disc		ZOI (mm) at 6.25 µg/disc		MIC (µg/disc)
	% growth inhibition		% growth inhibition			CZ	BZ	CZ	BZ	
Ch-458	98.7 ± 3.56*	1.58 ± 0.07	21.2 ± 1.57	14.8 ± 0.13‡	–	30 ± 1.2*	–	12 ± 1.25	31 ± 1.37*	0.195 ± 0.001
Ch-431	96.2 ± 2.23*	5.48 ± 0.16	42.7 ± 1.13	10.7 ± 1.17‡	–	31 ± 0.78*	33 ± 1.15*	10 ± 0.33	26 ± 0.16*	0.049 ± 0.002
Ch-450	98.5 ± 1.85*	2.81 ± 0.34	50.4 ± 2.63*	11.7 ± 0.05‡	–	32 ± 1.13*	–	–	28 ± 2.5*	0.195 ± 0.001
Ch-448	97.1 ± 2.34*	3.45 ± 0.63	43.1 ± 2.29	23.6 ± 1.07‡	–	31 ± 1.05*	–	–	25 ± 1.75*	0.781 ± 0.002
Ch-409	99.5 ± 3.15*	0.08 ± 0.001	19.4 ± 1.41	55.6 ± 2.32*‡	15.18 ± 0.75‡	30 ± 1.75*	31 ± 1.5*	12 ± 0.19	30 ± 1.17*	0.781 ± 0.002
Ch-459	96.5 ± 4.66*	0.62 ± 0.005	52.5 ± 0.99*	60.7 ± 1.68*	5.78 ± 0.34‡	35 ± 0.99*	–	–	30 ± 0.24*	0.391 ± 0.004
Ch-442	12.8 ± 1.37	–	44.6 ± 1.18	55.4 ± 1.74*‡	14.9 ± 0.25	40 ± 1.17*	–	10 ± 0.74	29 ± 0.78*	0.391 ± 0.006
Vincristine	–	–	100 ± 0.0*	76.3 ± 3.65*	6.66 ± 0.09	–	–	–	–	–
Doxorubicin	97.21 ± 1.14*	5.36 ± 0.75	–	–	–	–	–	–	–	–
Surfactin (10 µg/mL)	–	–	–	–	–	–	23 ± 1.98*	–	–	–
1% DMSO with PBS	0	–	0	0	–	0	0	0	0	–
DMSO	–	–	–	–	–	0	0	0	0	–

Data is Mean ± SD; $n = 3$; (–) indicates not applied; ZOI = zone of inhibition; (–) shows no ZOI; CZ = clear zone of inhibition; BZ = bald zone of inhibition; MIC = minimum inhibitory concentration; (*) means data is significantly different from HepG2 results; (‡) means $p < 0.05$ compared with negative control

Table 3 Antileishmanial activity of tributyltin (IV) compounds

Samples	Antileishmanial activity		ROS scavenging at 20 μg/mL		Photosensitizing effect			
	% growth inhibition at 20 μg/mL	LC50 μg/mL	% growth inhibition					
			NaN3 (0.1 mM)	Mannitol (1 mM)	Control	Sunlight	Sunlight with IR filter	Dark
Ch-458	97.8 ± 1.23*	0.256 ± 0.064	73.5 ± 2.78‡	60.3 ± 1.5‡	35.2 ± 1.78	42.7 ± 1.35	30.25 ± 0.17	36.7 ± 0.74
Ch-431	97.5 ± 2.75*	0.078 ± 0.002	66.2 ± 2.99‡	59.6 ± 0.19‡	50.7 ± 1.25	53.2 ± 1.55	47.5 ± 0.99	51.5 ± 1.35
Ch-450	97.4 ± 1.35*	0.361 ± 0.017	75.4 ± 1.75‡	62.8 ± 2.74‡	24.5 ± 1.63	32.12 ± 1.28	20.7 ± 0.43	26.34 ± 0.15
Ch-448	96.5 ± 2.67*	0.576 ± 0.088	77.9 ± 3.25‡	68.9 ± 0.75‡	54.65 ± 2.75	49.7 ± 0.89	52.9 ± 1.17	50.16 ± 1.19
Ch-409	97.5 ± 1.98*	0.954 ± 0.158	81.12 ± 1.63	82.5 ± 1.53	52.05 ± 1.98	57.63 ± 1.99	47.5 ± 1.56	56.9 ± 0.02
Ch-459	97.9 ± 3.99*	0.323 ± 0.002	63.52 ± 0.86‡	76.7 ± 1.17‡	20.1 ± 0.59	25.5 ± 1.75	30.14 ± 1.47	22.7 ± 1.05
Ch-442	95.8 ± 2.16*	0.088 ± 0.009	73.8 ± 1.36‡	57.6 ± 0.78‡	46.1 ± 0.56	40.5 ± 0.12	49.25 ± 0.63	44.18 ± 1.16
Amphotericin B	100 ± 0.0*	0.044 ± 0.001	84 ± 2.05	90 ± 1.85	--	--	--	--
1% DMSO with PBS	0	0	0	0	0	0	0	0

Data is Mean ± SD. (–) means not applied; (*) means $p < 0.05$ as compared with negative control. (‡) $p < 0.05$ compared with untreated control. Concentrations for photosensitizing assay are 0.55 μg/mL for Ch-409 and Ch-448; 0.092 μg/mL for Ch-431, Ch-442, Ch-458, Ch-459 and Ch-450

affinity of Ch-442 to target proteins in HepG2 cells causing no cytotoxicity.

In case of THP-1 cells, addition of naphthalene (Ch-450) and dimethylphenyl (Ch-459) might have enhanced binding of compounds to specific targets in THP-1 cells that vary from HepG2 and isolated lymphocytes. Nevertheless, the cytotoxicity is only around 50% at concentration of 20 µg/mL. Since, proteins and cellular components may vary between normal and cancer cells; therefore, activity of our compounds was pronounced against HepG2 cells with little/no effect against isolated lymphocytes. Substitutions of cyclohexyl ring (Ch-442), dimethylphenyl (Ch-459) and phenylenebis(oxy) diacetic acid (Ch-409) showed cytotoxicity against isolated lymphocytes. It is possible that these compounds gained access to biomarkers similar in normal and cancer cells. Since, Ch-459 showed cytotoxicity in all three cell types used; therefore, presence of dimethylphenyl group appears to be an important modulator of cytotoxicity.

Compounds were also highly cytotoxic against *leishmania* promastigotes. Ch-409 with phenylenebis(oxy) diacetic acid ligand was least potent among all compounds with LC50 0.954 µg/mL. Substitution of ethoxycarbonyl at position 4 on phenylamino group (Ch-431) gained maximum access to specific leishmania proteins and was 12.23-fold potent than Ch-409. Cyclohexyl moiety in Ch-442 showed targeted affinity for leishmania specific proteins or other biomolecules allowing selective cytotoxicity behavior with 10.84-fold higher potency than Ch-409 and 1.12-fold lower than Ch-431. Similarly, respective substitutions in Ch-458, Ch-459, Ch-450 and Ch-448 reduced potency by 3.28, 4.14, 4.62 and 7.38-folds compared with Ch-431. Reduction of a double bond at position 2 drastically decreased potency of Ch-448. Thus, tributylstannyl carboxylate backbone is highly cytotoxic against *leishmania* promastigotes and ligand modifications on it caused potency variations. Our results indicate dissimilarity in compounds' behavior against cancer cells, normal cells and *leishmania*. It depicts that these have different molecular targets as well as variable affinity against same biomolecules. This is supported by our *in-silico* molecular target prediction where both variable and overlapping interaction site have been predicted. Thus, these compounds have multimode cytotoxicity with potential for varied diseases.

Protein kinase inhibition activity

Protein kinases are essential modulators of cellular regulations and physiological processes [49]. Irregular activation of these kinases constitutes oncogenic signals. Cytoplasmic (Abl) or transmembrane (PDGFR, EGFR) protein kinases found in many cancer cells are targets for anticancer drugs to induce cytotoxicity [50]. Thus,

we assessed inhibition of protein kinases as possible mechanism of cytotoxicity in our study.

Being highly cytotoxic, initially clear zones were observed; however, compounds provided bald zones at lower doses with no cytotoxicity. Bald zone specify protein kinase inhibition by obstructing aerial hyphae formation whereas clear zones indicate complete inhibition of *Streptomyces* growth. Lowest MIC for PK inhibition was shown by Ch-431 (Table 2). MIC for PK inhibition is much lower than IC50 for HepG2 cytotoxicity and is somewhat comparable with LC50 for antileishmanial activity. It means that these compounds are effective in targeting protein kinase enzymes and other associated factors at lower doses that those which cause cytotoxicity.

Molecular target prediction predicted enzymes as likely targets. Although, *in-silico* target prediction shows little data on binding probability with kinases; however, we experimentally proved this fact that tributyltin (IV) carboxylate compounds used in our study significantly inhibited ($p < 0.001$) protein kinase activity in *Streptomyces*. Streptomyces requires protein kinase activity of RamC to convert pre-Sap B to Sap B, a surfactant important for aerial hyphae formation [51]. It has been found that RamC is a membrane associated receptor kinase [51], which supports binding of all our compounds with this motif including Ch-409 whose major targets are predicted to be receptors only. This indicates significance of tributyltin (IV) compounds in protein kinase inhibition that may be a reason for cytotoxicity in cancer cells and *leishmania*. Oncogenesis is mediated either directly or indirectly by transmembrane or cytoplasmic tyrosine/serine-threonine kinases [52]. Furthermore, MAPK MAPK-like kinases, cyclin-dependent kinase (Cdk) and glycogen synthase kinase 3 are implicated in growth, differentiation and infectivity of *leishmania* parasite [53]. Thus, our data suggests molecular level studies to further explore exact mechanism of these compounds.

Conclusions

Tributyltin (IV) carboxylate compounds are contenders of anticancer and antileishmanial drug development. *In-silico* analysis shows these compounds partially drug-like, permeable across GI membrane and blood brain barrier and mutagenic with possible risk of hERG inhibition. High PPB and rate of metabolism will provide very low free drug concentration in plasma that may reduce the risk of side effects, which can be further managed using targeted drug delivery system. Our new compounds are highly cytotoxic against HepG2 cells and *leishmania* parasite with lower cytotoxicity against normal isolated lymphocytes. These significantly inhibit protein kinase with very low IC50 values. These compounds can be evaluated further based on their risk benefit ratio.

Abbreviations

ADMET: Absorption, distribution, metabolism, elimination and toxicity; BZ: Bald zone; CZ: Clear zone; NOR: Normalized occurrence ration; ZOI: Zone of inhibition.

Acknowledgements

There are no acknowledgements in this manuscript.

Funding

This research did not receive any specific grant from funding agencies in the public, commercial, or not-for-profit sectors. However, indigenous scholarship for PhD studies from Higher Education Commission, Pakistan is acknowledged.

Authors' contributions

DW performed the experiments and was the major contributor in writing the manuscript. IH has made substantial contribution to the concept and design of study. AFB synthesized and provided the compounds. MHB and GMK facilitated in in vitro evaluation, data analysis and critically reviewed the manuscript for important intellectual comments. All authors read and approved the final manuscript.

Competing interests

The authors declare that they have no competing interests.

Author details

[1]Department of Pharmacy, Quaid-i-Azam University, Islamabad 45320, Pakistan. [2]Department of Chemistry, Allama Iqbal Open University, H-8, Islamabad 44000, Pakistan.

References

1. Clem A. A current perspective on leishmaniasis. J Glob Infect Dis. 2010;2(2):124–6.
2. Gazdar AF, Miyajima K, Reddy J, Sathyanarayana UG, Shigematsu H, Suzuki M, et al. Molecular targets for cancer therapy and prevention. Chest J. 2004; 125(5_suppl):97S–101S.
3. Gross S, Rahal R, Stransky N, Lengauer C, Hoeflich KP. Targeting cancer with kinase inhibitors. J Clin Invest. 2015;125(5):1780–9.
4. Singh N, Kumar M, Singh RK. Leishmaniasis: current status of available drugs and new potential drug targets. Asian Pac J Trop Med. 2012;5(6):485–97.
5. Xingi E, Smirlis D, Myrianthopoulos V, Magiatis P, Grant KM, Meijer L, et al. 6-Br-5methylindirubin-3′ oxime (5-Me-6-BIO) targeting the leishmanial glycogen synthase kinase-3 (GSK-3) short form affects cell-cycle progression and induces apoptosis-like death: exploitation of GSK-3 for treating leishmaniasis. Int J Parasitol. 2009;39(12):1289–303.
6. Martins P, Marques M, Coito L, Pombeiro AJ, Baptista PV, Fernandes AR. Organometallic compounds in cancer therapy: Past lessons and future directions. Anticancer Agents Med Chem. 2014;14(9):1199–212.
7. Sánchez-Delgado RA, Anzellotti A, Suárez L. Metal complexes as chemotherapeutic agents against tropical diseases: malaria, trypanosomiasis, and leishmaniasis. Met Ions Biol Syst. 2004;41:379–420.
8. Haldar AK, Sen P, Roy S. Use of antimony in the treatment of leishmaniasis: current status and future directions. Mol Biol Int. 2011;2011:1–23.
9. Dasari S, Tchounwou PB. Cisplatin in cancer therapy: molecular mechanisms of action. Eur J Pharmacol. 2014;740:364–78.
10. Sirajuddin M, Ali S, McKee V, Zaib S, Iqbal J. Organotin (IV) carboxylate derivatives as a new addition to anticancer and antileishmanial agents: design, physicochemical characterization and interaction with Salmon sperm DNA. RSC Adv. 2014;4(101):57505–21.
11. Frézard F, Demicheli C, Ribeiro RR. Pentavalent antimonials: new perspectives for old drugs. Molecules. 2009;14(7):2317–36.
12. McWhinney SR, Goldberg RM, McLeod HL. Platinum neurotoxicity pharmacogenetics. Mol Cancer Ther. 2009;8(1):10–6.
13. Hong M, Yang Y, Li C, Xu L, Li D, Li C-z. Study of the effect of molecular structure and alkyl groups bound with tin (IV) on their cytotoxicity of organotin (IV) 2-phenyl-4-selenazole carboxylates. RSC Adv. 2015;5(124):102885–94.
14. Hussain S, Ali S, Shahzadi S, Sharma SK, Qanungo K, Shahid M. Synthesis, characterization, semiempirical and biological activities of organotin (IV) carboxylates with 4-piperidinecarboxylic acid. Bioinorg Chem Appl. 2014; 2014:959203.
15. Lee SK, Chang GS, Lee IH, Chung JE, Sung KY, No KT: The PreADMET: PC-based program for batch prediction of ADME properties. EuroQSAR. 2004:9: 5–10.
16. Online SMILES Translator and Structure File Generator. National Institute of Health, USA. https://cactus.nci.nih.gov/translate/. Accessed 16 June 2016.
17. Daina A, Michielin O, Zoete V. iLOGP: a simple, robust, and efficient description of n-octanol/water partition coefficient for drug design using the GB/SA approach. J Chem Inf Model. 2014;54(12):3284–301.
18. Daina A, Zoete V. A BOILED-Egg to predict gastrointestinal absorption and brain penetration of small molecules. ChemMedChem. 2016;11(11):1117–21.
19. Boyer S, Arnby CH, Carlsson L, Smith J, Stein V, Glen RC. Reaction site mapping of xenobiotic biotransformations. J Chem Inf Model. 2007;47(2):583–90.
20. Boyer S, Zamora I. New methods in predictive metabolism. J Comput Aided Mol Des. 2002;16(5):403–13.
21. Gfeller D, Grosdidier A, Wirth M, Daina A, Michielin O, Zoete V. SwissTargetPrediction: a web server for target prediction of bioactive small molecules. Nucleic Acids Res. 2014;42(W1):W32–8.
22. Haq I-U, Ullah N, Bibi G, Kanwal S, Sheeraz Ahmad M, Mirza B. Antioxidant and cytotoxic activities and phytochemical analysis of euphorbia wallichii root extract and its fractions. Iran J Pharm Res. 2010;11(1):241–9.
23. Suman G, Jamil K. Application of human lymphocytes for evaluating toxicity of anti-cancer drugs. Int J Pharmacol. 2006;2(4):374–81.
24. Suman G, Naravaneni R, Jamil K. In vitro cytogenetic studies of cypermethrin on human lymphocyte. Indian J Exp Biol. 2006;44(3):233–9.
25. Mosmann T. Rapid colorimetric assay for cellular growth and survival: application to proliferation and cytotoxicity assays. J Immunol Methods. 1983;65(1-2):55–63.
26. Yao L, Fiona S, Ten-Jin K, Christophe W. Antileishmanial assay and antimicrobial activity on crude extracts of Melodinus eugeniifolus barks and leaves from Malaysia. Pharmacol Pharm. 2014;5:747–54.
27. Nadhman A, Nazir S, Khan MI, Arooj S, Bakhtiar M, Shahnaz G, et al. PEGylated silver doped zinc oxide nanoparticles as novel photosensitizers for photodynamic therapy against Leishmania. Free Radic Biol Med. 2014;77:230–8.
28. Fatima H, Khan K, Zia M, Ur-Rehman T, Mirza B, Haq I-U. Extraction optimization of medicinally important metabolites from Datura innoxia Mill.: an in vitro biological and phytochemical investigation. BMC Complement Altern Med. 2015;15(1):376.
29. Vistoli G, Pedretti A, Testa B. Assessing drug-likeness–what are we missing? Drug Discov Today. 2008;13(7):285–94.
30. Lalitha P, Sivakamasundari S. Calculation of molecular lipophilicity and drug likeness for few heterocycles. Orient J Chem. 2010;26(1):135–41.
31. Ramakrishnan P. The role of P-glycoprotein in the blood-brain barrier. Einstein Q J Biol Med. 2003;19(1):160–5.

32. van Noord C, Sturkenboom MC, Straus SM, Witteman JC, Stricker BHC. Non-cardiovascular drugs that inhibit hERG-encoded potassium channels and risk of sudden cardiac death. Heart. 2011;97(3):215–20.

33. Iyanagi T. Molecular mechanism of phase I and phase II drug-metabolizing enzymes: implications for detoxification. Int Rev Cytol. 2007;260:35–112.

34. Mimori K, Sadanaga N, Yoshikawa Y, Ishikawa K, Hashimoto M, Tanaka F, et al. Reduced tau expression in gastric cancer can identify candidates for successful Paclitaxel treatment. Br J Cancer. 2006;94(12):1894–7.

35. Rouzier R, Rajan R, Wagner P, Hess KR, Gold DL, Stec J, et al. Microtubule-associated protein tau: a marker of paclitaxel sensitivity in breast cancer. Proc Natl Acad Sci USA. 2005;102(23):8315–20.

36. Kawaguchi M, Kataoka H. Mechanisms of hepatocyte growth factor activation in cancer tissues. Cancers. 2014;6(4):1890–904.

37. Fish L, Pencheva N, Goodarzi H, Tran H, Yoshida M, Tavazoie SF. Muscleblind-like 1 suppresses breast cancer metastatic colonization and stabilizes metastasis suppressor transcripts. Genes Dev. 2016;30(4):386–98.

38. Cullen S, Brunet M, Martin S. Granzymes in cancer and immunity. Cell Death Differ. 2010;17(4):616–23.

39. Zhou XZ, Lu KP. The isomerase PIN1 controls numerous cancer-driving pathways and is a unique drug target. Nat Rev Cancer. 2016;16:463–78.

40. Pascale F, Bedouet L, Baylatry M, Namur J, Laurent A. Comparative chemosensitivity of VX2 and HCC cell lines to drugs used in TACE. Anticancer Res. 2015;35(12):6497–503.

41. Xiao X, Liang C, Zhao W. Organotin carboxylates: from structures to antitumour activities. Eur J BioMed Res. 2015;1(4):23–7.

42. Li Q, Yang P, Wang H, Guo M. Diorganotin (IV) antitumor agent. (C 2 H 5) 2 SnCl 2 (phen)/nucleotides aqueous and solid-state coordination chemistry and its DNA binding studies. J Inorg Biochem. 1996;64(3):181–95.

43. Pellerito L, Nagy L. Organotin (IV)$^{n+}$ complexes formed with biologically active ligands: equilibrium and structural studies, and some biological aspects. Coord Chem Rev. 2002;224(1):111–50.

44. Rocamora-Reverte L, Carrasco-García E, Ceballos-Torres J, Prashar S, Kaluđerović GN, Ferragut JA, et al. Study of the anticancer properties of tin (IV) carboxylate complexes on a panel of human tumor cell lines. ChemMedChem. 2012;7(2):301–10.

45. Vermeersch M, da Luz RI, Toté K, Timmermans J-P, Cos P, Maes L. *In vitro* susceptibilities of *Leishmania donovani* promastigote and amastigote stages to antileishmanial reference drugs: practical relevance of stage-specific differences. Antimicrob Agents Chemother. 2009;53(9):3855–9.

46. Bancirova M. Sodium azide as a specific quencher of singlet oxygen during chemiluminescent detection by luminol and Cypridina luciferin analogues. Luminescence. 2011;26(6):685–8.

47. Desesso JM, Scialli AR, Goeringer GC. D-mannitol, a specific hydroxyl free radical scavenger, reduces the developmental toxicity of hydroxyurea in rabbits. Teratology. 1994;49(4):248–59.

48. Carneiro PP, Conceição J, Macedo M, Magalhães V, Carvalho EM, Bacellar O. The role of nitric oxide and reactive oxygen species in the killing of leishmania braziliensis by monocytes from patients with cutaneous leishmaniasis. PloS One. 2016;11(2):e0148084.

49. Cheng H-C, Qi RZ, Paudel H, Zhu H-J. Regulation and function of protein kinases and phosphatases. Enzyme Res. 2011;2011:1–3.

50. Tsatsanis C, Spandidos DA. The role of oncogenic kinases in human cancer (Review). Int J Mol Med. 2000;5:583–90.

51. Hudson ME, Zhang D, Nodwell JR. Membrane association and kinase-like motifs of the RamC protein of Streptomyces coelicolor. J Bacteriol. 2002;184(17):4920–4.

52. Tsatsanis, Christos, Zafiropoulos, Alexandros, and Spandidos, Demetrios A. Oncogenic Kinases in Cancer. In: eLS. John Wiley & Sons Ltd, Chichester. 2007. http://www.els.net. [doi: 10.1002/9780470015902.a0006051.pub2].

53. Morales MA, Pescher P, Späth GF. Leishmania major MPK7 protein kinase activity inhibits intracellular growth of the pathogenic amastigote stage. Eukaryot Cell. 2010;9(1):22–30.

18

Application of nanostructured lipid carriers: the prolonged protective effects for sesamol in in vitro and in vivo models of ischemic stroke via activation of PI3K signalling pathway

Parichehr Hassanzadeh[1], Fatemeh Atyabi[1,2*], Rassoul Dinarvand[1,2], Ahmad-Reza Dehpour[3], Morteza Azhdarzadeh[1] and Meshkat Dinarvand[1]

Abstract

Background: Treatment of the ischemic stroke has remained a major healthcare challenge. The phenolic compound, sesamol, has shown promising antioxidant and neuroprotective effects, however, fast clearance may negatively affect its efficiency. This, prompted us to incorporate sesamol into the nanostructured lipid carriers (S-NLCs) and evaluate its therapeutic potential in in vitro and in vivo models of ischemic stroke.

Methods: S-NLCs formulations were prepared by high-pressure homogenization followed by physicochemical characterization, evaluation of the bioactivity of the optimal formulation in oxygen-glucose deprivation (OGD) and global cerebral ischemia/reperfusion (I/R) injury and implication of phosphatidylinositol 3-kinase (PI3K) pathway in this regard. Two- or three-way ANOVA, Mann-Whitney U test, and Student's t-test were used for data analysis.

Results: Formation of S-NLCs which exhibited a controlled release profile, was confirmed by scanning electron microscope and differential scanning calorimetry. 1- and 8-h OGD followed by 24 h re-oxygenation significantly reduced PC12 cell viability, increased lactate dehydrogenase activity and the number of condensed nuclei, and induced oxidative stress as revealed by increased malondialdehyde level and decreased glutathione content and superoxide dismutase and catalase activities. Sesamol (80 and 100 μM) reduced the cytotoxicity, oxidative stress, and cellular damage only after 1-h OGD, while, S-NLCs (containing 80 and 100 μM of sesamol) were effective at both time points. Intravenous injections of S-NLCs (20 and 25 mg/kg) into rats markedly attenuated I/R-induced neurobehavioural deficits, cellular damage, and oxidative stress, while, free sesamol failed. Pre-treatment with PI3K inhibitor, LY294002, abolished the protective effects against OGD or I/R.

Conclusions: S-NLCs improve the pharmacological profile of sesamol and provide longer lasting protective effects for this phenolic phytochemical. This nanoformulation by activating PI3K pathway may serve as a promising candidate for neuroprotection against the cerebral stroke or other neurodegenerative disorders.

Keywords: Sesamol, Nanostructured lipid carriers, Ischemic stroke, Phosphoinositide 3-kinase, PC12 cells, Rat

* Correspondence: atyabifa@tums.ac.ir
[1]Nanotechnology Research Center, Faculty of Pharmacy, Tehran University of Medical Sciences, Tehran, Iran
[2]Department of Pharmaceutics, Faculty of Pharmacy, Tehran University of Medical Sciences, Tehran, Iran
Full list of author information is available at the end of the article

Background

Ischemic stroke is one of the major causes of disability and death worldwide [1, 2]. Following the severe reduction or interruption of blood flow and oxygen in the cerebral arteries, a sequence of events including the inflammation, oxidative stress, mitochondrial dysfunction, and excessive release of excitatory amino acids may result in the neuronal death [2–4]. Based on the brain's requirement to a continuous supply of oxygen and glucose, it is the most susceptible organ to the oxygen-glucose deprivation and oxidative stress [5]. The limited efficiency of the currently available medications and their short therapeutic time windows [1], has provoked increasing research efforts to develop novel treatment strategies. During the last decade, antioxidant and neuroprotective effects of the phenolic compounds have been the focus of intense research. In this respect, sesamol, the major constituent of sesame seed oil (*Sesamum indicum*, Linn, Pedaliaceae) has attracted a growing interest due to its high safety profile and wide spectrum of pharmacological activities including the effects against the inflammation, oxidative stress, aging, and depression [6–9]. Moreover, sesamol has shown antithrombotic and neuroprotective properties [10–13] which might be of therapeutic value in the ischemic stroke. However, rapid elimination of sesamol [14, 15] may negatively affect its efficiency that necessitates the development of suitable drug delivery system to improve the stability and bioavailability of this phenolic compound. Over the last few decades, nanotechnology entities have been used to deliver compounds with poor solubility or short half-life [16–23]. There are reports demonstrating the efficiency of nanomaterials for detection or treatment of stroke [24–26]. In recent years, lipid-based colloidal drug delivery systems including the solid lipid nanoparticles (SLNs) and nanostructured lipid carriers (NLCs) as the alternative carrier systems to the liposomes, emulsions, and polymeric nanoparticles have attracted considerable attention. These biocompatible carriers protect the encapsulated active ingredients against the enzymatic degradation and are suitable for targeted drug delivery or controlled release [27]. SLNs have shown advantages of scale-up feasibility, sterility, and protection of incorporated compounds against the degradation, however, the risk of gelation, limited drug-loading capacity, and the possibility of drug leakage during the storage [27–29] led to the development of NLCs, a binary mixture of liquid and solid lipids which provides an imperfect matrix structure. Indeed, NLCs are a smarter generation of drug carriers with high biocompatibility, stability, and drug-loading capacity, prolonged drug residence in the target organ, and minimal drug expulsion during the storage [27, 30, 31]. This background prompted us to prepare sesamol-loaded NLCs (S-NLCs) and evaluate the therapeutic potential of this nanoformulation in both in vitro and in vivo models of ischemic stroke. As a mechanistic approach, we looked at the role of phosphatidylinositol 3-kinase (PI3K) pathway which is critically involved in the cell proliferation and survival [32, 33].

Methods

Materials

Cell culture materials were all purchased from GIBCO/Invitrogen, Germany. Cetyl palmitate and Tween 80 were provided by Merck (Darmstadt, Germany) and other chemicals or kits were purchased from Sigma Aldrich, Germany.

Preparation of sesamol-loaded NLCs (S-NLCs)

S-NLCs were prepared by high-pressure homogenization [34] with some modifications. Briefly, the lipid phase (cetyl palmitate and oleic acid; 85:15 or 70:30) was prepared at 75 °C and sesamol (3,4-methylenedioxyphenol) was added at 5, 10, 20, 40, or 100% w/w. The aqueous phase was prepared at 75 °C by dispersing poloxamer 188 (0.5 or 1%, w/v) and Tween 80 (1 or 2%, w/v) in double-distilled water and was subsequently added to the lipid phase under high-speed stirring (Ultra Turrax T25, IKA, Germany) at 8000 rpm for 30 s. The obtained pre-emulsion was subjected to high-pressure homogenization (Micron LAB 40, Germany) at 500 bar and 75 °C for ten cycles. For further size reduction, the emulsion was sonicated (Ultra sonic, tecno-Gaz Tecna 6, Italy) at 70% amplitude for 2, 4, 10, or 15 min. Afterwards, the nanoemulsion was cooled down to room temperature and then lyophilized (Freeze Drier, Christ, Germany) and stored at 4 °C. Blank NLCs were prepared by the same procedure.

Characterization of S-NLCs

Particle size, polydispersity index (PDI), and zeta potential (ZP)

NLCs dispersions were diluted by deionized water and the mean particle size, PDI, and ZP were analyzed at 25 °C by photon correlation spectroscopy (Zetasizer, Malvern Instruments, UK) ($n = 6$).

Morphological assessment

Scanning electron microscope (KYKY-EM3200, China) was used to evaluate the shape of nanoparticles.

Entrapment efficiency (EE) and drug loading capacity (DL)

S-NLC dispersion was placed in the upper chamber of an Amicon® centrifugal filter and centrifuged at 1500 g for 30 min. Then, the un-entrapped sesamol in the filtrate was analysed by high-performance liquid chromatography (HPLC) using Alliance 2695 system (Waters Corp, USA) with C18 column (250 × 4.6 mm, 5 μm) at room temperature. The mobile phase contained acetonitrile/

water/acetic acid (68:30:2, *v/v*) at flow rate of 1 ml/min and the sample injection volume was 50 µl. The limits of detection and quantification (LOD and LOQ) values were approximately 0.023 and 0.059 µg/ml, respectively, and the inter- and intra-day coefficients of variations were within ±5%. EE% and DL of S-NLCs were determined as follows:

$$EE\% = \frac{\text{The amount of sesamol encapsulated in NLCs}}{\text{Total amount of sesamol}} \times 100$$

$$DL\% = \frac{\text{The amount of sesamol encapsulated in NLCs}}{\text{Total amount of NLCs}} \times 100$$

Differential scanning calorimetry (DSC)

Thermal analysis of pure sesamol, cetyl palmitate, S-NLCs, or blank NLCs was performed by DSC apparatus (Mettler-Toledo, Switzerland). Each sample was placed in an aluminum pan and heated in the range 10–240 °C (10 °C/min) under a nitrogen purge (50 ml/min). Each experiment was carried out in triplicate.

In vitro release

The release profile of sesamol form NLCs was evaluated by dialysis membrane method [35]. Briefly, 5 ml of S-NLC solution was transferred into a dialysis bag with a molecular weight cut-off of 12 KD (Sigma laboratories, Osterode, Germany) which had been previously soaked in the release medium for 24 h. The dialysis bag was sealed at both ends and immersed in the receptor compartment containing 250 ml of phosphate-buffered saline (PBS, pH 7.4) in a shaking incubator (Heidolph Unimax 1010, Germany) at 37 °C and 100 rpm. At defined time intervals, 0.5-ml samples were collected from the receptor medium, replaced with pre-warmed fresh PBS of an equal volume, and assayed for sesamol content by HPLC. The percentage of dose released was plotted against the time and sesamol solution served as control. Experiments were carried out in triplicate.

Storage stability

Freeze-dried samples were kept at 4 °C. At defined time intervals (0, 1, 3, and 6 months), samples were resuspended in filtered water and analyzed for particle size, PDI, ZP, EE %, and DL %. The results were expressed as mean ± SEM ($n = 6$).

Evaluation of the bioactivity of S-NLCs
In vitro experiments

Cell culture

Rat pheochromocytoma-derived PC12 cells were grown in Dulbecco's modified Eagle's medium supplemented with fetal bovine serum (10%), horse serum (5%), streptomycin sulfate (100 µg/ml), penicillin G sodium (100 U/ml), and amphotericin B (0.25 µg/ml) in a humidified atmosphere with 5% CO_2 at 37 °C. The culture media were changed every day and experiments were carried out 72 h after seeding the cells.

In vitro model of ischemic stroke and treatments

Oxygen-glucose deprivation (OGD) is a well-recognized in vitro model of stroke and may also be used to develop novel neuroprotective agents or investigate the mechanisms underlying the brain ischemia [36]. PC12 cells were exposed to OGD insult as previously described [37]. In brief, the original culture medium was replaced with pre-warmed glucose-free Hepes buffer {in mM: Hepes (10), NaCl (150), KCl (5), $MgCl_2$ (1), $CaCl_2$ (2), pH 7.4} and antimycotic-antibiotic solution. Then, the cells were transferred into the anaerobic chamber flushed with 95% N_2 and 5% CO_2 for 1 and 8 h at 37 °C. The deoxygenation of media was monitored using the oxygen-sensing probes (dOxyBead™, Luxcel Biosciences, Cork, Ireland). In treatment groups, 20, 40, 80, and 100 µM of sesamol [6–10], S-NLCs (containing 20, 40, 80, and 100 µM of sesamol), vehicle, or blank NLCs were added to the cell cultures 24 h before and upon the OGD onset. In the case of any effect, cells were treated with specific PI3K inhibitor, LY294002, dissolved in 0.2% dimethyl sulfoxide (DMSO) at concentrations of 10, 20, and 50 µM [38, 39] 20 min before the application of the effective agent.

Cell viability assay

The viability of PC12 cells was assessed using MTT (3-[4,5-dimethylthiazol-2-yl]-2,5-diphenyl tetrazolium bromide) colorimetric assay [40]. 20 µl of MTT stock solution (5 mg/ml in PBS) was added to each well (1×10^4 cells/well) 4 h before the completion of re-oxygenation period. Then, the culture medium was aspirated and replaced with 100 µl of DMSO and the plate was shaken for 10 min in order to dissolve the crystals and the absorbance was determined at 570 nm (Anthos 2020, Anthos Labtec Instruments, Austria). Cell viability was expressed as the percentage of untreated control cells (assuming the survival rate of 100%) and presented as mean ± SEM of six independent experiments ($n = 6$).

Assessment of lactate dehydrogenase (LDH) activity

LDH activity is correlated to the lysed cell numbers [41]. In order to quantify LDH activity, the media were removed following the re-oxygenation period and to obtain the maximum LDH release values, cells were washed twice with PBS and lysed with 1% Triton X-100. The absorbance was recorded at 490 nm and the percentage of LDH release was calculated as follows; [LDH released into the media / (LDH released into the media + LDH released from the lysed cells)] × 100.

Morphological analysis

Following the re-oxygentaion period, PC12 cells were cultured in 24-well plates and fixed using 4% paraformaldehyde for 30 min at room temperature. Then, the cells were thoroughly washed with 0.02 M PBS and stained with 10 mg/ml of Hoechst 33,258 in the dark. Images were captured using a fluorescence microscope (Leica, Germany). The condensed nuclei were counted in six visual fields (~ 0.3 mm^2) in each group and the percentage of condensed nuclei over the total number of cells was calculated as previously described [42].

Assessment of the oxidative stress

PC12 cells (5×10^5) were homogenized and centrifuged at 3500 g for 20 min at 4 °C and the supernatant was collected for analysis of the reduced glutathione (GSH) and malondialdehyde (MDA) contents and catalase (CAT) and superoxide dismutase (SOD) activities by appropriate kits. Protein content of the supernatant was determined by Bradford method [43]. MDA and GSH contents were determined at 530 and 412 nm, respectively and expressed as nM/mg protein [44, 45]. SOD and CAT activities were evaluated at 560 and 240 nm, respectively and expressed as U/mg protein [46, 47].

In vivo experiments

Animals

Male Wistar rats (300–350 g) from our institution's laboratory animal centre were randomly assigned and housed under standard laboratory conditions with a 12-h light/dark cycle and food pellets and water provided ad libitum. The protocol for in vivo experiments was approved by the Institutional Animal Care and Use Committee.

Visualization of S-NLCs in rat brain

S-NLCs were labeled with coumarin-6 [(3-(2′-benzothiazolyl)-7-diethylaminocoumarin] as previously described [48]. 1 h after the intravenous (i.v.) injection of 25 mg/kg of the labelled S-NLCs, animals were deeply anaesthetized with intraperitoneal (i.p.) injection of ketamine/xylazine, perfused with 0.9% saline and 4% paraformaldehyde, and the brains were stored at –80 °C for 3 days. Afterwards, 20-μm cryosections were provided using a cryostat (Leica, Germany) and were observed under the fluorescence microscope.

Brain distribution study

Animals were sacrificed at 0.25, 0.5, 0.75, 1, 2, 4, 6, 8, 10, and 12 h following i.v. injection of 25 mg/kg of S-NLCs or free sesamol and then the brain tissue samples were collected, washed, and weighed for further sesamol analysis [49].

Animal groups, induction of ischemic stroke, and treatments

Rats were randomly assigned into the following groups; intact ($n = 6$), sham ($n = 10$), ischemia/reperfusion (I/R), I/R + vehicle, I/R + sesamol, I/R + S-NLCs, LY294002 + I/R + sesamol or S-NLCs, and I/R + blank NLCs ($n = 14$/group). Global cerebral ischemia was induced by a modified four-vessel occlusion (4-VO) method [50]. Animals exhibiting post-ischemic convulsions were excluded from the study. Sham-operated control group underwent the same surgical procedure without carotid ligation. Four days before and immediately after the stroke onset and during the reperfusion period, animals received once-daily i.v. injections of 5, 10, 20, and 25 mg/kg of sesamol (dissolved in 0.5% DMSO) [7–10], S-NLCs [containing the equivalent amounts of sesamol (5, 10, 20, and 25 mg/kg)], vehicle, or blank NLCs. In the case of any effect, LY294002 was dissolved in 3% DMSO and administered intracerebroventricularly (i.c.v.) at concentrations of 5, 10, and 25 μg/μl [51, 52] 20 min prior to the application of the effective agent.

Neurological deficit scoring

Post-ischemic neurological deficits were scored on a 5-point scale by an experimenter blinded to the treatment groups as follows, 0: no deficits, 1: difficulty in fully extending the contralateral forelimb, 2: unable to extend the contralateral forelimb, 3: mild circling to the contralateral side, 4: severe circling, and 5: falling to the contralateral side [53].

Behavioural assessments

Spatial learning and memory was assessed by Morris water-maze (MWM) test as previously described [54]. In order to assess the emotional memory, step-through passive avoidance test (STPAT) was performed [12].

Assessment of the brain infarcted area

Rats were anesthetized with 3.5% chloral hydrate and subjected to the intracardiac perfusion with 100 ml of isotonic saline. Then, animals were killed by decapitation and the brains were removed and sliced coronally at 2-mm intervals. Following the removal of dura mater and vascular tissue, slices were immersed into 2% 2,3,5-triphenyltetrazolium chloride (TTC, Sigma-Aldrich, Germany) solution in PBS (pH 7.4) for 30 min at 37 °C. Slices were turned over for several times and then washed twice in 10 ml of saline and kept in 10% phosphate buffered formalin (pH 7.4) overnight in a light-proof container for further photography. Infarcted areas of the brain sections were integrated and expressed as the percentage of total area [55].

Histological assessments

Neuronal loss in the hippocampal CA1 region was assessed as previously described [56]. Following the reperfusion period, animals were anesthetized with chloral hydrate (400 mg/kg, i.p.) and perfused intracardially with heparinized saline followed by 4% paraformaldehyde in 0.1 M PBS (pH 7.4). The brains were carefully removed, post-fixed in 4% paraformaldehyde for 24 h at 4 °C, and embedded in paraffin. For histological assessments which were performed by two observers blind to the experimental set-up, 5 μm-thick coronal sections from the dorsal hippocampus were prepared by a rotary microtome and stained with cresyl violet. Images were captured using a microscope (Olympus Optical Co, LTD, Japan) equipped with a digital camera system (Pixera 600CL-CU, Pixera Corporation, Japan). The survived neurons in CA1 regions of hippocampi were counted in 6 frames (1 mm^2/each) in five coronal sections and expressed as the percentage of total cell number.

Biochemical analysis

In other groups of animals, brains were removed and the hippocampi were immediately dissected on a frozen pad taken from a – 80 °C freezer [57], weighed, homogenized in ice-cold 0.1 M phosphate buffer (pH 7.4), sonicated for 30 s, and centrifuged at 12,000 g for 10 min. Then, the supernatants were collected to assess MDA and GSH contents and SOD and CAT activities as aforementioned. The protein contents of the supernatants were determined by Bradford method [43].

Statistical analysis

The normal distribution of data was verified by Shapiro-Wilk test. Two- or three-way ANOVA followed by Tukey's post hoc test were applied to analyse the cytotoxicity, behavioural, and biochemical data. Mann-Whitney U test was used to compare the neuron counts, brain infarcted area, and neurological deficit scores. Student's t-test was used in brain distribution study. Data are presented as mean ± SEM and the statistical significance was set at $P < 0.05$.

Results

Characterization of S-NLCs

S-NLCs dispersions were successfully prepared by a modified high-pressure homogenization technique without signs of phase separation or colour change during at least 1-month visual inspection. Using different ratios of solid and liquid lipids, sesamol and lipid, and surfactants or sonication time, various S-NLCs formulations with different physicochemical properties were prepared.

Application of the higher amount of oil lipid or surfactant resulted in the smaller particle size and higher entrapment efficiency (Table 1). Considering the EE%, DL%, and particle size, S-NLCs7 (Table 1) was selected as the optimal formulation for further experimental procedures. Based on the representative SEM images, the freshly-prepared S-NLCs (Fig. 1a) or those three months after freeze-drying (Fig. 1b) were spherical in shape and uniform in size. In DSC thermograms, pure sesamol showed a sharp endothermic peak around 64.59 °C (Fig. 2b) and the melting peak of cetyl palmitate was observed at 54.86 °C (Fig. 2c). The blank NLCs showed melting peak at 47.63 °C (Fig. 2d), while, S-NLCs displayed a melting peak at 43.81 °C three months after freeze drying (Fig. 2a). The release of sesamol from the solution was faster than S-NLCs formulation in which a controlled release pattern was observed (Fig. 3). In various S-NLCs formulations, the total release of 52.7 ± 4.8 to 77.8 ± 6.2% was achieved at the end of 48 h (Table 1). As shown in Table 2, the lyophilized nanoparticles remained stable at 4 °C without significant alterations in the particle size, PDI, ZP, EE or DL % during 6 months of storage ($P > 0.05$).

Evaluation of the bioactivity of S-NLCs

MTT assay

Following 1- and 8-h OGD insult, cell viability was significantly decreased (Fig. 4, $P < 0.001$ vs. control). Sesamol (80 and 100 μM) prevented the cell loss after 1-h OGD/R (Fig. 4a, P<0.05, $P < 0.01$ vs. OGD or OGD + vehicle group), while, it was ineffective after 8-h OGD/R (Fig. 4b, P>0.05). S-NLCs (containing 80 and 100 μM of sesamol) significantly prevented the cell loss after 1- and 8-h OGD/R (Fig. 4a and b, P<0.05, $P < 0.001$). Pretreatment with LY294002 (50 μM) prevented the cytoprotective effects of sesamol or S-NLCs (Figs 4a and b, P>0.05 vs. OGD or OGD + vehicle group). Pre-treatment with lower doses of LY294002 showed no effect and this antagonist had no effect by itself (data not shown). Sesamol or S-NLCs (20, 40, 80, and 100 μM) did not induce cytotoxicity in PC12 cells under the normal condition (not shown).

LDH release

LDH release was significantly increased in PC12 cells exposed to 1- or 8-h OGD/R (Fig. 5, $P < 0.001$ vs. control). Sesamol or S-NLCs (80 and 100 μM) prevented the enhancement of LDH activity due to 1-h OGD/R (Fig. 5a, P<0.01 and P < 0.001 vs. OGD or OGD + vehicle group). S-NLCs, but not sesamol, reduced LDH release following 8-h OGD/R (Fig. 5b, P<0.05 vs. OGD or OGD + vehicle group). Pretreatment with LY294002 (50 μM) reversed the effects of sesamol or S-NLCs (Fig. 5a and b, P>0.05 vs. OGD

Table 1 Physichochemical properties of sesamol-loaded NLCs

Formulation code	Particle size (nm)	PDI	ZP (mV)	EE (%)	DL (%)	DR after 48 h (%)
S-NLC1	137.4 ± 9.2	0.37 ± 0.04	−21.8 ± 0.51	41.4 ± 2.6	1.45 ± 0.14	52.7 ± 4.8
S-NLC2	123.6 ± 7.4	0.32 ± 0.01	−26.2 ± 0.37	47.7 ± 3.2	1.63 ± 0.08	57.3 ± 5.3
S-NLC3	104.3 ± 8.7	0.28 ± 0.03	−23.3 ± 0.63	66.3 ± 8.5	1.78 ± 0.12	68.5 ± 4.7
S-NLC4	66.3 ± 1.6	0.12 ± 0.07	−25.8 ± 0.58	94.3 ± 3.7	3.11 ± 0.06	82.3 ± 5.7
S-NLC5	73.8 ± 4.3	0.18 ± 0.07	−21.4 ± 0.47	92.7 ± 4.3	6.13 ± 0.17	77.8 ± 6.2
S-NLC6	81.6 ± 3.7	0.21 ± 0.05	−19.5 ± 0.53	89.2 ± 6.4	11.32 ± 3.4	74.6 ± 3.9
S-NLC7	92.3 ± 6.2	0.23 ± 0.04	−27.9 ± 0.56	94.2 ± 1.8	28.51 ± 1.2	69.8 ± 5.4
S-NLC8	124.7 ± 9.4	0.29 ± 0.09	−25.4 ± 0.45	91.4 ± 2.5	49.92 ± 3.7	60.3 ± 1.8
Blank NLCs	52.4 ± 6.7	0.13 ± 0.06	−18.7 ± 0.72	–	–	–

Data are represented as mean ± SEM ($n = 6$)

(*PDI* polydispersity index, *ZP* zeta potential, *EE* entrapment efficiency, *DL* drug loading, *DR* drug release, *S-NLCs* sesamol-loaded nanostructured lipid carriers)

or OGD + vehicle group), while, the lower doses of LY294002 showed no effect (data not shown). LY294002 showed no effect per se (not shown). Sesamol or S-NLCs (20, 40, 80, and 100 μM) did not significantly affect LDH release form PC12 cells under the normal condition (not shown).

Morphological alterations in PC12 cells induced by OGD
Exposure to 1- or 8-h OGD/R resulted in the reduced cell number and alteration in cellular morphology (Fig. 6b and c, respectively) as compared to the control (Fig. 6a). Sesamol (100 μM) attenuated the cellular damage due to 1-h OGD (Fig. 6d), however, it was ineffective

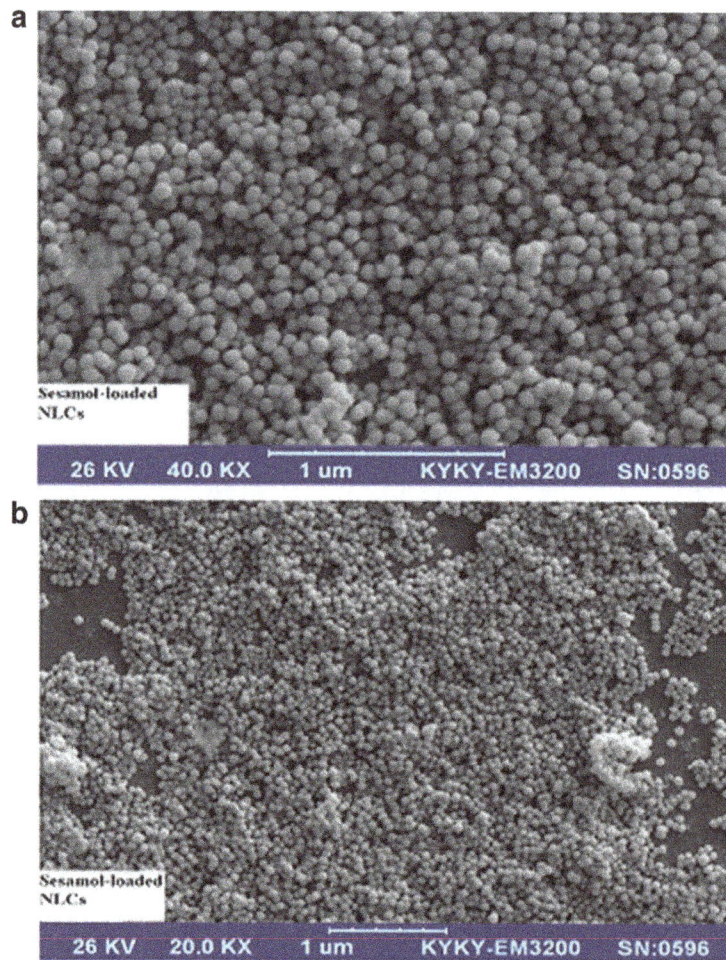

Fig. 1 Scanning electron micrographs of sesamol-loaded NLCs. The spherical shape and smooth surface with relatively uniform size are observed in highly-concentrated nanoparticles (formulation S-NLC7). **a** fresh sample with higher magnification, no pore on the nanoparticle surface is observed, **b** The non-aggregated and finely-dispersed nanoparticles three months after freeze drying

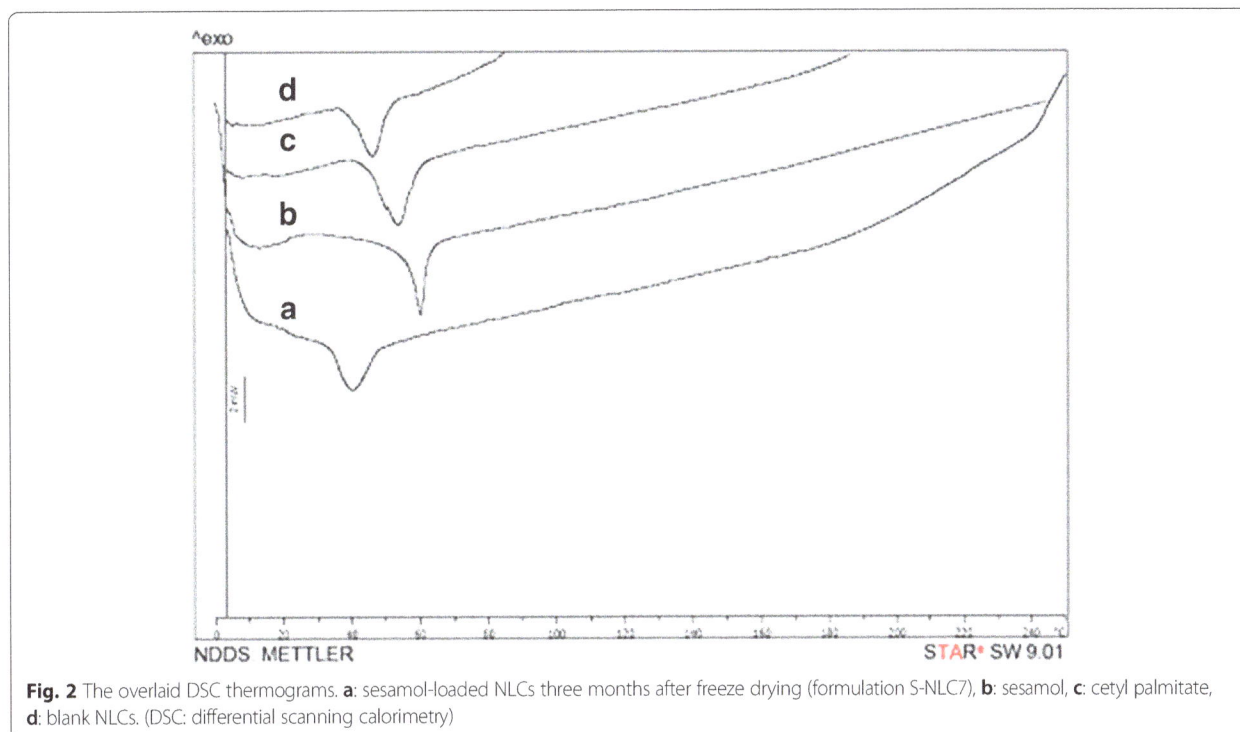

Fig. 2 The overlaid DSC thermograms. **a**: sesamol-loaded NLCs three months after freeze drying (formulation S-NLC7), **b**: sesamol, **c**: cetyl palmitate, **d**: blank NLCs. (DSC: differential scanning calorimetry)

following 8-h OGD insult (Fig. 6f). Cells treated with S-NLCs (containing 100 μM of sesamol) displayed improved morphology following both 1- and 8-h OGD (Fig. 6e and g, respectively). Pretreatment with LY294002 (50 μM) prevented the cytoprotective effect of S-NLCs (Fig. 6h). The significant enhancement of condensed nuclei induced by 1- or 8-h OGD (Fig. 6i and j, $P<0.001$ vs. the control) was prevented by 80 and 100 μM of sesamol or S-NLCs after 1-h OGD (Fig. 6i, $P<0.01$, $P < 0.001$). S-NLCs (containing 80

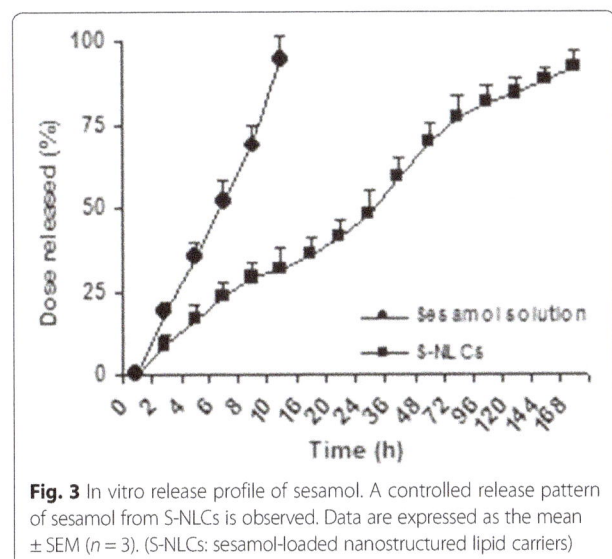

Fig. 3 In vitro release profile of sesamol. A controlled release pattern of sesamol from S-NLCs is observed. Data are expressed as the mean ± SEM ($n = 3$). (S-NLCs: sesamol-loaded nanostructured lipid carriers)

and 100 μM of sesamol), but not free sesamol, prevented the formation of condensed nuclei due to 8-h OGD insult (Fig. 6j, $P<0.001$). Pretreatment with LY294002 (50 μM) prevented the cytoprotective effects (Fig. 6i and j, $P>0.05$ vs. OGD or OGD + vehicle group), however, the lower doses of this antagonist were ineffective (not shown). LY294002 showed no effect by itself (not shown).

The effects of sesamol or S-NLCs on OGD-induced oxidative stress

As shown in Table 3, induction of OGD for 1 or 8 h resulted in a significant elevation of MDA level and reduction of GSH content and CAT and SOD activities in PC12 cells ($P < 0.001$ vs. control). Following 1-h OGD, 80 and 100 μM of free sesamol reduced MDA ($P < 0.05$ and $P < 0.01$ vs. OGD and OGD + vehicle groups), and elevated GSH content ($P < 0.05$) and activities of SOD ($P < 0.05$, $P < 0.01$) and CAT ($P < 0.001$), however, sesamol was ineffective following 8-h OGD ($P > 0.05$). S-NLCs (containing 80 and 100 μM of sesamol) showed antioxidant effects after both 1- and 8-h OGD (MDA: $P < 0.01$, $P < 0.001$; GSH: $P < 0.05$; SOD: $P < 0.05$, $P < 0.001$; and CAT: $P < 0.001$ vs. OGD or OGD + vehicle group). Pre-treatment with LY294002 (50 μM) prevented the antioxidant effects ($P > 0.05$ vs. OGD or OGD + vehicle group), while the lower doses were ineffective (not shown). LY294002 showed no effect by itself (not shown).

Table 2 The stability profile of sesamol-loaded NLCs

Initial					1st Month				
Size	PDI	ZP	EE%	DL%	Size	PDI	ZP	EE%	DL%
$92.3 \pm 6.2 \pm 1.2$	0.23 ± 0.04	-27.9 ± 0.5	94.2 ± 1.8	28.51	95.1 ± 4.9	0.19 ± 0.09	-25.3 ± 0.3	92.7 ± 5.4	26.84 ± 1.7
3rd Month					6th Month				
Size	PDI	ZP	EE%	DL%	Size	PDI	ZP	EE%	DL%
94.3 ± 4.1	0.21 ± 0.07	-26.5 ± 0.4	95.5 ± 2.4	28.03 ± 1.9	99.8 ± 3.3	0.19 ± 0.07	-23.7 ± 0.8	89.62 ± 4.7	25.86 ± 0.9

Data are represented as mean $\pm$ SEM (n = 6)

(*PDI* polydispersity index, *ZP* zeta potential, *EE* entrapment efficiency, *DL* drug loading, *S-NLCs* sesamol-loaded nanostructured lipid carriers)

In vivo experiments

Brain delivery of S-NLCs

Using coumarin-6-loaded nanoparticles, S-NLCs entry into the hippocampus was demonstrated (Fig. 7a). Based on the brain distribution study, administration of S-NLCs provided a significantly higher brain concentrations of sesamol as compared to the free sesamol (Fig. 7b, $P<0.001$).

The effects of sesamol solution or S-NLCs on I/R-induced neurobehavioral deficits

As shown Table 4, neurological deficit score was significantly increased in I/R or I/R + vehicle group ($P < 0.001$ vs. sham or intact group) and decreased in the groups treated with S-NLCs containing 20 or 25 mg/kg of sesamol ($P < 0.01$ and $P < 0.001$ vs. I/R or I/R + vehicle group). Furthermore, global ischemia impaired the learning and

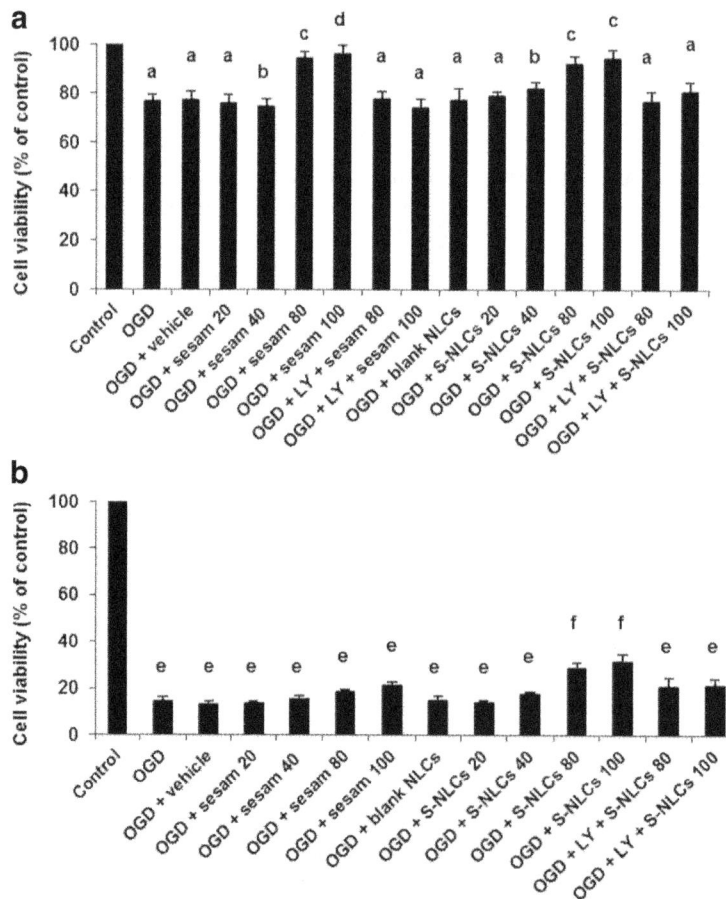

Fig. 4 Viability assay in PC12 cell culture. Following 1- and 8-h OGD insult (**a** and **b**, respectively), the viability of PC12 cells were assessed by MTT assay. As shown, S-NLCs elevate the cell viability for longer time period. Pre-treatment with LY294002 (50 μM) reversed the cytoprotective effects. Data are presented as mean $\pm$ SEM of six independent experiments. (OGD: oxygen-glucose deprivation, OGD + sesam 20, 40, 80, and 100: administration of 20–100 μM of sesamol 24 h before and upon the OGD insult, OGD + S-NLCs 20, 40, 80, and 100: administration of S-NLCs (containing 20–100 μM of sesamol) 24 h before and upon the OGD insult, LY: LY294002, S-NLCs: sesamol-loaded nanostructured lipid carriers). [a, e] $P < 0.001$ and [b] $P < 0.01$ vs. the control group, [c] $P < 0.05$ and [d] $P < 0.01$ vs. OGD and OGD + vehicle, [f] $P < 0.001$ vs. control, OGD, and OGD + vehicle

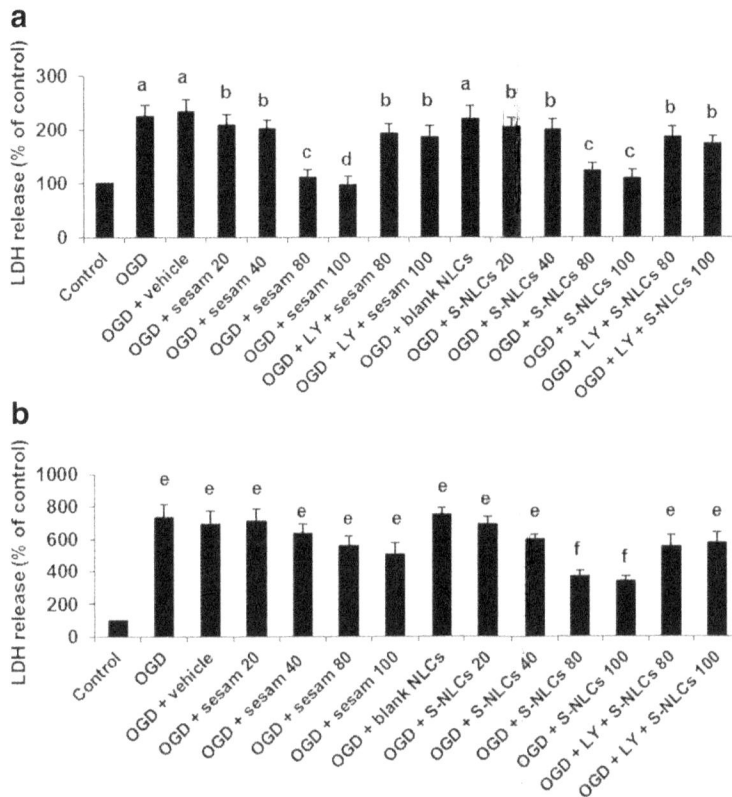

Fig. 5 The effect of OGD, sesamol, or S-NLCs on LDH release. S-NLCs effectively prevented the enhancement of LDH release after both 1-h (**a**) and 8-h OGD (**b**) that was reversed due to the pre-treatment with LY294002 (50 μM). Data are presented as the mean ± SEM of six independent experiments. [a, e] $P < 0.001$, and [b] $P < 0.01$ vs. the control, [c, d] $P < 0.01$ vs. OGD and OGD+ vehicle, [f] $P < 0.05$ vs. control and $P < 0.001$ vs. OGD and OGD + vehicle. (LDH: lactate dehydrogenase, OGD: oxygen-glucose deprivation, LY: LY294002, S-NLCs: sesamol-loaded nanostructured lipid carriers)

memory as revealed by MWMT or STPAT ($P < 0.001$ vs. sham or intact group). Treatment with S-NLCs (20 and 25 mg/kg) significantly improved the learning and memory ($P < 0.05$ and $P < 0.001$ vs. I/R or I/R + vehicle group). The free sesamol failed to affect I/R-induced neurobehavioral deficits at any dose tested ($P > 0.05$ vs. I/R or I/R + vehicle group). Pretreatment with LY294002 (25 μg/μl) abolished the ameliorative effects of S-NLCs ($P > 0.05$ vs. I/R or I/R + vehicle group). Pretreatment with lower doses of LY294002 showed no effect (not shown). LY294002 had no effect by itself (not shown).

The effects of S-NLCs or sesamol on the brain infarction induced by global cerebral I/R

TTC staining revealed the significantly increased infarcted areas in I/R group [Fig. 8b and f, $P<0.001$ vs. sham group (Fig. 8a and f)]. FA even at the highest dose tested (25 mg/kg) failed to prevent I/R-induced brain infarction (Fig. 8d and f, $P>0.05$ vs. I/R group), while, FA-NLCs (25 mg/kg) showed protective effect (Fig. 8c and f, $P<0.01$ vs. I/R group). Pre-treatment with LY294002 (25 μg/μl) abolished the protective effect of FA-NLCs (Fig. 8e and f, $P>0.05$ vs. I/R group). The lower doses of LY294002

were ineffective and the antagonist showed no effect by itself (not shown).

The effects of sesamol or S-NLCs on I/R-induced neuronal damage in the hippocampal CA1 region

Based on the histological evaluation, global cerebral ischemia induced the neuronal damage in the hippocampal CA1 region as revealed by the formation of dark-stained cells with dysmorphic shape (Fig. 9b) and less survived neurons (Fig. 9f, $P<0.001$ vs. sham or intact group) as compared to the sham group with closely arranged round cells including the distinct nucleus and nucleolus (Fig. 9a). Treatment with S-NLCs (25 mg/kg) improved the cell morphology (Fig. 9c) and significantly increased the number of survived cells (Fig. 9f, $P<0.001$ vs. I/R or I/R + vehicle group), while, free sesamol even at the highest dose tested (25 mg/kg) was ineffective against I/R-induced neuronal damage (Figs 9d and f, $P>0.05$). Pre-treatment with LY294002 (25 μg/μl) abolished the neuroprotective effect of S-NLCs (Figs. 9e and f, $P>0.05$ vs. I/R group or I/R + vehicle group), while, pretreatment with lower doses of LY294002 showed no

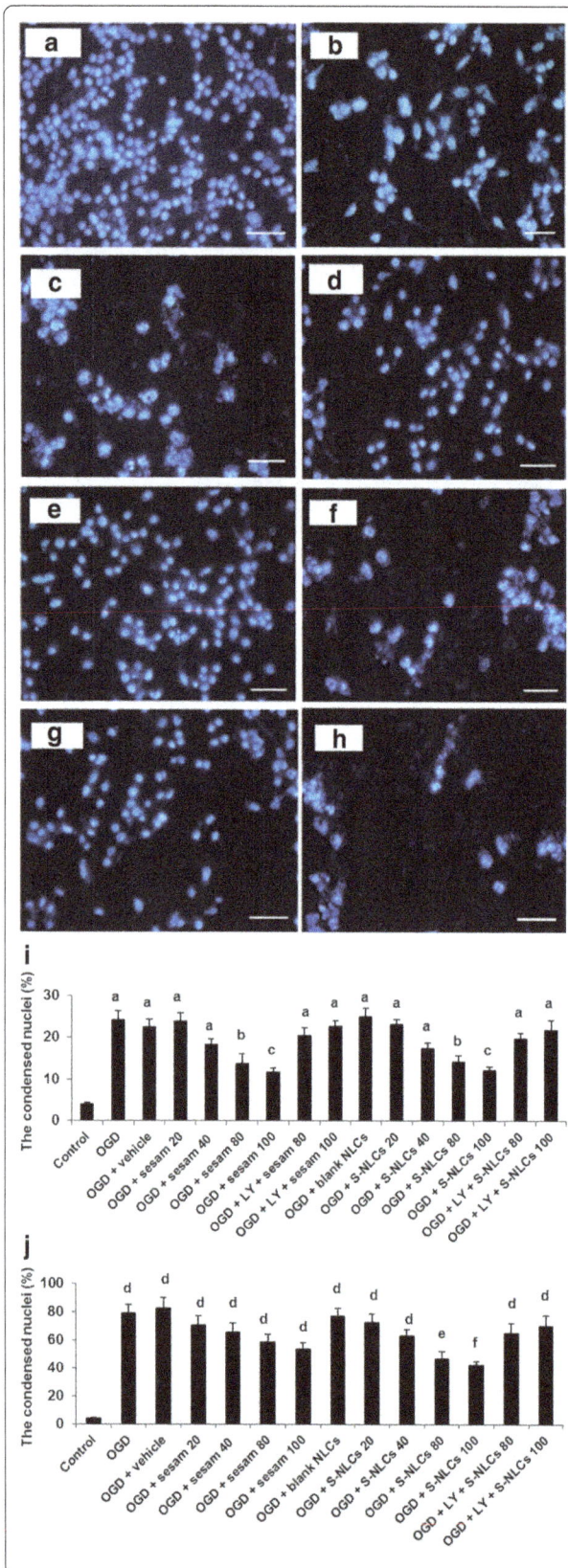

Fig. 6 Morphological alterations in PC12 cells exposed to OGD and quantitative analysis of the condensed nuclei. A high density of round cells is demonstrated in the control cells, while, alteration in the cellular morphology and enhancement of condensed nuclei occurred following 1- and 8-h OGD. Treatment of PC12 cells with sesamol or S-NLCs 24 h before and upon the exposure to 1-h OGD resulted in the ameliorative effects. Unlike free sesamol, S-NLCs preserved the protective effects following the longer exposure to OGD insult. Pre-treatment with LY294002 (50 μM) reversed the cytoprotective effects. **a**: control cells, **b**: 1-h OGD insult, **c**: 8-h OGD insult, **c**: sesamol (100 μM) + 1-h OGD, **e**: S-NLCs (100 μM) + 1-h OGD, **f**: sesamol (100 μM) + 8-h OGD, **g**: S-NLCs (100 μM) + 8-h OGD, **h**: LY294002 (50 μM) + S-NLCs (100 μM) + 8-h OGD (scale bars: 50 μm), **i**: (1-h OGD insult), **j** (8-h OGD insult). The numbers of condensed nuclei have been represented as the percentage of total number of nuclei counted. Data are mean ± SEM of six different cell culture preparations. [a, d] $P < 0.001$ vs. the control group, [b] $P < 0.01$ vs. control, OGD, and OGD + vehicle,[c] $P < 0.05$ vs. control, and $P < 0.001$ vs. OGD and OGD + vehicle, [e] $P < 0.001$ vs. control and $P < 0.01$ vs. OGD and OGD + vehicle, [f] $P < 0.001$ vs. control, OGD, and OGD + vehicle. (OGD: oxygen-glucose deprivation, LY: LY294002, S-NLCs: sesamol-loaded nanostructured lipid carriers)

effect (not shown). This PI3K antagonist showed no effect by itself (not shown).

The effects of sesamol or S-NLCs on I/R-induced oxidative stress in the hippocampus

As shown in Table 5, I/R led to the significant elevation of MDA ($P < 0.01$) and reduction of GSH ($P < 0.001$), SOD ($P < 0.001$), and CAT ($P < 0.001$) as compared to the sham or intact group. This, was prevented by 20 and 25 mg/kg of S-NLCs (MDA: $P < 0.01$; GSH: $P < 0.05$, $P < 0.01$; SOD: $P < 0.01$, $P < 0.001$; and CAT: $P < 0.01$ vs. I/R or I/R + vehicle.), while, free sesamol failed to prevent I/R-induced oxidative stress at any dose tested ($P > 0.05$ vs. I/R or I/R + vehicle). Pre-treatment with LY294002 (25 μg/μl) reversed the protective effect of S-NLCs against I/R-induced oxidative stress ($P > 0.05$ vs. I/R group or I/R + vehicle group), however, the lower doses of LY294002 were ineffective (not shown). LY294002 showed no effect by itself (not shown).

Discussion

Cerebral stroke has remained a major healthcare challenge. Recombinant tissue plasminogen activator (r-tPA) remains the sole medication, however, it should be administered in a short time after onset of symptoms [1]. Over the last decade, phenolic compounds such as sesamol have been the focus of intense research due to their antioxidant and neuroprotective properties, however, poor solubility or rapid metabolism may negatively affect their effectiveness [12, 13, 58–61]. In the present study, we have prepared S-NLCs as the nanoreserviors to provide longer-lasting therapeutic effects for sesamol in both in vitro and in vivo models of ischemic stroke. S-NLCs showed high stability profile during 6-month

Table 3 Effects of sesamol or S-NLCs on the biochemical parameters following the ischemic insult

Groups	MDA (nM/mg protein)		GSH (nM/mg protein)		SOD (U/mg protein)		CAT (U/mg protein)	
	1 h	8 h	1 h	8 h	1 h	8 h	1 h	8 h
Control	0.53 ± 0.04	0.57 ± 0.05	12.97 ± 1.19	12.71 ± 0.93	39.67 ± 2.94	38.29 ± 1.87	6.83 ± 0.44	6.88 ± 0.47
OGD	1.32 ± 0.10**	2.02 ± 0.25***	7.13 ± 0.49***	3.81 ± 0.36***	24.94 ± 2.38***	18.77 ± 1.14***	2.44 ± 0.19***	1.49 ± 0.18***
OGD + vehicle	1.37 ± 0.14**	1.91 ± 0.14***	7.29 ± 0.57***	3.65 ± 0.22***	23.63 ± 1.82***	19.35 ± 1.29***	2.32 ± 0.25***	1.53 ± 0.16***
OGD + sesamol (20 µM)	1.38 ± 0.23**	2.12 ± 0.21***	7.92 ± 0.48***	3.58 ± 0.17***	23.02 ± 2.11***	19.83 ± 1.82***	2.45 ± 0.14***	1.47 ± 0.13***
OGD + sesamol (40 µM)	1.22 ± 0.19**	1.76 ± 0.13***	7.22 ± 0.45***	3.81 ± 0.25***	26.83 ± 1.96**	18.22 ± 2.16***	2.76 ± 0.27**	1.64 ± 0.11***
OGD + sesamol (80 µM)	0.65 ± 0.06&	1.88 ± 0.11***	10.62 ± 0.83#	4.83 ± 0.28**	37.06 ± 1.89ω	21.63 ± 1.96***	4.28 ± 0.36Φ	1.59 ± 0.16***
OGD + sesamol (100 µM)	0.59 ± 0.03ᴨ	1.79 ± 0.09***	10.29 ± 0.52Δ	4.17 ± 0.13***	36.94 ± 2.14Ω	20.17 ± 1.07***	4.86 ± 0.19Q	1.73 ± 0.08***
LY + OGD + sesamol (80 µM)	1.43 ± 0.09**	1.94 ± 0.22**	7.56 ± 0.62**	4.33 ± 0.24***	25.17 ± 1.03***	18.73 ± 2.45***	2.34 ± 0.23**	1.29 ± 0.18**
LY + OGD + sesamol (100 µM)	1.28 ± 0.15**	1.67 ± 0.19**	8.19 ± 0.62**	4.61 ± 0.17***	23.86 ± 2.87**	21.08 ± 1.66***	2.69 ± 0.14***	1.55 ± 0.07***
OGD + blank NLCs	1.35 ± 0.16**	2.07 ± 0.17***	7.58 ± 0.67***	3.47 ± 0.18***	25.17 ± 2.34**	18.16 ± 1.01***	2.36 ± 0.15***	1.54 ± 0.12***
OGD + S-NLCs (20 µM)	1.15 ± 0.11*	1.98 ± 0.10***	7.38 ± 0.81***	4.26 ± 0.39***	27.70 ± 1.94**	17.38 ± 1.64***	2.23 ± 0.15***	1.71 ± 0.18***
OGD + S-NLCs (40 µM)	1.17 ± 0.08*	1.92 ± 0.16***	8.25 ± 0.89**	4.75 ± 0.17***	29.38 ± 1.33*	20.52 ± 2.02***	3.42 ± 0.24**	1.85 ± 0.21***
OGD + S-NLCs (80 µM)	0.58 ± 0.03*	1.02 ± 0.16Θ	10.87 ± 0.55$	6.67 ± 0.59@	35.33 ± 2.12ε	27.84 ± 2.14φ	4.86 ± 0.27β	2.83 ± 0.26ᵁ
OGD + S-NLCs (100 µM)	0.47 ± 0.04Σ	0.92 ± 0.07∞	11.03 ± 0.42©	7.49 ± 0.38£	34.52 ± 1.84	29.03 ± 1.23*	4.73 ± 0.14φφ	2.96 ± 0.23ᵁ
LY + OGD + S-NLCs (80 µM)	1.23 ± 0.07*	1.48 ± 0.33**	8.07 ± 0.24**	4.25 ± 0.19***	24.13 ± 1.08**	17.88 ± 1.13***	3.11 ± 0.19***	1.63 ± 0.09***
LY + OGD + S-NLCs (100 µM)	1.37 ± 0.19**	1.27 ± 0.08***	7.58 ± 0.13***	4.72 ± 0.22***	22.96 ± 1.85***	21.32 ± 1.89***	2.65 ± 0.27**	1.96 ± 0.16***

PC12 cells have been exposed to 1 and 8 h oxygen-glucose deprivation. Each value represents the mean ± SEM of six independent experiments

(*MDA* malondialdehyde, *GSH* reduced glutathione, *CAT* catalase, *SOD* superoxide dismutase, *OGD* oxygen-glucose deprivation, *S-NLCs* sesamol-loaded nanostructured lipid carriers, *LY* LY294002)

*$P < 0.05$, **$P < 0.01$, ***$P < 0.001$ vs. control, #, $, ©, &, €, Q, Δ, @, £, Ω $P < 0.05$ vs. OGD and OGD + vehicle, ᴨ, ¥, Σ, Θ, ω $P < 0.01$ vs. OGD and OGD + vehicle, ∞, Φ, Q, β, φ, *$P < 0.001$ vs. control, OGD, and OGD + vehicle, φ $P < 0.01$ vs. control and $P < 0.05$ vs. OGD and OGD + vehicle, ᵁ, ᵘ $P < 0.001$ vs. control and $P < 0.01$ vs. OGD and OGD + vehicle

follow up (Table 2) that might be due to the binary mixture of solid and liquid lipids which elevates the imperfection and minimizes the drug expulsion. The homogeneous S-NLCs with narrow particle size distribution and suitable ZP (Table 1), preserved their uniformity and spherical shape during the storage (Fig. 1) indicating the suitability of materials and preparation technique. In contrast to SLNs in which the aggregation or perikinetic flocculation may occur during the storage [27–29], the particles in highly-concentrated NLCs formed a network (Fig. 1b) that may not result in the collision of particles during the long-term storage.

Thermal behaviours of bulk materials, blank NLCs, and S-NLCs were determined by DSC (Fig. 2). The disappearance of sharp endothermic peak of pure sesamol in DSC thermogram of S-NLCs suggests that sesamol is distributed in an amorphous status. Furthermore, the melting peaks of blank- or S-NLCs shifted to the lower temperature indicating that the bulk materials have been transformed into the nanoparticulate forms. Small particle size and enhanced surface of nanoparticles may also result in the depression of melting point [62]. S-NLCs showed lower melting point as compared to the blank NLCs that might be due to the incorporation of sesamol into the lipid matrix.

A hyperbolic trend in the release profile (Fig. 3) indicates the controlled-release pattern of sesamol from NLCs which may be due to the partitioning of sesamol between the lipid and aqueous phases and interactions between the surfactant-lipid or sesamol-lipid molecules. The prolonged release may also be attributed to the diffusion of sesamol from the lipid core of NLCs. This kind of release pattern by providing a constant

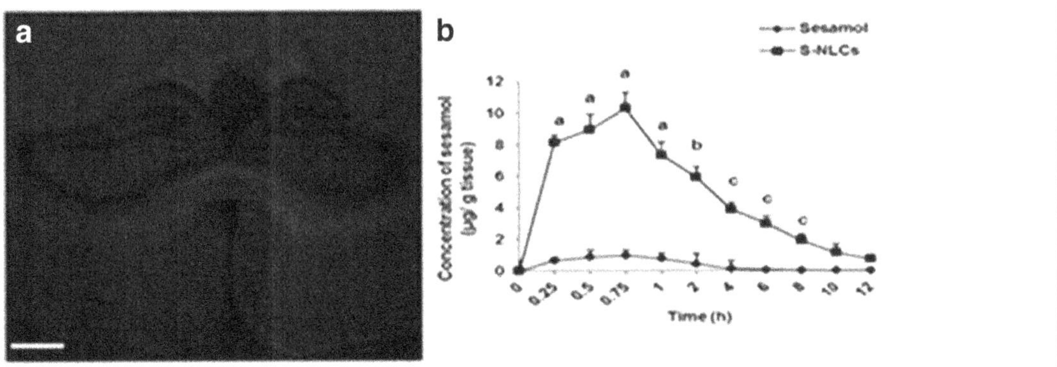

Fig. 7 The brain delivery of S-NLCs. **a**: The presence of coumarin-6-loaded S-NLCs in the hippocampus which is one of the most vulnerable brain regions in the ischemic stroke (scale bar: 500 µm), **b**: Brain distribution study shows that S-NLCs provide significantly higher concentrations of sesamol in the brain. ª $P < 0.001$, ᵇ $P < 0.01$, and ᶜ $P < 0.05$ vs. sesamol-treated group. (S-NLCs: sesamol-loaded nanostructured lipid carriers)

Table 4 The effects of sesamol or S-NLCs on I/R-induced neurobehavioral deficits

Groups scores	Neurological (1–5)	MWMT TSTQ (s)	STPAT Latency (s)
Sham	0	75.38 ± 6.26	283.17 ± 10.69
Intact	0	77.21 ± 4.23	278.42 ± 12.18
I/R	3.84 ± 0.36 [a]	16.33 ± 1.14 [a]	179.11 ± 9.46 [a]
I/R + vehicle	3.67 ± 0.44 [a]	14.83 ± 0.79 [a]	184.40 ± 11.32 [a]
I/R + sesamol (5 mg/kg)	3.44 ± 0.49 [a]	17.66 ± 1.02 [a]	176.61 ± 7.47 [a]
I/R + sesamol (10 mg/kg)	3.52 ± 0.23 [a]	15.79 ± 0.76 [a]	185.63 ± 11.33 [a]
I/R + sesamol (20 mg/kg)	3.74 ± 0.38 [a]	19.49 ± 1.31 [a]	183.57 ± 9.97 [a]
I/R + sesamol (25 mg/kg)	2.98 ± 0.29 [a]	16.65 ± 1.27 [a]	195.46 ± 12.68 [a]
I/R + blank NLCs	4.03 ± 0.26 [a]	18.33 ± 0.62 [a]	173.77 ± 7.63 [a]
I/R + S-NLCs (5 mg/kg)	3.57 ± 0.22 [a]	26.42 ± 2.41 [a]	189.27 ± 16.54 [a]
I/R + S-NLCs (10 mg/kg)	3.28 ± 0.17 [a]	23.79 ± 2.29 [a]	177.11 ± 11.13 [a]
I/R + S-NLCs (20 mg/kg)	1.76 ± 0.13 [b]	59.61 ± 3.76 [d]	217.50 ± 9.56 [e]
I/R + S-NLCs (25 mg/kg)	1.27 ± 0.07 [c]	66.27 ± 4.33[c]	237.33 ± 13.10 [c]
LY + I/R + S-NLCs (20 mg/kg)	3.55 ± 0.47 [a]	18.43 ± 1.75 [a]	180.16 ± 9.76 [a]
LY + I/R + S-NLCs (25 mg/kg)	3.21 ± 0.29 [a]	16.77 ± 2.93 [a]	191.45 ± 12.37 [a]

S-NLCs, but not free sesamol, significantly attenuated the neurobehavioral deficits induced by global ischemia. Data are presented as mean ± SEM ($n = 6$)

(I/R ischemia/reperfusion, S-NLCs sesamol-loaded nanostructured lipid carriers, LY LY294002 (25 µg/µl), MWMT Morris water maze test, TSTQ time spent in target quadrant, STPAT: step-through passive avoidance test, latency; time spent in crossing from the illuminated to the darkened compartment)

[a]$P < 0.001$ vs. sham or intact, [b]$P < 0.01$ vs. sham, intact, I/R, or I/R + vehicle, [c] $P < 0.001$ vs. I/R or I/R + vehicle, [d] $P < 0.01$ vs. sham or intact and $P < 0.001$ vs. I/R or I/R + vehicle, [e]$P < 0.05$ vs. I/R or I/R + vehicle

concentration of sesamol for longer time period might be of therapeutic value.

Since the cell internalization of nanoparticles is highly influenced by their size and surface properties, we selected S-NLCs7 as the optimal formulation due to the suitable EE%, DL%, and particle size (Table 1). These types of nanoparticles with particle diameter less than 100 nm and large surface area have shown unique biological effects such as the ability to bypass the reticuloendothelial system. Furthermore, the probability of destruction or phagocytosis is minimized [27–29] that may result in the enhanced retention time and efficiency. In this respect, these nanoparticles have been suggested as suitable carriers for effective drug delivery into the brain [27]. Regarding the bioactivity of S-NLCs in an in vitro model of ischemic stroke, MTT assay revealed that S-NLCs, but not free sesamol, exert dose-dependent

protective effects in longer exposure to OGD/R (Fig. 4) indicating the ability of this nanocarrier to provide a sustained concentration of sesamol. The cellular damage was also evaluated by measuring an indicator of cell toxicity, LDH, the cytoplasmic enzyme which is rapidly released into the cell culture medium following the damage of cell plasma membrane. In general, increased LDH activity has been recognized as a marker for the ischemic processes or cell death [39]. As shown in Fig. 5, sesamol solution failed to prevent the enhancement of LDH due to 8-h OGD, while, S-NLCs showed efficiency at both 1- and 8-h OGD indicating the ability of this nanocompound to protect sesamol against the rapid metabolism leading to the prolonged protective effects.

Unlike the free sesamol, S-NLCs protected PC12 cells, a model of neuron-like cells, against the morphological alterations due to 8-h OGD (Fig. 6) indicating the prolonged

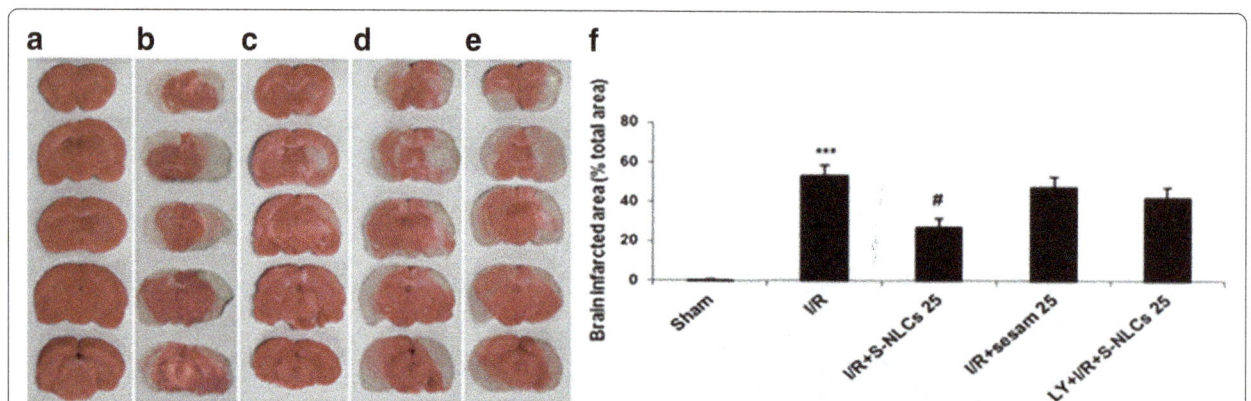

Fig. 8 Representative photographs of brain coronal sections stained with TTC. **a**: sham, **b**: I/R (infarcted areas have been shown in white), **c**: S-NLCs (containing 25 mg/kg of sesamol) + I/R, **d**: sesamol (25 mg/kg) + I/R, **e**: LY294002 (25 µg/µl) + S-NLCs (25 mg/kg) + I/R, **f**: The percentage of brain infarcted area with respect to the total area. Data are represented as mean ± SEM (n = 6). *** P < 0.001 vs. sham, # P < 0.01 vs. I/R group. (TTC: 2,3,5-triphenyltetrazolium chloride, I/R: ischemia/reperfusion, LY: LY294002, S-NLCs: sesamol-loaded nanostructured lipid carriers)

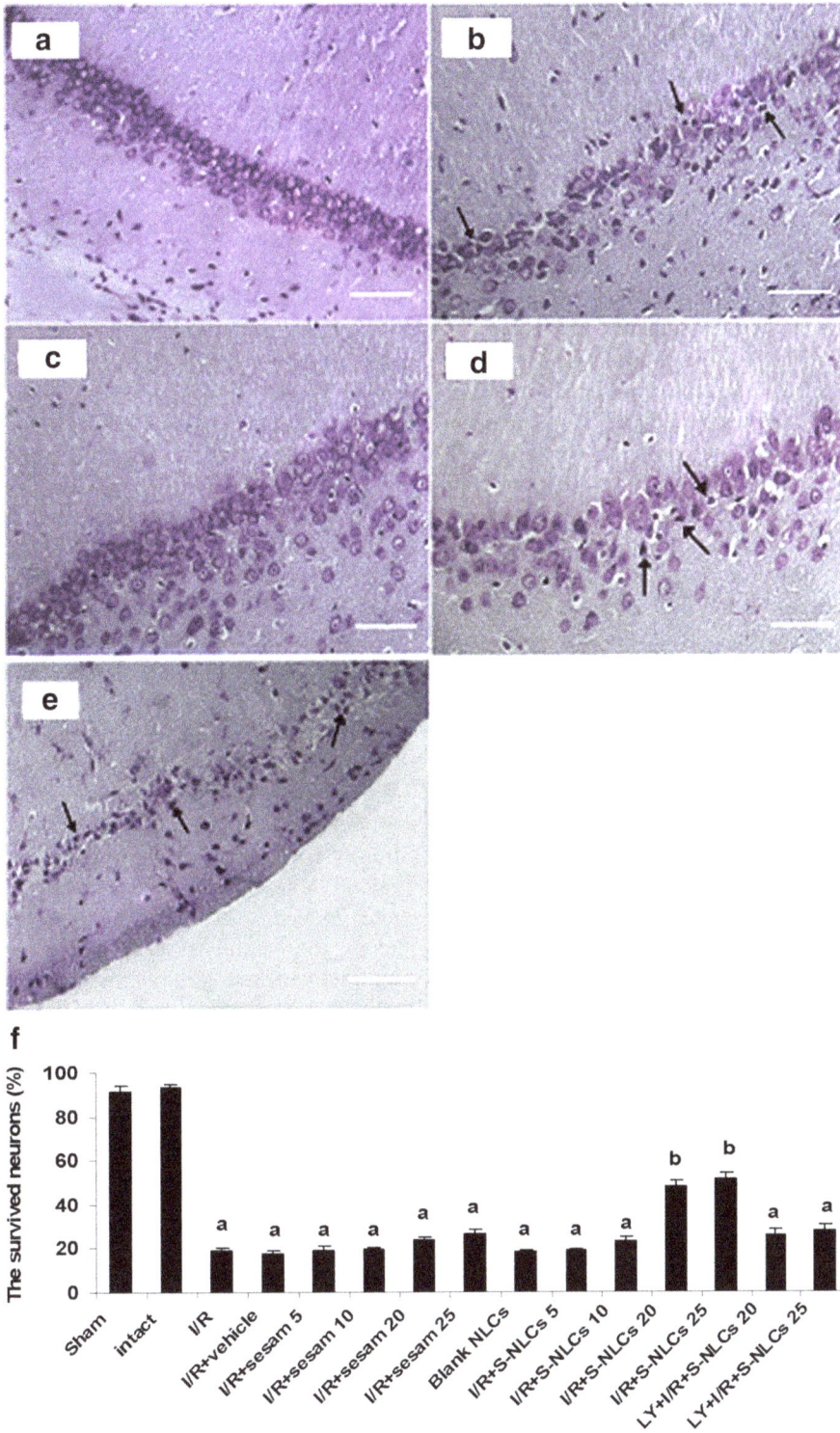

Fig. 9 (See legend on next page.)

(See figure on previous page.)

Fig. 9 Representative photomicrographs of hippocampal slices and quantitative analysis of the survived neurons in CA1 sub-regions. **a**: The viable round cells with distinct nucleus and nucleolus in sham-operated group, **b**: Dark-stained cells with dysmorphic or shrunken shape (black arrows) due to 10-min ischemia followed by 72 h reperfusion, **c**: Treatment with S-NLCs (containing 25 mg/kg of sesamol) attenuated I/R-induced neuronal damage, **d**: Free sesamol (25 mg/kg) failed to effectively prevent I/R-induced neuronal injury, **e**: Pre-treatment with LY294002 (25 µg/µl) abolished the ameliorative effects of S-NLCs (25 mg/kg), (scale bars: 50 µm). **f**: S-NLCs (20 and 25 mg/kg), but not sesamol, significantly increased the survived neurons in the hippocampal CA1 region. Pre-treatment with LY294002 (25 µg/µl) prevented the neuroprotective effects of S-NLCs. Data are expressed as mean ± SEM (n = 6). [a] P < 0.001 vs. sham or intact group, [b] P < 0.001 vs. sham, intact, I/R or I/R + vehicle groups. (I/R: ischemia/reperfusion, LY: LY294002, S-NLCs: sesamol-loaded nanostructured lipid carriers)

therapeutic effect of S-NLCs. As shown in Table 3, S-NLCs, but not sesamol, dose-dependently suppressed 8-h OGD-induced oxidative stress as revealed by the ability of this nanocarrier to reduce the production of MDA, an indicator of free radical generation, oxidative stress, and tissue injury [63], and enhance the content of GSH, a free radical scavenger and an essential component of cellular defence mechanism against the oxidative stress [64], and activities of SOD, an essential enzyme for the removal of superoxide radicals and protecting the cells against the oxidative injury [65], and CAT which is responsible for degradation of H_2O_2 and protects the cells against the oxidative stress [66]. These findings indicate the ability of NLCs to provide longer-lasting effects for sesamol. Based on the protective effects of sesamol against the neuronal injury [6–8, 11–13, 67], the extended activity of this phenolic compound might be of therapeutic significance against the cellular dysfunction in the acute or chronic forms of neural injury.

Besides the application of the visualization technique and brain distribution study (Fig. 7), evaluation of the bioactivity of S-NLCs in an in vivo model of ischemic strike confirmed the successful delivery of these nanoparticles into the rat brain. As shown in Table 4 and Fig. 8, S-NLCs effectively prevented I/R-induced neurobehavioral deficits.

S-NLCs, but not free sesamol, significantly attenuated I/R-induced histopathological alterations and cell loss in the CA1 hippocampal region (Fig. 9) which is one of the most vulnerable brain regions in the cerebral ischemia [68]. Even after a few minutes of global brain ischemia, the pyramidal cells of CA1 sub-region become irreversibly damaged [68, 69]. Therefore, S-NLCs by providing sustained concentrations of sesamol might be of therapeutic value in I/R-induced neuronal injury.

Because of its high rate of oxidative metabolic activity, brain is one of the most vulnerable tissues to the oxidative stress [69]. Antioxidant enzymes including the SOD and CAT by eliminating the free radicals protect the brain against the ischemic insult [70]. Furthermore, GSH which is involved in the maintenance of cell integrity, serves as a primary defensive agent against the oxidative stress in the brain [7, 65]. In this respect, S-NLCs by potentiating the antioxidant defense system and attenuation of I/R-induced oxidative stress in the hippocampal region (Table 5) may exert promising neuroprotective effects. Indeed, NLC-based formulations are promising therapeutic candidates against a variety of pathological conditions including the ophthalmic disorders [71, 72].

Sesamol even at the highest dose tested failed to significantly affect I/R-induced neurobehavioral deficits and

Table 5 Effects of sesamol or S-NLCs on the biochemical parameters in hippocampus following the global ischemia

Groups	MDA (nM/mg protein)	GSH (nM/mg protein)	SOD (U/mg protein)	CAT (U/mg protein)
Sham	0.92 ± 0.06	1.98 ± 0.09	5.77 ± 0.25	4.69 ± 0.32
Intact	0.87 ± 0.09	2.02 ± 0.18	5.83 ± 0.19	4.58 ± 0.54
I/R	2.12 ± 0.21**	0.96 ± 0.22***	3.31 ± 0.13***	2.49 ± 0.17***
I/R + vehicle	2.16 ± 0.19**	0.91 ± 0.15***	3.24 ± 0.21***	2.55 ± 0.22***
I/R + sesamol (5 mg/kg)	2.09 ± 0.20**	0.98 ± 0.17**	3.13 ± 0.15***	2.63 ± 0.24***
I/R + sesamol (10 mg/kg)	2.23 ± 0.18**	0.87 ± 0.15***	3.68 ± 0.25***	2.68 ± 0.18***
I/R + sesamol (20 mg/kg)	1.93 ± 0.20*	1.04 ± 0.06**	3.60 ± 0.37***	2.77 ± 0.12***
I/R + sesamol (25 mg/kg)	1.84 ± 0.19*	1.09 ± 0.13**	3.79 ± 0.19***	2.61 ± 0.15***
I/R + blank NLCs	2.03 ± 0.34*	1.01 ± 0.19**	3.31 ± 0.11***	2.83 ± 0.25***
I/R + S-NLCs (5 mg/kg)	2.14 ± 0.24**	0.98 ± 0.15**	3.19 ± 0.20***	2.80 ± 0.16***
I/R + S-NLCs (10 mg/kg)	1.95 ± 0.15*	0.93 ± 0.24***	2.77 ± 0.23***	3.13 ± 0.14**
I/R + S-NLCs (20 mg/kg)	1.29 ± 0.15$^\Omega$	1.63 ± 0.09$^¥$	4.68 ± 0.19$^\Delta$	4.06 ± 0.29$^\Phi$
I/R + S-NLCs (25 mg/kg)	1.08 ± 0.12$^\#$	1.81 ± 0.07$^\Sigma$	4.97 ± 0.14$^£$	4.29 ± 0.12$^€$
LY + I/R + S-NLCs (20 mg/kg)	2.13 ± 0.16**	0.93 ± 0.13***	3.07 ± 0.24**	2.66 ± 0.19***
LY + I/R + S-NLCs (25 mg/kg)	1.99 ± 0.22*	1.07 ± 0.09**	3.16 ± 0.11***	2.37 ± 0.98***

S-NLCs, but not free sesamol, significantly attenuated the oxidative stress induced by the global ischemia. Data are presented as mean ± SEM (n = 6)
(I/R ischemia/reperfusion, NLCs nanostructured lipid carriers, S-NLCs sesamol-loaded NLCs, MDA malondialdehyde, GSH reduced glutathione, SOD superoxide dismutase, CAT catalase)
*P < 0.05, **P < 0.01, ***P < 0.001 vs. sham or intact, $^¥$ P < 0.05, $^{\Phi, \Delta, \Omega, \#, \Sigma}$ $^€$P < 0.01, $^£$P < 0.001 vs. I/R or I/R + vehicle

oxidative stress (Figs 8 and 9, Tables 4 and 5) that might be due to the rapid metabolism and/or limited number of injections leading to the subtherapeutic concentrations in brain. In previous reports, sesamol has shown efficiency following 14–21 daily injections [9, 11, 12], while, in the present study, S-NLCs following the limited number of injections exhibited therapeutic effects indicating the enhanced bioavailability and efficiency of sesamol following its incorporation into the NLCs. Application of LY294002 abrogated the protective effects of S-NLCs (Figs. 4-6, 8 and 9, Tables 3-5) indicating that S-NLCs, like the classical neuroprotective agents, are able to recruit PI3K signalling pathway.

Conclusions

NLCs serve as promising carriers for sesamol, a phenolic compound with a wide spectrum of pharmacological activities. S-NLCs by improving the pharmacological profile of sesamol provide longer-lasting therapeutic effects in both in vitro and in vivo models of stroke. This nanoformulation through the activation of PI3K pathway might be a suitable controlled release drug carrier system against the ischemic injuries or other neurodegenerative pathologies.

Abbreviations

CAT: Catalase; DL: Drug loading; DMSO: Dimethyl sulfoxide; DSC: Differential scanning calorimetry; EE: Entrapment efficiency; GSH: Reduced glutathione; HPLC: High-performance liquid chromatography; I/R: Ischemia/reperfusion; LDH: Lactate dehydrogenase; MDA: Malondialdehyde; MTT: 3-[4,5-dimethylthiazol-2-yl]-2,5-diphenyl tetrazolium bromide; MWM: Morris watermaze; OGD: Oxygen-glucose deprivation; PBS: Phosphate buffered saline; PDI: Polydispersity index; PI3K: Phosphatidylinositol 3-kinase; S-NLCs: Sesamol-loaded nanostructured lipid carriers; SOD: Superoxide dismutase; STPAT: Step-through passive avoidance test; TBA: Thiobarbituric acid; TTC: 2,3,5-triphenyltetrazolium chloride; ZP: Zeta potential

Acknowledgements

Authors would like to thank Mrs. Faezeh Khosravi for technical assistance.

Funding

This research did not receive any specific grant from funding agencies in the public, commercial, or not-for-profit sectors.

Authors' contributions

FA, the chief instructor of the experiment, and PH performed the experiments, interpreted the data, and wrote the first draft of the manuscript. Other authors contributed to the experimental procedures. All authors read and approved the final manuscript.

Competing interests

The authors declare that they have no competing interests.

Author details

[1]Nanotechnology Research Center, Faculty of Pharmacy, Tehran University of Medical Sciences, Tehran, Iran. [2]Department of Pharmaceutics, Faculty of Pharmacy, Tehran University of Medical Sciences, Tehran, Iran. [3]Department of Pharmacology, Faculty of Medicine, Tehran University of Medical Sciences, Tehran, Iran.

References

1. Klijn CJ, Hankey GJ. Management of acute ischaemic stroke: new guidelines from the American Stroke Association and European stroke initiative. Lancet Neurol. 2003;2:698–701.
2. Moskowitz MA, Lo EH, Iadecola C. The science of stroke: mechanisms in search of treatments. Neuron. 2010;67:181–98.
3. Serteser M, Ozben T, Gumuslu S, Balkan S, Balkan E. The effects of NMDA receptor antagonist MK-801 on lipid peroxidation during focal cerebral ischemia in rats. Prog Neuro-Psychopharmacol Biol Psychiatry. 2002;26:871–7.
4. Xu L, Sun J, Lu R, Ji Q, Xu JG. Effect of glutamate on inflammatory responses of intestine and brain after focal cerebral ischemia. World J Gastroenterol. 2005;11:733–6.
5. Chen H, Yoshioka H, Kim GS, Jung JE, Okami N, Sakata H, et al. Oxidative stress in ischemic brain damage: mechanisms of cell death and potential molecular targets for neuroprotection. Antioxid Redox Signal. 2011;14:1505–17.
6. Wu XL, Liou CJ, Li ZY, Lai XY, Fang LW, Huang WC. Sesamol suppresses the inflammatory response by inhibiting NF-κB/MAPK activation and upregulating AMP kinase signaling in RAW 264.7 macrophages. Inflamm Res. 2015;64:577–88.
7. Kumar P, Kalonia H, Kumar A. Protective effect of sesamol against 3-nitropropionic acid-induced cognitive dysfunction and altered glutathione redox balance in rats. Basic Clin Pharmacol Toxicol. 2010;107:577–82.
8. Sharma S, Kaur IP. Development and evaluation of sesamol as an antiaging agent. Int J Dermatol. 2006;45:200–8.
9. Kumar B, Kuhad A, Chopra K. Neuropharmacological effect of sesamol in unpredictable chronic mild stress model of depression: behavioral and biochemical evidences. Psychopharmacology. 2011;214:819–28.
10. Changa CC, Luc WJ, Chiang CW, Jayakumarc T, Ong ET, Hsiaoc G, et al. Potent antiplatelet activity of sesamol in an in vitro and in vivo model: pivotal roles of cyclic AMP and p38 mitogen-activated protein kinase. J Nutr Biochem. 2010;21:1214–21.
11. Hassanzadeh P, Hassanzadeh A. Implication of NGF and endocannabinoid signalling in the mechanism of action of sesamol: a multi-target natural compound with therapeutic potential. Psychopharmacology. 2013;229:571–8.
12. Hassanzadeh P, Arbabi E, Rostami F. The ameliorative effects of sesamol against seizures, cognitive impairment and oxidative stress in the experimental model of epilepsy. Iran J Basic Med Sci. 2014;17:100–7.
13. Ahmad S, Yousuf S, Ishrat T, Khan MB, Bhatia K, Fazli IS, et al. Effect of dietary sesame oil as antioxidant on brain hippocampus of rat in focal cerebral ischemia. Life Sci. 2005;79:1921–8.
14. Jan KC, Ho CT, Hwang LS. Bioavailability and tissue distribution of sesamol in rat. J Agric Food Chem. 2008;56:7032–7.
15. Geetha T, Singh N, Deol PK, Kaur IP. Biopharmaceutical profiling of sesamol: physiochemical characterization, gastrointestinal permeability and pharmacokinetic evaluation. RSC Adv. 2015;5:4083–91.
16. Hassanzadeh P. New perspectives in biosensor technology. Gastroenterol Hepatol Bed Bench. 2010;3:105–7.
17. Hassanzadeh P, Fullwood I, Sothi S, Aldulaimi D. Cancer nanotechnology. Gastroenterol Hepatol Bed Bench. 2011;4:63–9.
18. Hassanzadeh P. Nanopharmaceuticals: innovative theranostics for the neurological disorders. Biomed Rev. 2014;25:25–34.
19. Hassanzadeh P, Arbabi E, Rostami F, Atyabi F, Dinarvand R. Carbon nanotubes prolong the regulatory action of nerve growth factor on the endocannabinoid signaling. Physiol Pharmacol. 2015;19:167–76.
20. Hassanzadeh P, Arbabi P, Atyabi F, Dinarvand R. Carbon nanotube-anandamide complex exhibits sustained protective effects in an in vitro model of stroke. Physiol Pharmacol. 2016;20:12–23.
21. Hassanzadeh P, Arbabi P, Atyabi F, Dinarvand R. Application of carbon nanotubes as the carriers of the cannabinoid, 2-arachidonoylglycerol: towards a novel treatment strategy in colitis. Life Sci. 2017;179:66–72.

22. Hassanzadeh P, Arbabi P, Atyabi F, Dinarvand R. Nerve growth factor-carbon nanotube complex exerts prolonged protective effects in an in vitro model of ischemic stroke. Life Sci. 2017;179:15–22.

23. Hassanzadeh P, Atyabi F, Dinarvand R. Application of carbon nanotubes for controlled release of growth factors or endocannabinoids: a breakthrough in biomedicine. Biomed Rev. 2016;27:19–27.

24. Kim D, Chun BG, Kim YK, Lee YH, Park CS, Jeon I, et al. In vivo tracking of human mesenchymal stem cells in experimental stroke. Cell Transplant. 2008;16:1007–12.

25. Marsh JN, Hu G, Scot MJ, Zhang H, Goette MJ, Gaffney PJ, et al. A fibrin-specific thrombolytic nanomedicine approach to acute ischemic stroke. Int J Nanomedicine. 2012;7:5137–49.

26. Ghosh A, Sarkar S, Mandal AK, Das N. Neuroprotective role of nanoencapsuled quercetin in combating ischemia-reperfusion induced neuronal damage in young and aged rats. PLoS One. 2013;8:e57735.

27. Müller RH. Lipid nanoparticles: recent advances. Adv Drug Deliv Rev. 2007;59:375–6.

28. Müller RH, Rühl D, Runge S, Schulze-Forster K, Mehnert W. Cytotoxicity of solid lipid nanoparticles as a function of the lipid matrix and the surfactant. Pharm Res. 1997;14:458–62.

29. Freitas C, Müller RH. Correlation between long-term stability of solid lipid nanoparticles (SLNs) and crystallinity of the lipid phase. Eur J Pharm Biopharm. 1999;47:125–32.

30. Li F, Wang WYL, He H, Yang J, Tang X. The efficacy and safety of bufadienolides loaded nanostructured lipid carriers. Int J Pharm. 2010;393:203–11.

31. Kumbhar DD, Pokharkar VB. Engineering of a nanostructured lipid carrier for the poorly water-soluble drug, bicalutamide: physicochemical investigations. Colloids Surf A Physicochem Eng Asp. 2013;416:32–42.

32. Cantley LC. The phosphoinositide 3-kinase pathway. Science. 2002;296:1655–7.

33. Mullonkal CJ, Toledo-Pereyra LH. Akt in ischemia and reperfusion. J Investig Surg. 2007;20:195–203.

34. Beloqui A, Solinís MÁ, Gascón AR, del Pozo-Rodríguez A, des Rieux A, Préat V. Mechanism of transport of saquinavir-loaded nanostructured lipid carriers across the intestinal barrier. J Control Release. 2013;166:115–23.

35. Yang R, Zhang S, Kong D, Gao X, Zhao Y, Wang Z. Biodegradable polymercurcumin conjugate micelles enhance the loading and delivery of low potency curcumin. Pharm Res. 2012;29:3512e25.

36. Mehta SL, Manhas N, Raghubir R. Molecular targets in cerebral ischemia for developing novel therapeutics. Brain Res Rev. 2007;54:34–66.

37. Larsen EC, Hatcher JF, Adibhatla RM. Effect of tricyclodecan-9-yl potassium xanthate (D609) on phospholipid metabolism and cell death during oxygen–glucose deprivation in PC12 cells. Neuroscience. 2007;146:946–61.

38. Koha SH, Kwon H, Parka KH, Ko JK, Kim JH, et al. Protective effect of diallyl disulfide on oxidative stress-injured neuronally differentiated PC12 cells. Mol Brain Res. 2005;133:176–86.

39. Zakharova IO, Sokolova TV, Bayunova LV, Vlasova YA. α-Tocopherol at nanomolar concentration protects PC12 cells from hydrogen peroxide-induced death and modulates protein kinase activities. Int J Mol Sci. 2012;13:11543–68.

40. Carmichael J, DeGraff WG, Gazdar AF, Minna JD, Mitchell JB. Evaluation of a tetrazolium-based semiautomated colorimetric assay: assessment of chemosensitivity testing. Cancer Res. 1987;47:936–41.

41. Decker T, Lohmann-Matthes ML. A quick and simple method for the quantitation of lactate dehydrogenase release in measurements of cellular cytotoxicity and tumor necrosis factor (TNF) activity. J Immunol Methods. 1988;115:61–9.

42. Zhao J, Bai Y, Zhang C, Zhang X, Zhang YX, Chen J, et al. Cinepazide maleate protects PC12 cells against oxygen–glucose deprivation-induced injury. Neurol Sci. 2014;35:875–81.

43. Bradford MM. A rapid and sensitive method for the quantitation of microgram quantities of protein utilizing the principle of protein-dye binding. Anal Biochem. 1976;72:248–54.

44. Ohkawa H, Ohishi N, Yagi K. Assay for lipid peroxides in animal tissues by thiobarbituric acid reaction. Anal Biochem. 1979;95:351–8.

45. Jollow DJ, Mitchell JR, Zampaglione N, Gillette JR. Bromobenze induced liver necrosis: protective role of glutathione and evidence for 3,4-bromobenzenoxide as the hepatotoxic intermediate. Pharmacology. 1974;11:151–69.

46. Kakkar P, Das B, Viswanathan PN. A modified spectrophotometric assay of superoxide dismutase. Ind J Biochem Biophys. 1984;21:130–2.

47. Aebi H. Catalase in vitro. Methods Enzymol. 1984;105:121–6.

48. Zhaoa C, Fana T, Yanga Y, Wua M, Li L, Zhoua Z, et al. Preparation, macrophages targeting delivery and anti-inflammatory study of pentapeptide grafted nanostructured lipid carriers. Int J Pharm. 2013;450:11–20.

49. Wang MT, Jin Y, Yang YX, Zhao CY, Yang HY, Xu XF, et al. In vivo biodistribution, anti-inflammatory, and hepatoprotective effects of liver targeting dexamethasone acetate loaded nanostructured lipid carrier system. Int J Nanomedicine. 2010;5:487–97.

50. Pulsinelli WA, Brierley JB. A new model of bilateral hemispheric ischemia in the unanesthetized rat. Stroke. 1979;10:267–72.

51. Hu X, Xie C, He S, Zhang Y, Li Y, Jiang L. Remifentanil postconditioning improves global cerebral ischemia induced spatial learning and memory deficit in rats via inhibition of neuronal apoptosis through the PI3K signaling pathway. Neurol Sci. 2013;34:1955–62.

52. Zhang R, Yang G, Wang Q, Guo F, Wang H. Acylated ghrelin protects hippocampal neurons in pilocarpine-induced seizures of immature rats by inhibiting cell apoptosis. Mol Biol Rep. 2013;40:51–8.

53. Longa EZ, Weinstein PR, Carlson S, Cummins R. Reversible middle cerebral artery occlusion without craniectomy in rats. Stroke. 1989;20:84–91.

54. Morris R. Developments of a water-maze procedure form studying spatial learning in the rat. J Neurosci Methods. 1984;11:47–60.

55. Goldlust EJ, Paczynski RP, He YY, Hsu CY, Goldberg MP. Automated measurement of infarct size with scanned images of triphenyltetrazolium chloride-stained rat brains. Stroke. 1996;27:1657–62.

56. Zhang W, Miao Y, Zhou S, Jiang J, Luo Q, Qiu Y. Neuroprotective effects of ischemic postconditioning on global brain ischemia in rats through upregulation of hippocampal glutamine synthetase. J Clin Neurosci. 2011;18:685–9.

57. Paxinos G, Watson C. The rat brain in stereotaxic coordinates. San Diego: Academic; 2007.

58. Habauzit V, Morand C. Evidence for a protective effect of polyphenols-containing foods on cardiovascular health: An update for clinicians. Ther Adv Chronic Dis. 2011;3:87–106.

59. Hassanzadeh P, Atyabi F, Dinarvand R. Resvertrol: more than a phytochemical. Biomed Rev. 2015;26:13–21.

60. Hassanzadeh P, Arbabi E, Atyabi F, Dinarvand R. The endocannabinoid system and NGF are involved in the mechanism of action of resveratrol: a multi-target nutraceutical with therapeutic potential in neuropsychiatric disorders. Psychopharmacology. 2016;233:1087–96.

61. Manach C, Williamson G, Morand G, Scalbert A, Rémésy C. Bioavailability and bioefficacy of polyphenols in humans. I. Review of 97 bioavailability studies. Am J Clin Nut. 2005;81:230S–42S.

62. Siekmann B, Westesen K. Thermoanalysis of the recrystallization process of melt-homogenized glyceride nanoparticles. Colloids Surf B: Biointerfaces. 1994;3:159–75.

63. Draper HH, Hadley M. Malondialdehyde determination as index of lipid peroxidation. Methods Enzymol. 1990;186:421–31.

64. Spitz DR, Sullivan SJ, Malcolm RR, Roberts RJ. Glutathione dependent metabolism and detoxification of 4-hydroxy-2-nonenal. Free Radic Biol Med. 1991;11:415–23.

65. Warner DS, Sheng H, Batinic-Haberle I. Oxidants, antioxidants and the ischemic brain. J Exp Biol. 2004;207:3221–31.

66. Michiels C, Raes M, Toussaint O, Remacle J. Importance of glutathione peroxidase, catalase, and cu/Zn-SOD for cell survival against oxidative stress. Free Radic Biol Med. 1994;17:235–48.

67. Chopra K, Tiwari V, Arora V, Kuhad A. Sesamol suppresses neuro-inflammatory cascade in experimental model of diabetic neuropathy. J Pain. 2010;11:950–7.

68. Schmidt-Kastner R, Freund TF. Selective vulnerability of the hippocampus in brain ischemia. Neuroscience. 1991;4:599–636.

69. White BC, Sullivan JM, DeGracia DJ, O'Neil BJ, Neumar RW, Grossman LI, et al. Brain ischemia and reperfusion: molecular mechanisms of neuronal injury. J Neurol Sci. 2000;179:1–33.

70. Cui K, Luo X, Xu K, Murthy MRV. Role of oxidative stress in neurodegeneration: recent developments in assay methods for oxidative stress and nutraceutical antioxidants. Prog NeuroPsychopharm Biol Psych. 2004;28:771–99.

71. Balguri SP, Adelli GR, Majumdar S. Topical ophthalmic lipid nanoparticle formulations (SLN, NLC) of indomethacin for delivery to the posterior segment ocular tissues. Eur J Pharm Biopharm. 2016;109:224–35.

72. Balguri SP, Adelli GR, Janga KY, Bhagav P, Majumdar S. Ocular disposition of ciprofloxacin from topical, PEGylated nanostructured lipid carriers: effect of molecular weight and density of poly (ethylene) glycol. Int J Pharm. 2017;529:32–43.

19

Inhibition of mirtazapine metabolism by Ecstasy (MDMA) in isolated perfused rat liver model

Sanaz Jamshidfar, Yalda H. Ardakani, Hoda Lavasani and Mohammadreza Rouini[*]

Abstract

Background: Nowadays MDMA (3,4-methylendioxymethamphetamine), known as ecstasy, is widely abused among the youth because of euphoria induction in acute exposure. However, abusers are predisposed to depression in chronic consumption of this illicit compound.

Mirtazapine (MRZ), an antidepressant agent, may be prescribed in MDMA-induced depression. MRZ is extensively metabolized in liver by CYP450 isoenzymes. 8-hydroxymirtazapine (8-OH) is mainly produced by CYP2D6. N-desmethylmirtazapine (NDES) is generated by CYP3A4.

MDMA is also metabolized by the mentioned isoenzymes and demonstrates mechanism-based inhibition (MBI) in association with CYP2D6. Several studies revealed that MDMA showed inhibitory effects on CYP3A4.

In the present study, our aim was to evaluate the impact of MDMA on the metabolism of MRZ in liver. Therefore, isolated perfused rat liver model was applied as our model of choice in this assessment.

Methods: The subjects of the study were categorized into two experimental groups. Rats in the control group received MRZ-containing Krebs-Henselit buffer (1 μg/ml). Rats in the treatment group received aqueous solution of 1 mg/ml MDMA (3 mg/kg) intraperitoneally 1 hour before receiving MRZ. Perfusate samples were analyzed by HPLC.

Results: Analyses of perfusate samples showed 80% increase in the parent drug concentrations and 50% decrease in the concentrations of both metabolites in our treatment group compared to the control group. In the treatment group compared to the control group, $AUC_{(0-120)}$ of the parent drug demonstrated 50% increase and $AUC_{(0-120)}$ of 8-OH and NDES showed 70% and 60% decrease, respectively.

Observed decrease in metabolic ratios were 83% and 79% for 8-OH and NDES in treatment group compared to control group, respectively.

Hepatic clearance (CL_h) and intrinsic clearance (Cl_{int}) showed 20% and 60% decrease in treatment group compared to control group.

Conclusion: All findings prove the inhibitory effects of ecstasy on both CYP2D6 and CYP3A4 hepatic isoenzymes.

In conclusion, this study is the first investigation of MRZ metabolism in presence of MDMA in isolated perfused rat liver model.

Keywords: Mirtazapine, Ecstasy, Metabolism, Isolated perfused rat liver model

* Correspondence: rouini@tums.ac.ir
Biopharmaceutics and Pharmacokinetic Division, Department of Pharmaceutics, Faculty of Pharmacy, Tehran University of Medical Sciences, Tehran, Iran

Background

Nowadays, hallucinogens and stimulants are profoundly abused by the youth due to their primary effects to elevate energy levels, to induce euphoria, and to reach higher levels of pleasure and empathy. MDMA (3,4-methylenedioxymethamphetamine), known as ecstasy, is one of these illicit drugs that acts as both releaser and reuptake inhibitor of central neurotransmitters and causes a large number of adverse effects not only in acute encounter but also in long-term abuse [1].

Major metabolic pathways involved in the bioactivation of MDMA are N-dealkylation and O-demethylenation. N-dealkylation of MDMA, catalyzed by CYP2B6, CYP1A2, and CYP2C19, produces the metabolite 3,4-methylendioxyamphetamine (MDA). O-demethylenation of MDMA and MDA, mediated by CYP2D6, CYP3A4, and CYP2C19, produces 3,4-dihydroxymethamphetamine (HHMA) and 3,4-dihydroxyamphetamine (HHA), respectively. HHMA and HHA metabolism generates 4-hydroxy-3-methoxymethamphetamine (HMMA) and 4-hydroxy-3-methoxyamphetamine (HMA) by the activity of catechol-O-methyltransferase (COMT) [2, 3].

MDMA demonstrates non-linear pharmacokinetics; the non-linearity is due to mechanism-based inhibition (MBI), observed in chemical structures containing methylendioxy group [1, 4]. Previous studies revealed that MDMA exhibited MBI in association with CYP2D6 isoenzyme. It is hypothesized that CYP2D6 forms an orthoquinone intermediate with methylenedioxyphenyl ring of MDMA. This complex attacks macromolecular structures as a nucleophile and interferes with their functions [4, 5]. These events result in irreversible inhibition of CYP2D6 isoenzyme, which resembles CYP2D6 inhibition by paroxetine [4, 6]. This phenomenon involves most of CYP2D6 isoenzymes and is demonstrated within 1 h of MDMA administration [7].

Chronic abuse of MDMA is associated with a wide variety of complications such as serotonergic and dopaminergic nerve deterioration, cognitive disorders, and psychological problems [8]. Among these adverse effects, depression is one of the most common psychiatric problems associated with long-term consumption of ecstasy. Treatment of MDMA-induced depression is, therefore, of great value.

Mirtazapine (MRZ), a piperazinoazepine compound, belongs to noradrenergic and specific serotonergic antidepressants (NaSSA) [9]. Its pharmacological activity is virtually associated with presynaptic-α2 receptor blockade, which results in an increase in both serotonin and norepinephrine levels and contributes to antidepressant activities [10]. In clinical practice, MRZ is particularly indicated for treatment of major depressive disorder (MDD) [11].

Previous clinical studies have shown that MRZ is superior to placebo and some selective serotonin reuptake inhibitors (SSRIs) such as fluoxetine. MRZ also has equal efficacy as some tricyclic antidepressants (TCAs) such as amitriptyline and clomipramine in treatment of depression. Moreover, MRZ is better tolerated during the treatment process since it does not induce nausea and has less anticholinergic side effects. MRZ exhibits more rapid onset of action compared with TCAs and SSRIs [11].

MRZ demonstrates linear pharmacokinetics in the therapeutic dosage regimen (15 to 80 mg/day). Good absorption via oral route and elimination half-life of 20 to 40 h, that is in favor of once daily dosing, are of notable pharmacokinetic parameters of MRZ [12].

MRZ is mostly excreted in urine and is extensively metabolized in liver by means of CYP450 isoenzymes. CYP3A4, CYP2D6 and CYP1A2 are involved in biotransformation of MRZ. 8-hydroxymirtazapine (8-OH), the major metabolite, is mainly produced by CYP2D6 and to a lesser extent by CYP1A2. N-desmethylmirtazapine (NDES), the only pharmacologically active metabolite, and N-oxidemirtazapine are generated by CYP3A4 [13, 14].

In this study we focused on the possible interaction between MRZ and MDMA, considering both CYP2D6 and CYP3A4 isoenzymes. We assessed the impact of MDMA on the metabolism of MRZ in liver. Therefore, isolated perfused rat liver model was applied as our model of choice in this assessment.

Materials and methods
Materials

MRZ, 8-OH and NDES were kindly supplied by Mario Georgi (University of Pisa, Italy).

MDMA.HCl powder was synthesized in Medicinal Chemistry Department of Tehran University of Medical Sciences according to the previously reported [15] method that showed the acceptable purity compared to standard sample purchased from Lipomed Pharmaceutical (Switzerland). The structure was confirmed by IR, H-NMR and Mass spectra.

HPLC grade acetonitril and methanol, and analytical grade salts such as potassium dihydrogen phosphate were all from Merck (Darmstadt, Germany).

Standard solutions

Primary stocks of MRZ and its two major metabolites were prepared by dissolving pure powders in methanol to make concentration of 1 mg/ml. Final dilution for QC and calibration samples was done using Krebs-Henselit buffer. MRZ and NDES concentrations were between 5 and 150 ng/ml. Concentrations used for 8-OH were between 2.5 and 75 ng/ml (Fig. 1). All the above solutions

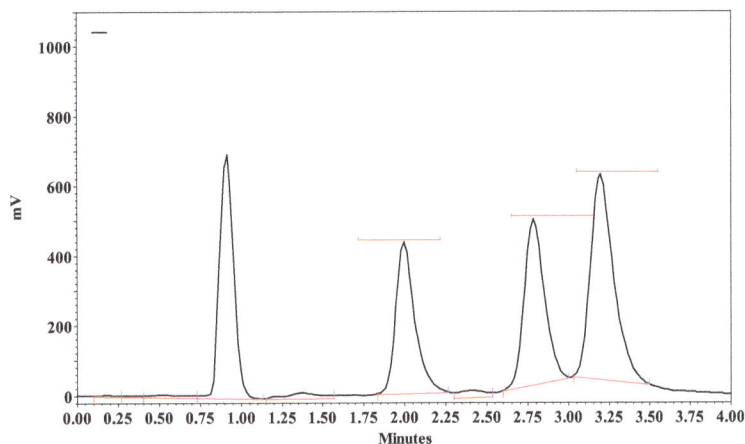

Fig. 1 Chromatogram of standard solution (40 ng/ml of 8OHand 80 ng/ml of NDES and MRZ). Retention time:(8-OH: 2 min, NDES: 2.75 min, MRZ: 3.25 min)

were kept at 4 °C. Aqueous stock of MDMA (1 mg/ml) was prepared by dissolving in double distilled water.

Animals
Twelve healthy male Sprague-Dawley rats (divided into two experimental groups called control and treatment) weighting between 250 and 300 g were applied in this assessment. They were kept under 12-h light-dark cycle with controlled environment temperature and without any limit in access to standard laboratory chow and water.

The present study was approved by the Institutional Review Board of Tehran University of Medical Sciences. Ethical approval code number was [253066].

Rat liver perfusion
The rats were anesthetized via intraperitoneal (IP) injection of xylazine/ketamine mixture (15/75 mg/kg). Cannulation of portal vein and inferior vena cava was done using previously heparinized intravenous catheters (guage of 16, 18 respectively). After inserting catheters, the Krebs-Henselit buffer (118 mM NaCl, 4.5 mM KCl,2.75 mM $CaCl_2$, 1.19 mM KH_2PO_4, 1.18 mM $MgSO_4$, and 25 mM $NaHCO_3$) adjusted to the physiological pH (using 95% O_2/5%CO_2) was passed through the portal vein employing peristaltic pump set on the constant flow rate of 500 ml/h for 10 min. Then MRZ-containing medium (inlet concentration of 1 μg/ml) was delivered into the portal vein for 120 min and the perfusate samples were collected immediately after wash and then every 10 min from the inferior vena cava to calculate outlet concentrations of parent drug and both metabolites.

Earlier rat liver perfusion studies with MRZ in our lab revealed that 8-OH metabolite of MRZ was not detectable in low parent drug concentrations while NDES was measurable even in low concentrations of MRZ, so, a 1 μg/ml concentration of MRZ was selected as exposure concentration for control ($n = 6$) and treatment ($n = 6$) group.

Previous studies showed that single dose administration of MDMA (3 mg/kg) to rats resembles the plasma concentration following the ordinary MDMA dosage taken in humans [16].

So, treatment group were received freshly prepared aqueous solution of 1 mg/ml MDMA (3 mg/kg) intraperitoneally 1 hour before receiving MRZ-containing medium (1 μg/ml) through the single pass mode of liver perfusion.

Perfusion pressure (15 mmHg), temperature, and pH (7.4) were monitored continuously during the procedure and remained constant till the end. Liver viability tests were carried out intermittently and were passed. Normal range for AST and ALT are 0–46(U/L) and 0–49(U/L) respectively (Figs. 2 and 3).

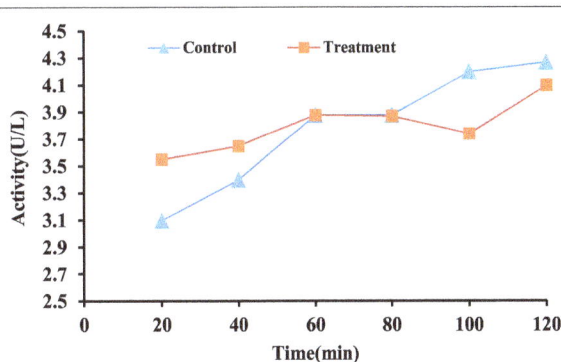

Fig. 2 Mean profile of AST during the perfusion study in control and treatment groups ($n = 6$)

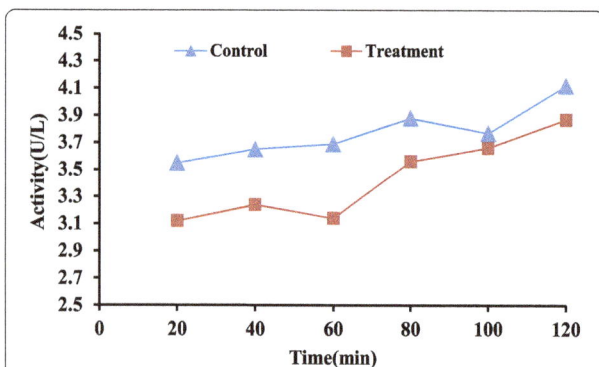

Fig. 3 Mean profile of ALT during the perfusion study in control and treatment groups (n = 6)

$$F = \frac{\text{mean outlet concentration of MRZ at four latest samples}}{\text{inlet concentration of MRZ}} \quad (1)$$

$$E = 1-F \quad (2)$$

$$CL_h = Q \times E \quad (3)$$

$$CL_{int} = E \times \frac{Q}{F} \quad (4)$$

Q, in the above equation, is the constant perfusion flow rate of 500 ml/h that equals 8.3 ml/min.

Since concentrations of MRZ and its two metabolites reach the plateau at four latest time intervals, mean concentration of these samples were used in the equation.

All data in this study were reported as Mean ± SD.

Statistics
The t-test was applied in this study in order to determine differences between means of groups (*P* value <0.05).

Results
According to our results, analyses of four latest sample intervals taken from treatment group showed 80% enhancement in parent drug concentration (236.8 ± 44.7 vs 131.9 ± 56.9 ng/ml) in comparison to control group (*P* value < 0.05) (Fig. 4).

Similarly, the AUC $_{(0-120)}$ of parent compound also showed 50% enhancement in treatment group comparing to control group (1792.5 ± 2871.7 vs 1184.8 ± 3655.2 ng.min/ml), (*P* value < 0.05) (Table 1).

Contrary to parent drug, concentrations of both metabolites, 8-OH and NDES, showed 50% decrease in treatment group at four latest sampling time intervals compared to control group (4.7 ± 2.9 vs 10.3 ± 3.2 ng/ml) and (98.5 ± 64.3 vs 188.6 ± 63.44 ng/ml), (*P* value < 0.05) respectively (Figs. 5, 6 and 7).

Collected samples (in 10 min intervals) were centrifuged for 15 min at 12000 rpm and the clear solutions were separated and were stored at –20 °C until use.

Apparatus and chromatographic condition
The chromatographic apparatus consisted of a low pressure gradient HPLC pump coupled with fluorescence detector (290 nm–370 nm), a 100μlit loop, and a Rheodyne model 7725i injector, all from Knauer (Berlin, Germany).

A Chromolith™Performance RP-8e 100 mm × 4.6 column (Knauer, Berlin, Germany) attached to a protective Chromolith™ guard cartridge RP-18e 5 mm × 4.6 mm was applied for chromatographic separation (Merck, Darmstadt, Germany).

A mixture of 0.025 M KH_2PO_4 buffer, adjusted to pH = 3 using ortho-phosphoric acid, and acetonitril (83:17, *v/v*) was employed as mobile phase and was delivered through the column with the constant flow rate of 2 ml/min [17]. Data acquisition and analyses were achieved by ChromGate chromatography software (Knauer, Berlin, Germany).

Pharmacokinetic parameters
The analytes concentrations were determined using standard calibration curves. Based on concentrations of MRZ and its two metabolites, the areas under the concentration versus time curves AUC $_{(0-120)}$ were acquired using trapezoidal rule. The metabolic ratios at different times for both metabolites were calculated using metabolite concentration divided by MRZ concentration at specific times.

Availability (F), extraction ratio (E), clearance (CL$_h$) and intrinsic clearance (CL$_{int}$) were of hepatic pharmacokinetic parameters determined in this study using following equations [18].

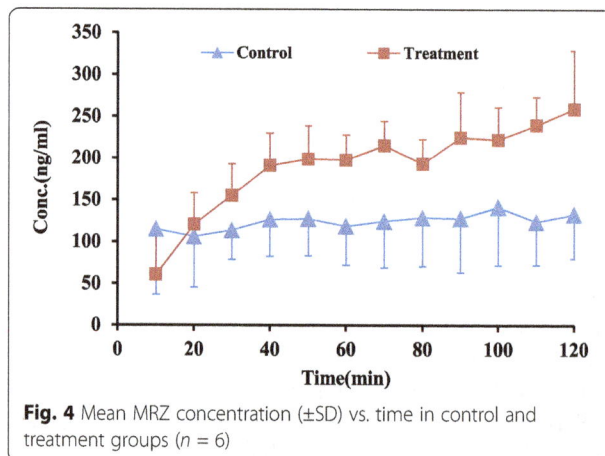

Fig. 4 Mean MRZ concentration (±SD) vs. time in control and treatment groups (n = 6)

Table 1 AUC $_{(0-120)}$ MRZ, NDES, and 8-OH in control and treatment groups ($n = 6$)

	MRZ		8-OH		NDES	
	Control	Treatment	Control	Treatment	Control	Treatment
1	15,530.1	24,053.4	2124.9	287.5	28,525.2	593.7
2	9928.7	18,031.1	1398.9	398.6	22,505.4	12,111.8
3	16,443.6	17,675.6	1960.2	449.2	15,171.6	15,346.2
4	10,611.4	23,553.7	1674.1	415.4	18,839.8	5860.1
5	13,295.1	23,063.4	610.9	371.3	11,195.2	10,613.3
6	19,497.1	22,680.5	588.2	920.5	12,075.7	3605.2
MEAN	14,217.7	21,509.6*	1392.9	473.7*	18,052.1	8021.7*
SD	3655.2	2871.7	662.7	225.6	6650.9	5593.7
CV	25.7	13.4	47.6	47.6	36.8	69.7

P value < 0.05, significant difference between control and treatment groups

In accordance with decreasing in both metabolite concentrations in perfusate buffer at four latest sampling time intervals, the AUC $_{(0-120)}$ of both metabolites showed 70% and 60% decrease for 8-OH and NDES respectively in treatment group in comparison to control group (473.7 ± 225.6 vs 1392.9 ± 662.7 ng.min/ml) and (8021.7 ± 5593.7 vs 18,052.1 ± 6650.8 ng.min/ml), (P value < 0.05) respectively (Table 1).

Based on pharmacokinetic equations, CL_h and CL_{int} demonstrated 20% and 60% decrease respectively in treatment group compared to control group (6.3 ± 0.4vs 7.2 ± 0.5 ml/min) and (27.7 ± 6.3 vs 63.4 ± 25.8 ml/min), (P value < 0.05), respectively (Table 2).

Metabolic ratios for 8-OH, main metabolite of CYP2D6, and NDES, main metabolite of CYP3A4, at four latest sampling time intervals showed 83% and 79% decrease respectively in treatment group compared to control group (0.02 ± 0.008 vs 0.1 ± 0.05) and (0.45 ± 0.3 vs 1.7 ± 0.8), (P value < 0.05), respectively (Figs. 8 and 9).

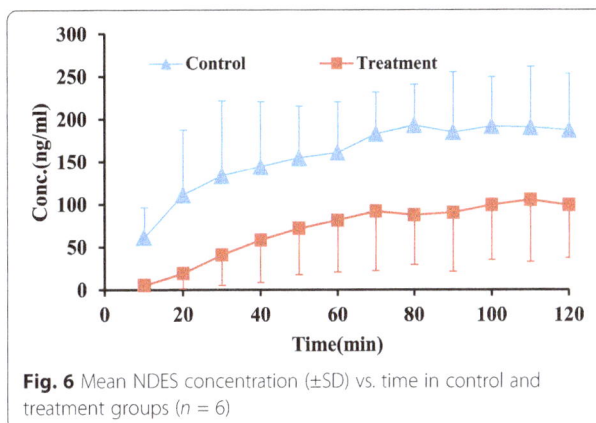

Fig. 6 Mean NDES concentration (±SD) vs. time in control and treatment groups ($n = 6$)

Discussion

Hepatic metabolism appears to play an important role in the toxicity induced by MDMA consumption [19]. MDMA is metabolized by various cytochrome P450 enzymes. The primary pathway is O-demethylenation by CYP2D6; however, it has been shown that CYP3A4 is effectively involved in bioactivation of MDMA. Although several studies were focused on MDMA as a potent mechanism-based inhibitor of CYP2D6, a number of investigations proposed that inhibitory effects of MDMA on CYP3A4 could also be of great clinical value [20, 21].

Since both CYP3A4 and CYP2D6 are involved in many drugs metabolism, simultaneous use of MDMA and other substances could be of high concern.

In order to extend the desirable effects and cut down the undesirable ones such as depression or anxiety, most ecstasy users are interested in using other pharmaceutical drugs concurrently.

Previous studies have focused mostly on the pharmacodynamic interactions between MDMA, on one hand, and SSRIs and MAO inhibitors, on the other hand.

In a clinical study, after pretreatment of subjects with 20 mg/day of paroxetine (a potent inhibitor of CYP2D6 and an SSRI) for 3 days before MDMA administration,

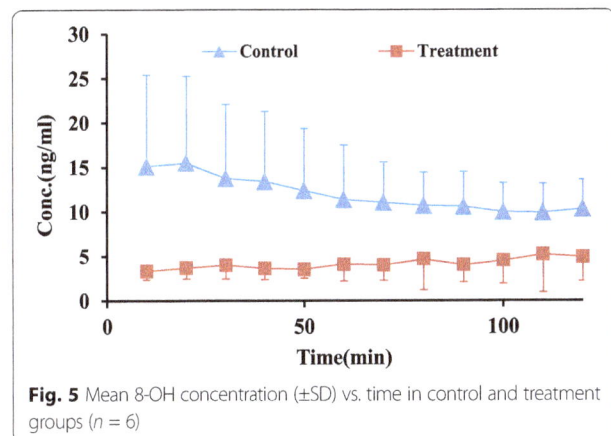

Fig. 5 Mean 8-OH concentration (±SD) vs. time in control and treatment groups ($n = 6$)

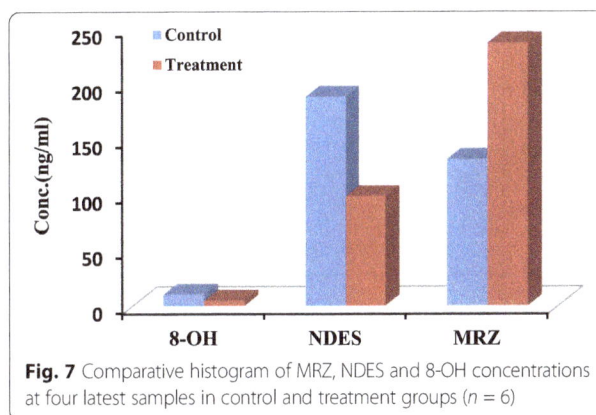

Fig. 7 Comparative histogram of MRZ, NDES and 8-OH concentrations at four latest samples in control and treatment groups ($n = 6$)

Table 2 Comparison of availability, extarction ratio, clearance and intrinsic clearance (±SD) in control and treatment groups (n = 6)

	F	E	CL$_h$(ml/min)	CL$_{int}$(ml/min)
Control	0.13 ± 0.06	0.87 ± 0.06	7.21 ± 0.47	63.4 ± 25.81
Treatment	0.24 ± 0.04	0.76 ± 0.06	6.33 ± 0.37	27.71 ± 6.26
P value	0.005	0.004	0.005	0.008

thirty hundred percent enhancement in MDMA plasma concentrations was observed. In spite of this concentration enhancement, psychological effects of MDMA were attenuated due to pharmacodynamic interactions [22].

Co-administration of moclobemide (a selective MAO A inhibitor) and MDMA caused several reported deaths due to serotonin syndrome [23].

MRZ can be prescribed in MDMA-induced depression [24]. Moreover, MDMA may be abused in patients suffering from depression who are under treatment with MRZ as a mood elevator [25]. The present study was, therefore, proposed to evaluate the pharmacokinetics of MRZ and its two main metabolites after MDMA administration.

As recent studies revealed that MBI could occur shortly after a single dose administration of MDMA, 1-hour interval was chosen between rat IP injection of MDMA and exposure of liver to MRZ.

Our findings prove the inhibitory effects of MDMA not only on CYP2D6 but also on CYP3A4 hepatic isoenzymes.

Although the inhibitory mechanism of MDMA on CYP2D6 is known as MBI, the mechanisms that have been proposed to justify the inhibitory effects of ecstasy intake on other CYPs include increased levels of neurotransmitters, impairment of mitochondrial function, oxidation of biogenic amines, and metabolic bioactivation. Among these, it has been shown that biotransformation of MDMA has a significant role in its

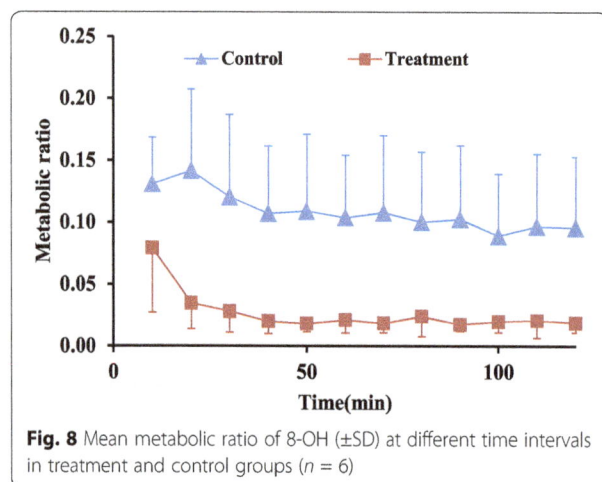

Fig. 9 Mean metabolic ratio of NDES (±SD) at different time intervals in control and treatment groups (n = 6)

hepatotoxicity because of its oxidative metabolites corresponding to the formation of ortho-quinones. These ortho-quinone compounds are able to enter a redox cycle that has been proposed to be the reason of cytotoxicity in several tissues such as liver, brain, kidney, and heart [2, 5–7, 20, 21, 26].

While several studies have focused on the interaction of MDMA with CYP2D6, the interaction of MDMA with CYP3A4 would also be of great clinical relevance because of the potential hepatotoxicity in MDMA abusers, which results from the reaction between oxidative metabolites and other essential intracellular macromolecules.

Another finding of this study, i.e., 80% enhancement in outlet perfusate concentration of MRZ in treatment group in comparison to control group, may propose the importance of dose adjustment in clinic. This finding is in line with two case reports [27] concerning the interactions between MRZ and fluvoxamine (an inhibitor of both CYP2D6 and CYP3A4 isoenzymes), that had reported 3 to 4 fold increase in serum concentrations of MRZ manifested by increased anxiety in patients under treatment [28].

Conclusion

In conclusion, this study is the first investigation of the metabolism of MRZ in presence of MDMA in isolated perfused rat liver model. To our knowledge, only few studies have been carried out on this subject. Complementary studies with higher amounts of MDMA or with different time intervals between IP injection of MDMA and liver perfusion are suggested to be designed.

Abbreviations
8-OH: 8-hydroxymirtazapine; COMT: Catechol-O-methyltransferase; HHA: 3, 4-dihydroxyamphetamine; HHMA: 3, 4-dihydroxymethamphetamine; HMA: 4-hydroxy-3-methoxyamphetamine; HMMA: 4-hydroxy-3-methoxymethamphetamine; MBI: Mechanism-based inhibition; MDA: 3, 4-methylendioxyamphetamine; MDMA: 3, 4-methylenedioxymethamphetamine; MRZ: Mirtazapine; NDES: N-desmethylmirtazapine

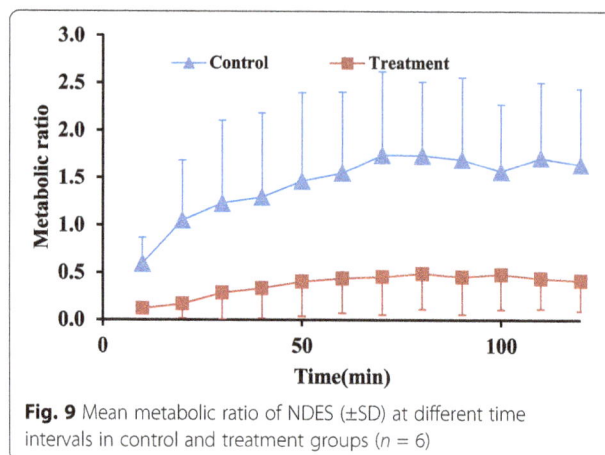

Fig. 8 Mean metabolic ratio of 8-OH (±SD) at different time intervals in treatment and control groups (n = 6)

Acknowledgements
Not applicable.

Funding
No funding was received.

Authors' contributions
MR R participated in research design. SJ conducted the experiments. HL contributed new reagents or analytical tools. YH A performed data analysis. Both SJ and YH A wrote or contributed to the writing of the manuscript. All authors read and approved the final manuscript.

Competing interests
The authors declare that they have no competing interests.

References
1. De la Torre R, Farré M, Roset PN, Pizarro N, Abanades S, Segura M, et al. Human pharmacology of MDMA: pharmacokinetics, metabolism, and disposition. Ther Drug Monit. 2004;26(2):137–44.
2. Antolino-Lobo I, Meulenbelt J, Nijmeijer SM, Scherpenisse P, van den Berg M, van Duursen MB. Differential roles of phase I and phase II enzymes in 3, 4-methylendioxymethamphetamine-induced cytotoxicity. Drug Metab Dispos. 2010;38(7):1105–12.
3. Jamali B, Ardakani YH, Foroumadi A, Kobarfard F, Rouini M-R. Determination of MDMA and Its Three Metabolites in the Rat Perfused Liver. J Anal Toxicol. 2013.
4. Bertelsen KM, Venkatakrishnan K, Von Moltke LL, Obach RS, Greenblatt DJ. Apparent mechanism-based inhibition of human CYP2D6 in vitro by paroxetine: comparison with fluoxetine and quinidine. Drug Metab Dispos. 2003;31(3):289–93.
5. Heydari A, Yeo KR, Lennard M, Ellis SW, Tucker G, Rostami-Hodjegan A. Mechanism-based inactivation of CYP2D6 by methylenedioxymethamphetamine. Drug Metab Dispos. 2004;32(11):1213–7.
6. Venkatakrishnan K, Obach R, Rostami-Hodjegan A. Mechanism-based inactivation of human cytochrome P450 enzymes: strategies for diagnosis and drug–drug interaction risk assessment. Xenobiotica. 2007;37(10–11):1225–56.
7. Yang J, Jamei M, Heydari A, Yeo KR, de la Torre R, Farré M, et al. Implications of mechanism-based inhibition of CYP2D6 for the pharmacokinetics and toxicity of MDMA. J Psychopharmacol. 2006;20(6):842–9.
8. Green AR, Mechan AO, Elliott JM, O'Shea E, Colado MI. The pharmacology and clinical pharmacology of 3, 4-methylenedioxymethamphetamine (MDMA,"ecstasy"). Pharmacol Rev. 2003;55(3):463-508.
9. Delbressine L, Moonen M, Kaspersen F, Wagenaars G, Jacobs P, Timmer C, et al. Pharmacokinetics and biotransformation of mirtazapine in human volunteers. Clin Drug investig. 1998;15(1):45–55.
10. Puzantian T. Mirtazapine, an antidepressant. Am J Health Syst Pharm. 1998; 55(1):44–9.
11. Kasper S, Praschak-Rieder N, Tauscher J, Wolf R. A risk-benefit assessment of mirtazapine in the treatment of depression. Drug Saf. 1997;17(4):251–64.
12. Anttila SA, Leinonen EV. A review of the pharmacological and clinical profile of mirtazapine. CNS Drug Rev. 2001;7(3):249–64.
13. Störmer E, von Moltke LL, Shader RI, Greenblatt DJ. Metabolism of the antidepressant mirtazapine in vitro: contribution of cytochromes P-450 1A2, 2D6, and 3A4. Drug Metab Dispos. 2000;28(10):1168–75.
14. Timmer CJ, Sitsen JA, Delbressine LP. Clinical pharmacokinetics of mirtazapine. Clin Pharmacokinet. 2000;38(6):461–74.
15. Pizarro N, de la Torre R, Farré M, Segura J, Llebaria A, Joglar J. Synthesis and capillary electrophoretic analysis of enantiomerically enriched reference standards of MDMA and its main metabolites. Bioorg Med Chem. 2002; 10(4):1085–92.
16. Baumann MH, Zolkowska D, Kim I, Scheidweiler KB, Rothman RB, Huestis MA. Effects of dose and route of administration on pharmacokinetics of (±)-3, 4-methylenedioxymethamphetamine in the rat. Drug Metab Dispos. 2009;37(11):2163–70.
17. Lavasani H, Giorgi M, Sheikholeslami B, Hedayati M, Rouini MR. A rapid and sensitive hplc-fluorescence method for determination of mirtazapine and its two major metabolites in human plasma. Iran J Pharm Res. 2014;13(3):853.
18. Mehvar R, Vuppugalla R. Hepatic disposition of the cytochrome P450 2E1 marker chlorzoxazone and its hydroxylated metabolite in isolated perfused rat livers. J Pharm Sci. 2006;95(7):1414–24.
19. Downey C, Daly F, O'Boyle K. An in vitro approach to assessing a potential drug interaction between MDMA (ecstasy) and caffeine. Toxicol in Vitro. 2014;28(2):231–9.
20. Antolino-Lobo I, Meulenbelt J, Nijmeijer SM, Maas-Bakker RF, Meijerman I, van den Berg M, et al. 3, 4-Methylenedioxymethamphetamine (MDMA) interacts with therapeutic drugs on CYP3A by inhibition of pregnane X receptor (PXR) activation and catalytic enzyme inhibition. Toxicol Lett. 2011; 203(1):82–91.
21. Zhou S, Chan SY, Goh BC, Chan E, Duan W, Huang M, et al. Mechanism-based inhibition of cytochrome P450 3A4 by therapeutic drugs. Clin Pharmacokinet. 2005;44(3):279–304.
22. Farré M, Abanades S, Roset PN, Peiró AM, Torrens M, O'Mathúna B, et al. Pharmacological interaction between 3, 4-methylenedioxymethamphetamine (ecstasy) and paroxetine: pharmacological effects and pharmacokinetics. J Pharmacol Exp Ther. 2007; 323(3):954–62.
23. Vuori E, Henry JA, Ojanperä I, Nieminen R, Savolainen T, Wahlsten P, et al. Death following ingestion of MDMA (ecstasy) and moclobemide. Addiction. 2003;98(3):365–8.
24. Fetter JC. Letter to the Editor: Mirtazepine for MDMA-induced Depression. Am J Addict. 2005;14(3):300–1.
25. Mohamed WM, Hamida SB, Cassel J-C, de Vasconcelos AP, Jones BC. MDMA: interactions with other psychoactive drugs. Pharmacol Biochem Behav. 2011;99(4):759–74.
26. Baumann MH, Rothman RB. Neural and cardiac toxicities associated with 3, 4-methylenedioxymethamphetamine (MDMA). Int Rev Neurobiol. 2009;88: 257–96.
27. Greenblatt DJ, von Moltke LL, Harmatz JS, Shader RI. Human cytochromes and some newer antidepressants: kinetics, metabolism, and drug interactions. J Clin Psychopharmacol. 1999;19(5):23S–35S.
28. Anttila SA, Rasanen I, Leinonen EV. Fluvoxamine augmentation increases serum mirtazapine concentrations three-to fourfold. Ann Pharmacother. 2001;35(10):1221–3.

Sustained-release study on Exenatide loaded into mesoporous silica nanoparticles: in vitro characterization and in vivo evaluation

Cuiwei Chen[1], Hongyue Zheng[2], Junjun Xu[3], Xiaowei Shi[1], Fanzhu Li[1*] and Xuanshen Wang[4*]

Abstract

Background: Exenatide (EXT), the first glucagon-like peptide-1 receptor agonist, has been approved as an adjunctive therapy for patients with type 2 diabetes. Due to EXT's short half-life, EXT must be administrated by continuous subcutaneous (s.c.) injection twice daily. In previous studies, many studies on EXT loaded into polymer materials carriers for sustained release had been reported. However, these carriers have some defects, such as hydrophobicity, low surface energy, low mechanical strength, and poor chemical stability. Therefore, this study aims to develop a novel drug delivery system, which is EXT loaded into well-ordered hexagonal mesoporous silica structures (EXT-SBA-15), to control the sustainability of EXT.

Methods: SBA-15 was prepared by hydrothermal method with uniform size. Morphology of SBA-15 was employed by transmission electron microscopy. The pore size of SBA-15 was characterized by N_2 adsorption–desorption isotherms. The in vitro drug release behavior and pharmacokinetics of EXT-SBA-15 were investigated. Furthermore, the blood glucose levels of diabetic mice were monitored after subcutaneous injection of EXT-Sol and EXT-SBA-15 to evaluate further the stable hypoglycemic effect of EXT-SBA-15.

Results: EXT-SBA-15 showed a higher drug loading efficiency ($15.2 \pm 2.0\%$) and sustained-release features in vitro. In addition, pharmacokinetic studies revealed that the EXT-SBA-15 treatment group extended the half-life $t_{1/2(\beta)}$ to 14.53 ± 0.70 h compared with that of the EXT solution (EXT-Sol) treatment group (0.60 ± 0.08 h) in vivo. Results of the pharmacodynamics study show that the EXT-SBA-15 treatment group had inhibited blood glucose levels below 20 mmol/L for 25 days, and the lowest blood glucose level was 13 mmol/L on the 10th day.

Conclusions: This study demonstrates that the EXT-SBA-15 delivery system can control the sustainability of EXT and contribute to improve EXT clinical use.

Keywords: Exenatide, Type 2 diabetic, Mesoporous silica nanoparticles, Sustained release, Pharmacokinetics/Pharmacodynamics

* Correspondence: lifanzhu@zcmu.edu.cn; 542695603@qq.com
[1]Department of Pharmaceutics, Zhejiang Chinese Medical University, Hangzhou 311042, China
[4]Department of Pharmacy, The Second Hospital of Dalian Medical University, Dalian 116027, China
Full list of author information is available at the end of the article

Background

Exenatide (EXT), a 39-amino acid peptide, is the synthetic version of exendin-4 isolated from salivary secretions of *Heloderma horridum lizard* venom [1, 2]. EXT shares approximately 53% sequence homology with the mammalian glucagon-like peptide-1 (GLP-1), which exhibits obvious advantages developed as a glucose-lowering agent with similar functions as GLP-1 [3, 4]. In currently, EXT is available in the market (Byetta™) as adjunctive therapy to improve glucose homeostasis in type 2 diabetic patients [5]. However, the twice daily subcutaneous (s.c.) injections of EXT have posed clear shortcomings, such as inconvenience for the administration, local pain and irritation during the injection [6]. Sustained-release drug delivery system for exenatide (EXT) must be developed to solve the problem of long-term medication and overcome the inconvenience of injection.

Many studies had reported EXT loaded into carriers for sustained release [7–9]. The US FDA has approved a long-acting formulation of EXT dispersed in poly-(D,L-lactide-co-glycolide) polymer microspheres in 2012 [10]. However, these polymer-material carriers have defects, such as hydrophobicity, low surface energy, low mechanical strength, and poor chemical stability. In this study, we selected well-ordered hexagonal mesoporous silica structures (SBA-15) to load EXT This drug carrier material presents several beneficial properties for sustained-release drug delivery, including controllable size and pore morphology to obtain the desired rate of drug release, large internal surface area to allow the adsorption and delivery of high drug payloads within the nanopores, proper in vivo stability preventing premature drug degradation, biodegradability and biocompatibility [11–14]. Moreover, SBA-15 has the potential for the delivery of peptides and proteins. For example, cytochrome c, xylanase, and heme proteins have been loaded into SBA-15 [15–17]. Favorably, peptides and proteins loading into SBA-15 avoid stressful procedures that can protect the molecules from bioinactivation, and the stable inorganic oxide framework of mesoporous silica nanoparticles shelters the peptides and proteins from chemical and thermal exposure and harmful species; thus, the electrochemical activity of proteins and peptides would be retained or even increased. Additionally, studies on EXT loaded into SBA-15 are few.

In this study, we have developed EXT loaded into SBA-15 (EXT-SBA-15) delivery system to control the sustainability of EXT. EXT-SBA-15 showed a high drug-loading efficiency. Morphology and pore size of SBA-15 was characterized. The obtained results indicated that EXT-SBA-15 has a significant sustained-release effect and can improve EXT's pharmacokinetic features. Furthermore, EXT-SBA-15 exhibited long-lasting and remarkable glucose-lowering effects. The present study demonstrates the therapeutic potential of EXT-SBA-15 for clinical applications.

Methods

Materials and animals

Exenatide (mw. 4186.63, 98%) was provided by GL Biochem Ltd. (Shanghai, China). Poly(ethylene oxide)–poly (propylene oxide)–poly(ethylene oxide) (PEO_{20}-PPO_{70}-PEO_{20}) (P-123), Tetraethyl orthosilicate (TEOS) and streptozotocin (STZ) were purchased from Sigma-Aldrich Co., Ltd. (St. Louis, MO, USA). Exendin-4 ELISA kit (EK-070-94) was purchased from Phoenix Pharmaceuticals Inc. (USA). Sprague-Dawley (SD) rats (250 ± 20 g) and ICR mice (25 ± 5 g) were supplied by SLRC Laboratory Animal Ltd. (Shanghai, China). All experimental protocols and animal handling procedures were performed in accordance with the guidelines for the care and use of laboratory animals and approved by the Committees for Animal Experiments at Zhejiang University.

Preparation of EXT-SBA-15

SBA-15 was prepared by hydrothermal method according to the existing methods [18]. SBA-15 used in this study was synthesized according to the following procedure: We mixed 4 g P-123 in 129.6 g double distilled water and 19.3 mL of hydrochloric acid (HCl 37%). Stirring the mixture intensively at 50 °C for 2 h was needed to ensure a homogeneous emulsion. Then TEOS (8.65 g) was added and the system was stirred for another 20 h at 80 °C. The resultant particles were collected by centrifugation (Optima MAX Ultracentrifuge, Beckman-Coulter Co. Ltd., California, USA) (5590×g, 30 min) after washing with 1000 mL of distilled water. The precipitate was dried in a vacuum at 100 °C for 12 h, and then SBA-15 was obtained by calcination at 550 °C for 6 h.

Dispersing 20 mg SBA-15 with 10 mL aqueous solution of EXT (1 mg/mL) and stir at a rate of 300 r/min at room temperature for 24 h. The loading solution was treated with ultrasound 3 times to guarantee homogeneity [19]. The nanoparticles were collected by centrifugation (5590×g, 30 min), followed by washing with double distilled water for three times. Then, EXT-SBA-15 was dried for 3 h at room temperature in vacuum.

EXT loading degree was detected by thermogravimetric (TG) analysis (20 °C/min, 25 °C–800 °C N_2 gas purge 200 mL/min, TGA, SDT Q600, TA instrument). Three batches of EXT-SBA-15 were used in the experiments.

In vitro characterization

Morphological evaluation of blank SBA-15 was performed on transmission electron microscopy (TEM, H-7650, Jeol, Tokyo, Japan). Samples were prepared by dispersing the powder products as slurry in water, which was then deposited and dried on a holey carbon film on a copper grid. A low-exposure technique was used to reduce the effect of beam damage and sample drift. The micrographs of SBA-15 were recorded digitally with TEM operating at 200kv. The particle size (mean diameter, nm) and Zeta potential (mV) were determined by Zetasizer Nano-ZS (Malvern Instruments, Malvern, UK) at room temperature.

The mesostructure ordering was recorded on a small angle X-ray diffractometer (SAXRD) analyzer (D8-AD-VANCE, Bruker, Karlsruhe, Germany) with the scattering angle (2θ) range from 0.5° to 6° and scanning speed of 0.02°/min.

Surface area, pore size and pore volume were calculated by N_2 adsorption-desorption isotherms and structure parameters were determined with multi-channel automatic specific surface area analyzer (TriStar II 3020, Micromeritics Instrument Corp, USA). The surface area and pore size of MSNs were calculated by the BET and the Barrett Joyner Halenda (BJH) methods respectively. The pore volume was determined from the absorption branch of the N_2 isotherm curve at the P/P_0 = 0.983 signal point, STP, standard temperature and pressure.

In vitro release study
5 mg EXT-SBA-15 nanoparticles were placed in an Eppendorf tube and suspended in 1.5 mL phosphate-buffered saline (PBS, pH 7.4). Eppendorf tubes were placed in a water bath with orbital shaking at a frequency of 150 shakes/min at 37 °C. The release medium was removed at each time point (0.04, 0.08, 0.17, 0.25, 0.42, 0.67, 1, 2, 3, 5, 7, 10, 14 d) after centrifugation at 5590×g for 15 min. Supernatants were collected for the High Performance Liquid Chromatograph (HPLC) analysis of the EXT concentration. The system was consisted of an Agilent 1200 (Agilent, USA) equipped with UV detector. The analytical column was a TSKgel G2000SWXL column (300 mm × 7.8 mm, 5 μm) maintained at 25 °C. The mobile phase consisted of 0.13 mol/L sodium sulfate (Na_2SO_4) and acetonitrile (75:25) containing 0.1% trifluoroacetic acid (TFA) at a flow rate of 0.8 mL/min, and EXT was detected at 283 nm.

Pharmacokinetics study
Pharmacokinetic studies of EXT-Sol and EXT-SBA-15 were conducted in healthy male SD rats. Sixteen rats were randomly divided into two groups (n = 8) and fasted overnight with free access to water before administration. SD rats were received s.c. administration of EXT-Sol and EXT-SBA-15 at a single EXT dose of 50 μg/kg, respectively [20, 21]. The blood samples (0.5 mL) of EXT-Sol treatment group were collected from the rat's orbit and at specific time 0, 0.25, 0.5, 1, 1.5, 2, 3, 4, 6, 8 h after injection [21]. The blood samples (0.5 mL) of EXT-SBA-15 treatment group (0.5 mL) were

collected at 0, 0.5, 1, 1.5, 2, 3, 5, 8, 12, 24, 36, 48, 72, 120 h. The collected blood samples were centrifuged at 503×g for 10 min to obtain the plasma, which were stored at –80 °C for further analysis. The plasma concentrations of EXT were measured by Exendin-4 ELISA kit according to the instructions supplied by the manufacturer [22–24]. The relevant pharmacokinetic parameters were analyzed by PKSolver 2.0 [25].

In vivo Pharmacodynamics study
Type 2 diabetes model was induced by STZ with multiple injection method into ICR mice. Each mouse was injected intraperitoneally with 30 mg/kg·d STZ in 0.1 mol/L citric acid buffer (pH 5.0) [26, 27]. One week after the injection, mice were fasted for 12 h (with free access to water) before their blood glucose was measured by glucometer (Accu-Chek Performa, Germany). Diabetic mice were considered by fasting blood glucose above 11.1 mmol/L. Six healthy normal ICR mice were used as the blank control group (A). Twenty-four mice that had developed type 2 diabetes were randomly divided into four experimental groups and received s.c. administration of saline (B), EXT-Sol (C), EXT-SBA-15 (D) and SBA-15 (E), respectively. Group A and B received saline twice daily via s.c. administration. Group C received EXT-Sol twice daily with a dose of EXT (3 μg/kg/d). Group D and E were administrated a single injection of EXT-SBA-15 (600 μg/kg) and SBA-15 via s.c. administration, respectively [28]. The blood sample (about 0.2 ml) was collected from the tail-vein on days 0, 1, 5, 10, 15, 20, 25 for all groups, and blood glucose levels were determined measured simultaneously with a glucometer before administration.

Statistical analysis
Statistical analysis using one way analysis of variance (ANOVA) with SPSS software (version 19, IBM Inc., Chicago, IL, USA) and a value of $p < 0.05$ was considered to be statistically significant.

Results
In vitro characterization
Figure 1 a, b, c, d shows that SBA-15 has a rod-like morphology with uniform size and less aggregation. The well-ordered hexagonal arrays of mesoporous on SBA-15 are shown in the highly magnified TEM image (Fig. 1e, f) and confirm that SBA-15 has a 2D p6mm hexagonal structure. The prepared SBA-15 exhibited an average diameter of 920 ± 120 nm with a narrow size distribution, and the Zeta potential is –8.19 ± 2.96 mV. Figure 2a displays the N_2 adsorption–desorption patterns of SBA-15 exhibiting the characteristic type IV isotherm, and a clear type-H1 hysteresis loop was observed; this observation further proves that mesoporous were

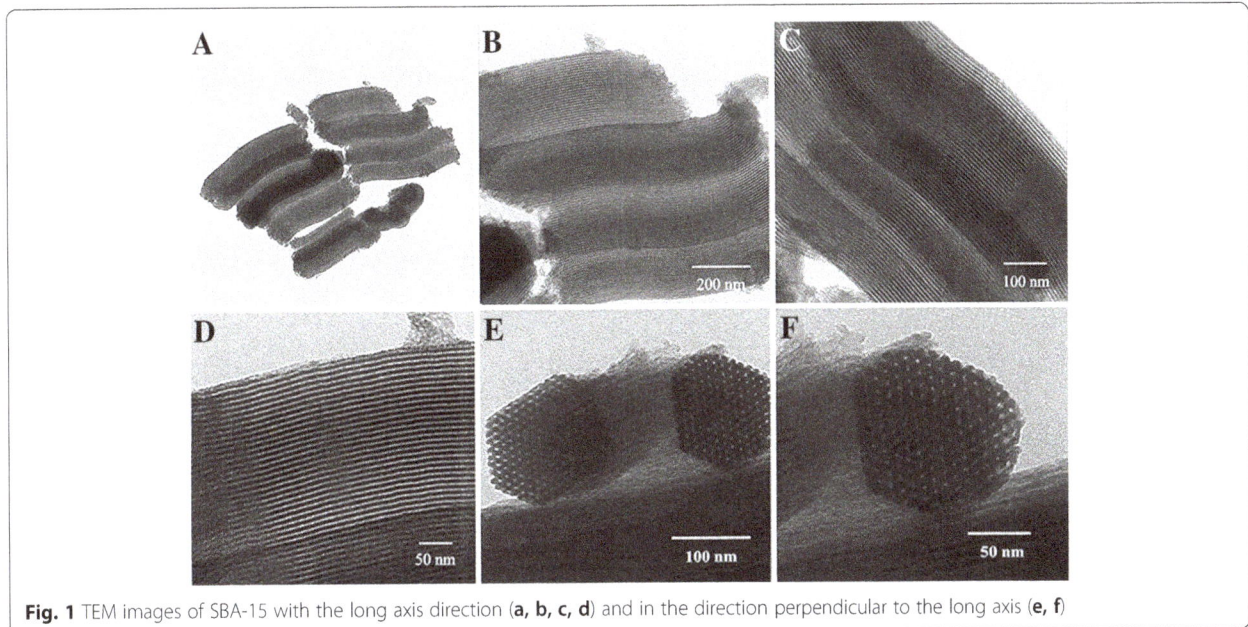

Fig. 1 TEM images of SBA-15 with the long axis direction (**a, b, c, d**) and in the direction perpendicular to the long axis (**e, f**)

regular and uniform. In addition, SBA-15 was yielded with a Barrett Joyner Halenda pore volume of 0.94 ± 0.03 cm^3/g and a Brunauer Emmett Teller surface area of 701.4 ± 0.70 m^2/g. The pore size distribution of SBA-15 shows a narrow distribution with a mean value of 6.0 ± 0.2 nm (Fig. 2b). The SAXRD of SBA-15 is shown in Fig. 2c; a strong diffraction peak occurred around 1°, indicating that the internal structures of nanoparticles were in ordered arrangement. On the contrary, the diffraction peak became weak in 1–2°. Three well-resolved peaks are indexable as (100), (110), and (200) reflections associated with a P6mm hexagonal symmetry. TGA method was applied to calculate the drug-loading efficiency ($15.2 \pm 2.0\%$).

In vitro release study

The in vitro release profiles of EXT-SBA-15 in 2 weeks were illustrated in Fig. 3. The release rate was relatively rapid, with approximately 33% of the encapsulated drug released at day 1. The rapid initial release of the cargo can be explained by wake bonding between the drug and the surface of the nanoparticles through electrostatic absorption and Van der Waals Forces. Then the drug released more slowly and moderately than before. The cumulative release is about 67% in 14 days. The in vitro release study of EXT-SBA-15 enhanced its sustained-release characteristics and can control the concentration within a narrow range.

Pharmacokinetics study

The pharmacokinetics of EXT-SBA-15 was evaluated in SD rats through s.c. administration to investigate the in vivo behavior of EXT-SBA-15. The plasma concentration–time profiles of rats are shown in Fig. 4. After SD rats were injected with EXT-Sol at a dose of 50 μg/kg, the plasma concentration of EXT increased rapidly, reached the peak within 0.5 h, followed by a rapid decrease to baseline after 8 h. In contrast, in the group treated with EXT-SBA-15, the absorption and elimination of EXT in vivo were very slow. Sustained-release characteristics can be observed in EXT-SBA-15. The EXT concentration–time curves for EXT-Sol and

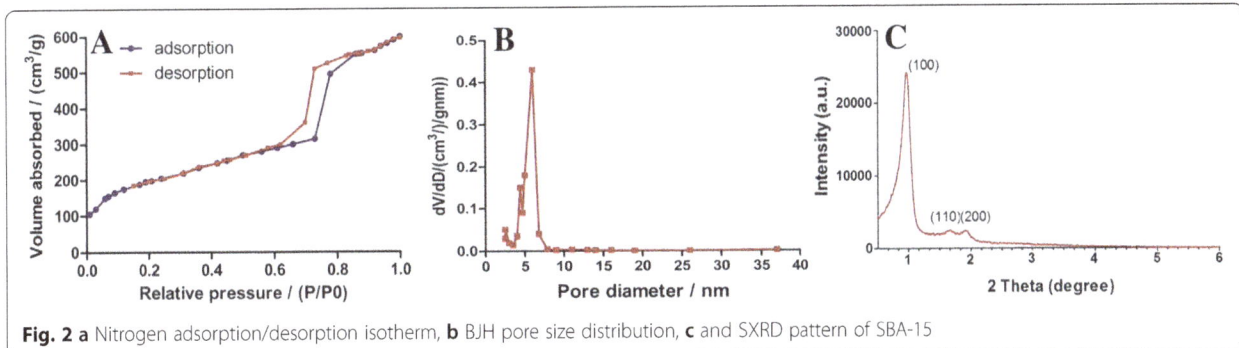

Fig. 2 a Nitrogen adsorption/desorption isotherm, **b** BJH pore size distribution, **c** and SXRD pattern of SBA-15

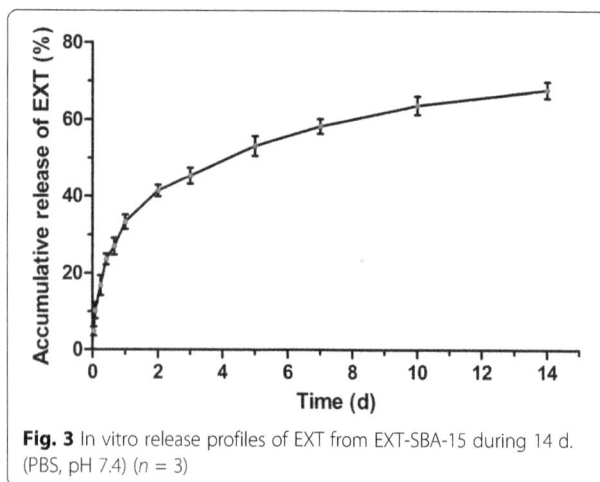

Fig. 3 In vitro release profiles of EXT from EXT-SBA-15 during 14 d. (PBS, pH 7.4) (n = 3)

Table 1 Pharmacokinetics parameters of EXT-Sol and EXT-SBA-15 after s.c. injection in SD rats (Mean ± SD, $n = 8$)

Parameters	EXT-Sol	EXT-SBA-15
$t_{1/2(\alpha)}$/h	0.22 ± 0.03	0.26 ± 0.05*
$t_{1/2(\beta)}$/h	0.60 ± 0.08	14.53 ± 0.70**
t_{max}/h	0.46 ± 0.02	1.38 ± 0.22*
c_{max}/ng·ml^{-1}	1.16 ± 0.09	0.39 ± 0.01*
$AUC_{0\rightarrow t}$/ng·ml^{-1}·h	1.71 ± 0.07	8.60 ± 0.57**
$AUC_{0\rightarrow\infty}$/ng·ml^{-1}·h	1.71 ± 0.07	8.77 ± 0.76**
MRT/h	1.14 ± 0.07	21.30 ± 0.99**

*$p < 0.05$, **$p < 0.01$, EXT-SBA-15 compared to EXT-Sol
$t_{1/2(\alpha)}$ half-life of distribution, $t_{1/2(\beta)}$ half-life of elimination, t_{max} time to peak concentration, c_{max} peak concentration, $AUC_{0\rightarrow t}$ area under concentration-time curve from 0 to final time, $AUC_{0\rightarrow\infty}$ area under concentration-time curve from 0 to infinite time, MRT mean residence time of drug in body

EXT-SBA-15 were all fitted with the two-compartment model; the pharmacokinetic parameters are listed in Table 1. The plasma concentration of the sustained-release EXT-SBA-15 attained C_{max} of 0.39 ng/mL at T_{max} of 1.38 h. The EXT-SBA-15 treatment group extended the half-life $t_{1/2(\beta)}$ to 14.53 ± 0.70 h compared with that of the EXT solution (EXT-Sol) treatment group (0.60 ± 0.08 h) in vivo. Remarkably, a prolonged MRT ($p < 0.01$) indicated the extended circulation time of EXT-SBA-15; the $AUC_{0\rightarrow\infty}$ of EXT-SBA-15 was significantly larger than that of EXT-Sol; these results implicated that EXT-SBA-15 possess an enhanced sustained-release characteristics and improves the pharmacokinetic behavior of EXT in rats by prolonging the retention time in circulation.

In vivo Pharmacodynamics study
As shown in Fig. 5a, during the first 8 h after treatment, the blood glucose levels of saline-treated diabetic mice (model control treatment group) were at 20 mmol/L,

whereas the group treated with EXT-Sol effectively lowered blood glucose within 2 h and EXT-Sol was kept effective for another 2 h, and then blood glucose gradually returned to the original level. By contrast, the group treated with EXT-SBA-15 slowly reduced the blood glucose levels to 14 mmol/L, which exhibited long-lasting and remarkable glucose-lowering effects. These results indicated a prolonged duration of action in the case of EXT-SBA-15 treatment. In addition, the blood glucose concentration in the blank SBA-15 treatment group was kept greater than 20 mmol/L after s.c. treatment; this result indicates that blank SBA-15 had no effect in lowering glucose. During further measurements, up to 25 days (Fig. 5b), the effect on glucose lowering was not observed in the EXT-Sol treatment group in spite of twice daily injection. However, the EXT-SBA-15 treatment group continued to inhibit glucose level after administration and had a significant difference with the model control treatment group (*$p < 0.001$, **$p < 0.01$, compared with model control treatment group). The

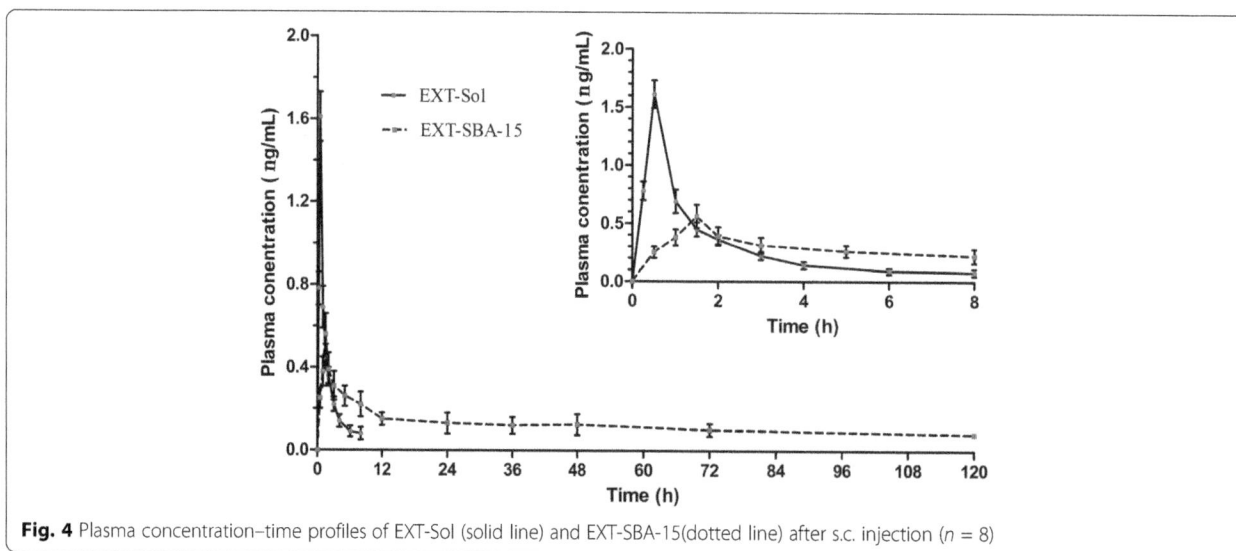

Fig. 4 Plasma concentration–time profiles of EXT-Sol (solid line) and EXT-SBA-15(dotted line) after s.c. injection ($n = 8$)

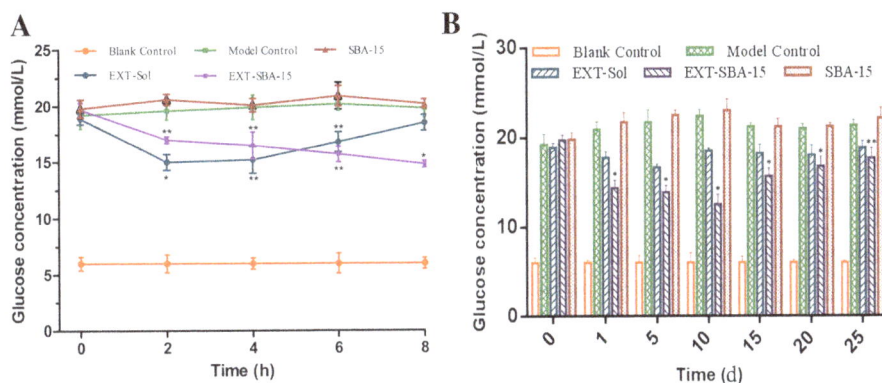

Fig. 5 The anti-diabetes effects of EXT-Sol and EXT-SBA-15 on diabetic mice (n = 6). **a** The short-term glucose regulating effects of EXT-Sol and EXT-SBA-15 on diabetic mice (s.c. EXT 3 μg/kg/d, twice daily; EXT-SBA-15 600 μg/kg, single injection, n = 6). **b** The long-term glucose regulating effects of EXT-Sol and EXT-SBA-15 on diabetic mice (s.c. EXT 3 μg/kg/d, twice daily; EXT-SBA-15 600 μg/kg, single injection, n = 6). *$P < 0.001$ and **$P < 0.01$ compared to model control

lowest blood glucose level was 13 mmol/L on the 10th day. Similarly, the SBA-15 treatment group did not have an effect of lowered glucose level.

Discussion

EXT is a very promising drug for the treatment of type 2 diabetes. However, due to the rapid degradation of EXT in vivo via elimination in the kidneys, it must be administered continuously twice-daily s.c. injection. The need for EXT has continued to fuel attempts to develop it with long-acting pharmacodynamic and pharmacokinetic properties. Therefore, SBA-15 might offer a solution to the obstacles of EXT administration. In the present study, the large-pore SBA-15 had high payloading (15% w/w), though EXT is a large-molecule drug. Nanoporous structure and large surface area of SBA-15 contributes to its great capability to adsorb and deliver high amounts of EXT that has been a problem with traditional polymer materials (3.65% w/w) [29]. Furthermore EXT consists of a 39-amino acid, which might be loaded into nanoporous SBA-15 in the form of a chain structure. Hence, the rod-like SBA-15 is a potential to load EXT. EXT adsorption into nanoporous SBA-15 is caused by a complex interplay of different mechanisms, such as the electrostatic interaction, counterion release, and Van der Waals Forces [30]. The protein molecules bind to the negative-charged silica via charged amino acid residues on the protein's surface. In addition, as the concentration of EXT outside was much higher than that inside, EXT tended to diffuse into the channel of the nanoparticles. Therefore, only by combining different mechanisms are we able to explain the load behavior of EXT into SBA-15.

The in vitro drug release of EXT-SBA-15 exhibited biphasic drug release patterns, which is a burst release at the initial stage and a prolonged release afterwards. The

initial burst release of EXT, which benefits by quickly reaching the effective treatment concentration, was due to the presence of EXT in the external pores of SBA-15. EXT in the pores inside SBA-15 were released slowly into the release medium and maintained the effective concentration. As mentioned earlier, the release of drug stored in mesoporous silica nanoparticles occurs only after the release medium has penetrated into the channels and the drug has been dissolved. This is then followed by diffusion along aqueous pathways into the medium. The mechanism of release is a combination of diffusion and dissolution processes [31, 32]. EXT molecules, which are loaded in large-pore SBA-15, had much more opportunity of escaping from pore channels and diffusing into the release medium. Furthermore, the release rate of EXT from SBA-15 may depend on the degradation of the silica nanoparticles. Silica nanoparticles degrade over time in the body, which is available to be material for drug delivery [33]. The in vitro release and pharmacokinetics studies demonstrate sustained EXT release from the nanoporous SBA-15. Pharmacokinetics results suggest that EXT-SBA-15 significantly improved the absolute bioavailability of EXT from that of the EXT-Sol. These results suggest that a complete absorption of subcutaneous EXT requires a sustained release process instead of an immediate release process. Combined with the in vitro drug release study, the cumulative release rate (F_r) was the independent variable, and the in vivo absorption percentage (F_a) was the dependent variable. The correlation equation was $F_a = 1.152F_r - 3.137$, $r = 0.8161$. EXT-SBA-15 showed certain correlation between in vitro cumulative release rate and in vivo absorption percentage. Generally, the pharmacokinetics results indicate that the investigated SBA-15 nanocarriers are compatible with the peptide and do not compromise its biological activity, as the method used here for determining EXT plasma concentrations is a specific ELISA-detecting active EXT molecules.

The pharmacological activity of EXT, which was administered via SBA-15 nanoparticles in vivo, was examined by measuring the glucagon level. In agreement, sustained effects on glucagon inhibition were obtained with EXT-SBA-15 nanoparticles. The short-term glucose-regulating effects of EXT-Sol and EXT-SBA-15 on diabetic mice confirmed a more rapid and immediate decrease in the blood glucose after EXT-Sol administration compared with EXT-SBA-15 administration. However, the effect of EXT gradually weakened after 2 h. EXT-SBA-15 exhibited efficacy that is comparable to EXT-Sol on 5 h. Finally, EXT-Sol returned to the original glucagon level after 10 h; this result shows that EXT has been metabolized completely in vivo and has no ability to control blood glucose for a long time. The long-term glucose-regulating effects of EXT-SBA-15 administration showed that on the first day, a relatively rapid decrease in the blood glucose level was observed. This result indicates that the initial release rate of EXT-SBA-15 is adequate for its pharmacological efficacy. In the first week after EXT-SBA-15 administration, glucose level is maintained at a lower concentration level, and the lowest blood glucose level was 13 mmol/L on the 10th day. Afterwards, the blood glucose concentration started to increase; however, the glucose level was significantly lower than that of the model control group (>20 mmol/L). These results clearly indicate that EXT-SBA-15 provides adequate initial release and sustained release in vivo to maintain blood glucose levels.

Conclusion

In conclusion, EXT was successfully loaded into SBA-15 mesoporous silica nanoparticles with a high loading degree, as much as 15% *w*/w. In vitro release and pharmacokinetics studies EXT showed sustained release from the nanoporous of SBA-15. It exhibited prolonged circulation time and significantly increased the bioavailability of EXT. In addition, EXT-SBA-15 showed a prolonged hypoglycemic effect compared with EXT solution. These works contribute to improve EXT clinical use, and further develop the SBA-15 as drug carriers for achieving controlled proteins and peptides drug delivery.

Acknowledgements
Not applicable.

Funding
This work was financially supported by the National Natural Science Foundation of China (No. 81274089, No. 81473361), the Natural Science Foundation of Zhejiang Province (No. LZ13H280001, LY12H280004) and the Traditional Chinese Medicine Science and Technology Plan of Zhejiang Province (2016ZA130).

Authors' contributions
All authors have participated sufficiently in this work to take public responsibility for it; and have reviewed the final version of the manuscript and approve it for publication.

Competing interests
The authors declare that they have no competing interests.

Author details
[1]Department of Pharmaceutics, Zhejiang Chinese Medical University, Hangzhou 311042, China. [2]Libraries of Zhejiang Chinese Medical University Zhejiang Chinese Medical University, Hangzhou 310053, China. [3]Department of Pharmacy, The Second Affiliated Hospital, School of Medicine, Zhejiang University, Hangzhou 310052, China. [4]Department of Pharmacy, The Second Hospital of Dalian Medical University, Dalian 116027, China.

References
1. Davidson MB, Bate G, Kirkpatrick P. Exenatide. Nat Rev Drug Discov. 2005;4:713–4.
2. Nielsen LL, Young AA, Parkes DG. Pharmacology of exenatide (synthetic exendin-4): a potential therapeutic for improved glycemic control of type 2 diabetes. Regul Pept. 2004;117:77–88.
3. Hui H, Zhao X, Perfetti R. Structure and function studies of glucagon-like peptide-1 (GLP-1): the designing of a novel pharmacological agent for the treatment of diabetes. Diabetes Metab Res. 2005;21:189–96.
4. Gentilella R, Bianchi C, Rossi A, et al. Exenatide: a review from pharmacology to clinical practice. Diabetes Obes Metab. 2009;11:544–56.
5. Scheen AJ, Van Gaal LF. Exenatide (Byetta) incretinomimetic in the treatment of type 2 diabetes after failure and as add-on therapy to oral agents. Rev Med Lieg. 2008;63:158–65.
6. Gedulin BR, Smith PA, Jodka CM, et al. Pharmacokinetics and pharmacodynamics of exenatide following alternate routes of administration. Int J Pharm. 2008;356:231–8.
7. Kwak HH, Shim WS, Son MK, et al. Efficacy of a new sustained-release microsphere formulation of exenatide, DA-3091, in Zucker diabetic fatty (ZDF) rats. Eur J Pharm Sci. 2010;40:103–9.
8. Kwak HH, Shim WS, Hwang S, et al. Pharmacokinetics and efficacy of a biweekly dosage formulation of exenatide in Zucker diabetic fatty (ZDF) rats. Pharm Res. 2009;26:2504–12.
9. Xuan J, Lin Y, Huang J, et al. Exenatide-loaded PLGA microspheres with improved glycemic control: in vitro bioactivity and in vivo pharmacokinetic profiles after subcutaneous administration to SD rats. Peptides. 2013;46:172–9.
10. Larue S, Malloy J. Evaluation of the dual-chamber pen design for the injection of exenatide once weekly for the treatment of type 2 diabetes. J Diabetes Sci Technol. 2015;9:815–21.
11. Mamaeva V, Sahlgren C, Lindén M. Mesoporous silica nanoparticles in medicine-recent advances. Adv Drug Deliv Rev. 2013;65:689–702.
12. Niu D, Liu Z, Li Y, et al. Monodispersed and ordered large-pore mesoporous silica nanospheres with tunable pore structure for magnetic functionalization and gene delivery. Adv Mater. 2014;26:4947–53.
13. Wu SH, Mou CY, Lin HP. Synthesis of mesoporous silica nanoparticles. Chem Soc Rev. 2013;42:3862–75.
14. Chen Y, Chen H, Shi J. In vivo bio-safety evaluations and diagnostic/therapeutic applications of chemically designed Mesoporous silica Nanoparticles. Adv Mater. 2013;25:3144–76.
15. Deere J, Magner E, Wall JG, et al. Mechanistic and structural features of protein adsorption onto mesoporous silicates. J Phys Chem B. 2002;106:7340–7.
16. Slowing II, Trewyn BG, Lin VS. Mesoporous silica nanoparticles for intracellular delivery of membrane-impermeable proteins. J Am Chem Soc. 2007;129:8845–9.
17. Miyahara M, Vinu A, Hossain KZ, et al. Adsorption study of heme proteins on SBA-15 mesoporous silica with pore-filling models. Thin Solid Films. 2006;499:13–8.
18. Zhao D, Feng J, Huo Q, et al. Triblock copolymer syntheses of mesoporous silica with periodic 50 to 300 angstrom pores. Science. 1998;279:548–52.
19. Jia L, Shen J, Li Z, et al. In vitro and in vivo evaluation of paclitaxel-loaded mesoporous silica nanoparticles with three pore sizes. Int J Pharm. 2013;445:12 9.

20. Nguyen HN, Wey SP, Juang JH, et al. The glucose-lowering potential of exendin-4 orally delivered via a pH-sensitive nanoparticle vehicle and effects on subsequent insulin secretion in vivo. Biomaterials. 2011;32:2673–82.

21. Zhang B, He D, Fan Y, et al. Oral delivery of exenatide via microspheres prepared by cross-linking of alginate and hyaluronate. PLoS One. 2014;9:e86064.

22. Zhu Z, Luo H, Lu W, et al. Rapidly dissolvable microneedle patches for Transdermal delivery of Exenatide. Pharm Res. 2014;31:3348–60.

23. Ahn S, Lee IH, Lee E, et al. Oral delivery of an anti-diabetic peptide drug via conjugation and complexation with low molecular weight chitosan. J Control Release. 2013;170:226–32.

24. Liang R, Li X, Zhang R, et al. Acylation of exenatide by glycolic acid and its anti-diabetic activities in db/db mice. Pharm Res. 2014;31:1958–66.

25. Zhang Y, Huo M, Zhou J, et al. PKSolver: an add-in program for pharmacokinetic and pharmacodynamic data analysis in Microsoft excel. Comput Meth Prog Bio. 2010;99:306–14.

26. Mcanuff-Harding MA, Omoruyi FO, Asemota HN. Intestinal disaccharidases and some renal enzymes in streptozotocin-induced diabetic rats fed sapogenin extract from bitter yam (Dioscorea Polygonoides). Life Sci. 2006;78:2595–600.

27. Arnés L, Moreno P, Nuche-Berenguer B, et al. Effect of exendin-4 treatment upon glucose uptake parameters in rat liver and muscle, in normal and type 2 diabetic state. Regul Pept. 2008;153:88–92.

28. Liu B, Dong Q, Wang M, et al. Preparation, characterization, and pharmacodynamics of exenatide-loaded poly(DL-lactic-co-glycolic acid) microspheres[J]. Chem Pharm Bull. 2010;58:1474–9.

29. Qi F, Wu J, Hao D, et al. Comparative studies on the influences of primary emulsion preparation on properties of uniform-sized exenatide-loaded PLGA microspheres. Pharm Res. 2014;31:1566–74.

30. Moerz ST, Huber P. Protein adsorption into mesopores: a combination of electrostatic interaction, counterion release, and van der Waals forces. Langmuir. 2015;30:2729–37.

31. Li X, Zhang L, Dong X, et al. Preparation of mesoporous calcium doped silica spheres with narrow size dispersion and their drug loading and degradation behavior. Micropor Mesopor Mat. 2007;102:151–8.

32. Barbé C, Bartlett J, Kong L, et al. Silica particles: a novel drug-delivery system. Adv Mater. 2004;16:1959–66.

33. Hudson SP, Padera RF, Langer R, et al. The biocompatibility of mesoporous silicates. Biomaterials. 2008;29:4045–55.

Linagliptin versus sitagliptin in patients with type 2 diabetes mellitus

Khosro Keshavarz[1], Farhad Lotfi[1], Ehsan Sanati[2], Mahmood Salesi[3], Amir Hashemi-Meshkini[2], Mojtaba Jafari[1], Mohammad M. Mojahedian[2], Behzad Najafi[4] and Shekoufeh Nikfar[5*]

Abstract

Background: Diabetes is one of the most common chronic and costly diseases worldwide and type 2 diabetes is the most common type which accounts for about 90% of cases with diabetes. New medication-therapy regimens such as those containing linagliptin alone or in combination with other medications (within the category of DDP-4 inhibitors) must be evaluated in terms of efficacy and compared with other currently used drugs and then enter the medication list of the country. Hence, this study aimed to compare the clinical efficacy of the two drugs, i.e. linagliptin and sitagliptin, in patients with type 2 diabetes.

Methods: A systematic review was conducted to identify all clinical trials published by 2015 which compared the two drugs in patients with type 2 diabetes. Using keywords such as "linagliptin", "type 2 diabetes mellitus", "sitagliptin" and related combinations, we searched databases including Scopus, PubMed, and Web of Science. The quality of the selected studies was evaluated using the Jadad score. Considering primary and secondary outcomes extracted from the reviewed studies, a network meta-analysis was used to conduct a systematic comparison between the two studied drugs.

Results: This network meta-analysis included 32 studies (Linagliptin vs PLB: $n = 8$, Sitagliptin vs PLB: $n = 13$, Linagliptin + MET vs PLB + MET: $n = 4$, and Sitagliptin + MET vs PLB + MET: $n = 7$) and a total of 13,747 patients. The results showed no significant difference between linagliptin and sitagliptin in terms of key efficacy and safety outcomes such as HbA1c changes from baseline, body weight change from baseline, percentage of patients achieving HbA1c <7, and percentage of patients experiencing hypoglycemic events ($p > 0.05$). The results showed that the efficacy of the two drug regimens was the same.

Conclusions: Based on the results, there was no significant difference between the two drugs, i.e. linagliptin and sitagliptin, in terms of efficacy; in other words, the efficacy of the two drugs was the same. Therefore, the use of these two drugs depends on their availability and cost.

Keywords: Linagliptin, Type 2 diabetes mellitus, Sitagliptin, Network meta-analysis

* Correspondence: shekoufeh.nikfar@gmail.com
[5]Department of Pharmacoeconomics and Pharmaceutical Administration, Faculty of Pharmacy and Evidence-Based Medicine Group, Pharmaceutical Sciences Research Center, Tehran University of Medical Sciences, Tehran, Iran
Full list of author information is available at the end of the article

Background

The incidence and prevalence of diabetes has been rapidly increasing in the last century and morbidity and mortality from these two pandemic diseases have caused massive problems for the health of human communities [1, 2]. Diabetes is one of the most common and a costly chronic disease worldwide, which is considered as a latent epidemic disease one of the health sector challenges around the world. Based on the statistical data published by the International diabetes Federation (IDF), currently 415 million people worldwide have diabetes and this number is predicted to reach 642 million people by 2040. In Iran, more than 4.6 million people were affected by the disease in 2015 [3]. Recent estimates suggest that diabetes mellitus causes 59,258,034 disability adjusted life years (DALYs) in 2012 with a 89.7% increase in deaths from diabetes since 1990 to 2013 [4].

Among different types of diabetes, type 2 diabetes is the most common type which accounts for about 90% of the cases [5]. Although the prevalence of both types of diabetes, i.e. type 1 and type 2, is increasing in the world, type 2 diabetes is more prevalent and the genetic background and environmental factors can be very effective in increasing the incidence of the disease [6–8].

Diabetes has many complications which can severely affect the quality of life of the patients and impose a high economic burden on individuals and community [9, 10].

Among available diabetes treatments, DPP4 inhibitors are one of the new generation classes with good efficacy and safety profile [11–13]. As though in a Meta- analyze study including 62 RCT studies was indicated these kind of drugs decrease HbA1c about 76% in comparison placebo [14], In other meta-analyze including 8 RCT studies, the result was shown DPP-4 decrease the risk of heart diseases in comparison MET. It seems some drugs such as linagliptin, sitagliptin and etc. can be a suitable alternatives for patients who don't reply to MET [15].

Also, According to published clinical studies, linagliptin in this class seems to be more advantageous for patients with renal insufficiency [16]. Using evidence based approach in order to optimize resource utilization in pharmaceutical policy making has started from 2013 in Iran [17, 18]. The aim of this study was also to compare the clinical efficiency of linagliptin and sitagliptin in patients with type 2 diabetes to provide scientific evidences to policy makers for an appropriate decision making.

Methods

Data resources and search strategy

In order to evaluate the efficacy of the two drugs, linagliptin and sitagliptin, we conducted a systematic review of the studies published by the end of 2015. Using keywords such as "linagliptin", "type 2 diabetes mellitus",

"sitagliptin" and related combinations, we searched databases including Scopus, PubMed, and Web of Science (Additional file 1: Appendix).

Study selection and inclusion and exclusion criteria

Based on the inclusion criteria for this systematic review, we reviewed randomized clinical trial studies published in English that compared the clinical efficacy of linagliptin and sitagliptin. It is important to remind that these medicines had some alternatives for comparing such as placebo and metformin as shown in Tables 2 and 3. Exclusion criteria were animal studies, non-controlled trial studies, observational studies, review studies, and economic evaluation studies.

Study selection and data extraction

PRISMA guideline was used for this systematic review, and after the initial search the duplicates were eliminated. The titles and abstracts of the remaining papers were independently evaluated by two researchers to detect and eliminate unrelated articles and those which did not meet the inclusion criteria. The results obtained by the two researchers were compared with each other and the discrepancies were resolved by referring to the articles. Then, the full-text of the selected articles was studied and the papers that met the mentioned criteria were selected.

Quality assessment

The quality of the trials was evaluated using the Jadad score system; accordingly, each study was evaluated in terms of the three indicators, including "randomized, double blinded, and withdrawal or dropout" and scored between 0 and 5. The studies with a score more than or equal to 3 had an acceptable quality while those with a score less than 3 met the exclusion criteria. Therefore, the studies which met the intended criteria, had an acceptable quality (based on the table of Jadad score), and had the same methodology were entered into the network meta-analysis.

Data analysis

After searching and investigating the mentioned databases, we did not find any study which directly compared the two drugs; hence, we decided to find and review clinical trials which investigated DPP-4 drugs, extract the data on their efficiency, and compare the data extracted from independent studies. Therefore, in order to integrate the results of the studies, we used network meta-analysis. To carry out the analysis, we used STATA and Excel softwares.

Thus, as noted above, in this study first we used a systematic review approach to collect studies on the efficiency of the two drugs, i.e. sitagliptin and linagliptin, which are among DPP-4 category. Then, using network meta-analysis, we analyzed the data and compared the efficacy of the drugs. In this study, we not only evaluated the efficacy of the monotherapy using each of the drugs, but also assessed the efficacy of combination therapy using the drugs together with metformin. However, due to the lack of sufficient studies, we did not assess combination therapy with other drugs, such as sulfonylureas, insulin, and glitazones.

Moreover, in order to include a study in meta-analysis, it had to meet the following PICO criteria:

P (Population): Patients with type 2 diabetes.

I (Intervention): linagliptin.

C (Comparators): sitagliptin.

O (Outcomes): The desired outcomes were: "HbA1c change from baseline", "Percentage of patients achieving HbA1c < 7%", "Percentage of patients experiencing hypoglycemic events", and "Body weight change from baseline".

To carry out this network meta-analysis, we analyzed the data using random effect approach. In this approach, first the researcher conducted a meta-analysis of the existing comparisons and combined the results via indirect meta-analysis and finally made its own comparison.

For calculating indirect effect, Bucher et al. method was used [19]. In this method the effects of lina relative to sita can be estimated indirectly as follows, using the direct estimators for the effects of PLB relative to Lina (effect$_{Lina,PLB}$) and PLB relative to sita (effect$_{Sita,PLB}$):

$$Effect_{Lina,Sita} = effect_{Lina,PLB} - effect_{Sita,PLB}$$

The indirect estimator variance of Effect$_{Lina,Sita}$ is the sum of the direct estimators variances:

$$variance_{Lina,Sita} = variance_{Lina,PLB} + variance_{Sita,PLB}$$

for indirect effects of Lina + MET or Sita + MET vs PLB + MET, the same formula were used.

In this study, two tables were provided for every outcome. In the first table, it was considered that the monotherapy and combination therapy studies were not similar, while in the second table the effects of monotherapy and combination therapy were considered to be similar. For each parameter in the first table, we combined the results of the meta-analysis of the existing combinations and indirectly compared linagliptin 5 mg with sitagliptin 100 mg and also compared LIN 5 mg + MET with SIT 100 mg + MET. In the second table, it was assumed that the results of comparisons between drugs with and without MET were the same; thus, we compared linagliptin 5 mg (with and without MET) with sitagliptin 100 mg (with and without MET). For the first two outcomes, we compared the changes

from the baseline and for the second two outcomes we compared the Log of odds ratios.

Results

Study screening, characteristics and quality of the selected studies

After searching the electronic databases and reviewing the references of articles, a total of 3711 articles was obtained. All the obtained articles were carefully assessed to find the articles which met the intended criteria and finally a total of 32 articles which had an acceptable level of quality were selected for the meta-analysis. Table 1 presents the data on the selected papers (Fig. 1). It presents a summary of the characteristics of the selected studies, including the core of comparison, study period, and the number of patients. Moreover, using the Jadad score, we assessed the quality of all the selected studies; as the results showed, the all the selected studies which underwent quality assessment obtained a score equal to or more than three.

Outcomes

Network meta-analysis was used to compare different groups in terms of HbA1c changes from baseline, body weight change from baseline, percentage of patients achieving HbA1c <7, and percentage of patients experiencing hypoglycemic events. Figure 2 presents a schematic of the various comparisons between the groups. Figures 2a–d, respectively, show the number of studies which presented outcomes for HbA1c changes from baseline, body weight change from baseline, percentage of patients achieving HbA1c <7, and percentage of patients experiencing hypoglycemic events; these figures compare linagliptin and sitagliptin groups with the placebo group and compare LIN 5 mg + MET and SIT 100 mg + MET groups with PLB + MET group. The maximum total number of studies was 32; HbA1c changes from baseline was the outcome with the largest number of studies (32 studies) while body weight change from baseline was the outcome with the least number of studies (18 studies).

HbA1c change from baseline

Based on the results of the meta-analysis presented in Table 2, the two groups of linagliptin and sitagliptin were significantly different from the placebo group in terms of HbA1c changes from baseline, as these two drugs, respectively, reduced HbA1c by 0.644 and 0.284 units as compared with the placebo (comparisons 1 and 2). In addition, there was no significant difference between the LIN 5 mg + MET group and PLB + MET group in terms of HbA1c changes from baseline (comparison 3). However, it showed a significant

Table 1 Summarized characteristics of the selected studies in the network meta-analysis

Study identifier References	Treatment 1	Treatment 2	N	Weeks	Age Mean (s.d.)	Sex (males) N (%)
Linagliptin Mono. (8 RCTs)						
Del Prato et al. (2011) [31]	LIN 5 mg	PLB	503	24	55.7 (10.2)	243 (48.3)
Haak et al. (2012) [32]	LIN 5 mg	PLB	214	24	55.95 (10.9)	116 (54.2)
Kawamori (2012) [33]	LIN 5 mg	PLB	239	12	60.0 (9.1)	168 (70.2)
Barnett et al. (2012) [34]	LIN 5 mg	PLB	227	18	56.5 (10.3)	88(38.7)
Lajara (2014) [35]	LIN 5 mg	PLB	202	24	69.1(10.0)	122 (60.4)
Chen et al. (2015) [36]	LIN 5 mg	PLB	299	24	54.3 (9.7)	175 (58.5)
Taskinen (2011) [37]	LIN 5 mg	PLB	700	24	56.5 (10.3)	379 (54.1)
Inzucchi (2015) [38]	LIN 5 mg	PLB	247	24	74.3 (3.9)	126 (51.0)
Sitagliptin Mono. (13 RCTs)						
Barzilai et al. (2011) [39]	SIT 100 mg	PLB	206	24	72.0 (6.0)	97(47.1)
Nonaka et al. (2008) [40]	SIT 100 mg	PLB	151	12	55.3 (8.3)	95 (62.9)
Aschner et al. (2006) [41]	SIT 100 mg	PLB	491	24	–	–
Goldstein et al. (2007) [42]	SIT 100 mg	PLB	355	24	–	–
Hanefeld et al. (2007) [43]	SIT 100 mg	PLB	221	12	56.0 (8.5)	131 (59.2)
Scott (2008) [44]	SIT 100 mg	PLB	186	18	55.2 (9.5)	106 (57.9)
Raz (2008) [45]	SIT 100 mg	PLB	190	30	54.8 (9.5)	88(46.3)
Charbonnel (2006) [46]	SIT 100 mg	PLB	701	24	–	–
Pe'rez-Monteverde et al. (2011) [47]	SIT 100 mg	PLB	492	12	–	–
Russell-Jones et al. (2012) [48]	SIT 100 mg	PLB	409	26	54	59
Nauck 2007 [49]	SIT 100 mg	PLB	1172	52	56.7 (9.5)	694 (59.2)
Arechavaleta 2011 [50]	SIT 100 mg	PLB	1035	30	56.2 (9.9)	563(54.4)
Bergenstal (2010) [51]	SIT 100 mg	PLB	331	26	52.5 (10.5)	165 (49.8)
Linagliptin Com. (4 RCTs)						
Forst et al. (2010) [52]	LIN 5 mg + MET	PLB+ MET	137	12	59.8 (8.9)	81 (59.1)
Gallwitz et al. (2012) [53]	LIN 5 mg + MET	PLB+ MET	1551	104	59.8 (9.4)	933 (60.1)
Taskinen et al. (2011) [37]	LIN 5 mg + MET	PLB+ MET	700	24	56.5 (10.3)	379 (54.1)
Ross et al. (2012) [54]	LIN 5 mg + MET	PLB+ MET	268	12	59.1 (10.6)	142 (52.9)
Sitagliptin Com. (7 RCTs)						
Aaboe et al. (2010) [55]	SIT 100 mg + MET	PLB+ MET	24	12	59.8	17(70.8)
Arechavaleta et al. (2011) [50]	SIT 100 mg + MET	PLB+ MET	1035	30	56.2 (9.9)	563 (54.4)
Charbonnel et al. (2006) [46]	SIT 100 mg + MET	PLB+ MET	678	24	–	–
Derosa et al. (2012) [56]	SIT 100 mg + MET	PLB+ MET	178	52	55.4 (8.4)	86(48.3)
Raz et al. (2008) [45]	SIT 100 mg + MET	PLB+ MET	190	30	54.8 (9.5)	88(46.3)
Scott et al. (2008) [44]	SIT 100 mg + MET	PLB+ MET	186	18	55.2 (9.5)	106 (56.9)
Hermansen et al. (2007) [57]	SIT 100 mg + MET	PLB+ MET	229	24	57.1 (8.8)	120 (52.4)

difference in SIT 100 mg + MET group, as compared with PLB + MET group, so that the drug reduced HbA1c by 0.555 units in PLB + MET group (comparison 4). Then, the results of the reported meta-analyses were combined and an indirect comparison showed a significant difference in HbA1c from baseline in linagliptin group, as compared with the sitagliptin group; in other words, linagliptin decreased HbA1c by 0.359 units, as compared with sitagliptin (comparison 5). However, the changes in LIN 5 mg + MET

group, as compared with SIT 100 mg + MET group, did not show a significant difference (comparison 6).

Body weight change from baseline

Table 2 shows no significant difference between the linagliptin and placebo groups (comparison 1) and between sitagliptin groups and placebo group (comparison 2) in terms of body weight changes from baseline. However, it had a significant difference in LIN 5 mg + MET

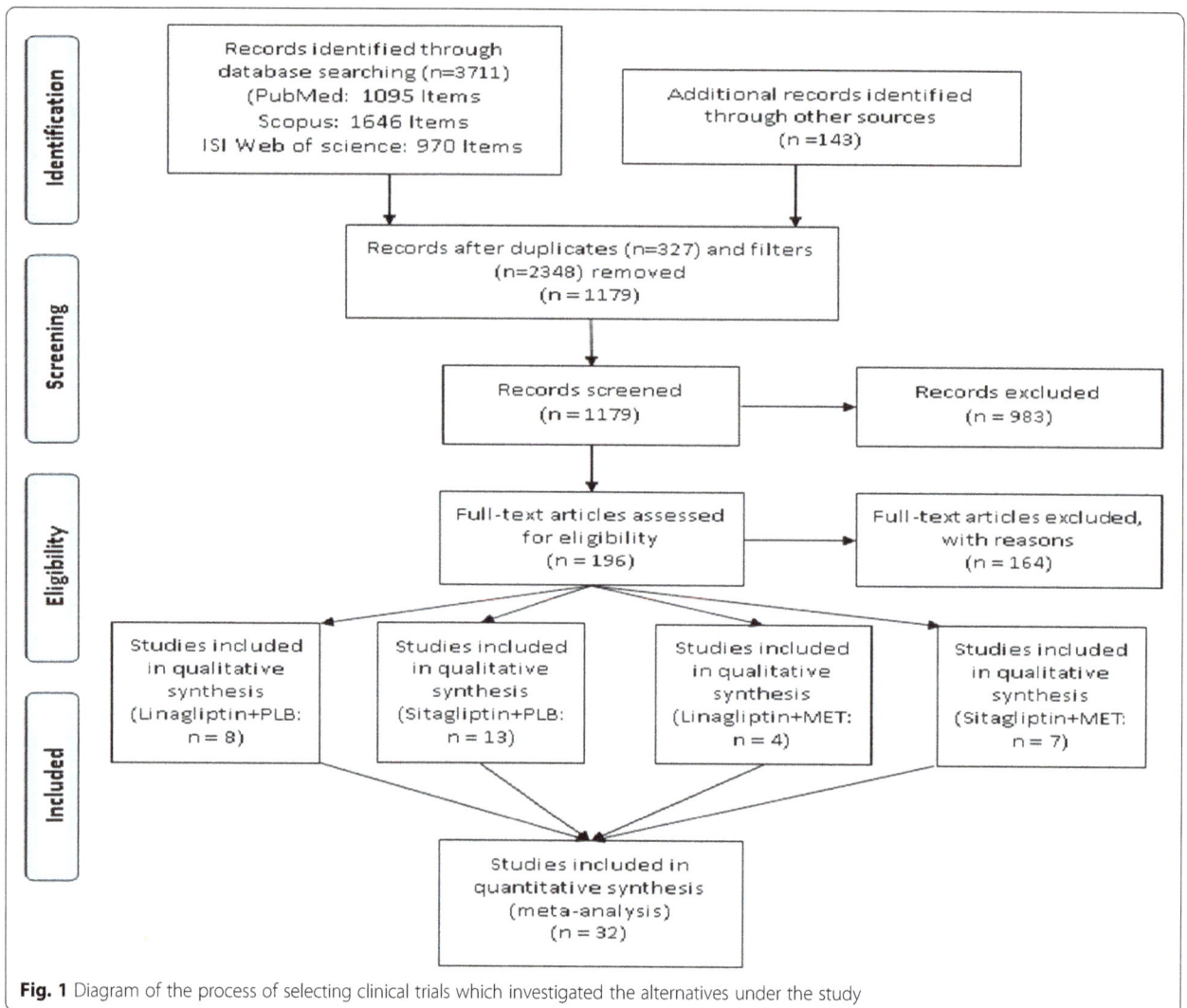

Fig. 1 Diagram of the process of selecting clinical trials which investigated the alternatives under the study

group, as compared with the PLB + MET group, so that the drug reduced the body weight by 2.489 units, as compared with the PLB + MET group (comparison 3). On the other hand, there was no significant difference in the SIT 100 mg + MET group, as compared with the PLB + MET group (comparison 4).

Then, the results of reported meta-analyses were combined and an indirect comparison showed no significant difference between linagliptin and sitagliptin groups in terms of body weight changes from baseline (comparison 5). However, it showed a significant difference in the LIN 5 mg + MET group as compared with the SIT 100 mg + MET groups, so that LIN 5 mg + MET decreased body weight by 2.288 units, as compared with SIT 100 mg + MET (comparison 6).

Percentage of patients achieving HbA1c <7
As shown in Table 2, the percentage of patients achieving HbA1c <7 significantly increased in the linagliptin group,

as compared with the placebo group; the odds ratio of HbA1c <7 in this group was 2.04 times more than that in the placebo group (comparison 1). However, it did not show a significant difference in the sitagliptin group, as compared with the placebo group (comparison 2). In addition, comparing the percentage of HbA1c <7 showed that there was no significant difference between the LIN 5 mg + MET group and PLB + MET group (comparison 3) and between the SIT 100 mg + MET group and PLB + MET group (comparison 4). Then, the results of reported meta-analyses were combined and an indirect comparison of the percentage of HbA1c <7 showed no significant difference between the linagliptin group and sitagliptin group (comparison 5) and between the LIN 5 mg + MET group and SIT 100 mg + MET group (comparison 6).

Percentage of patients experiencing hypoglycemic events
As shown in Table 2, the percentage of patients experiencing hypoglycemic events significantly decreased in

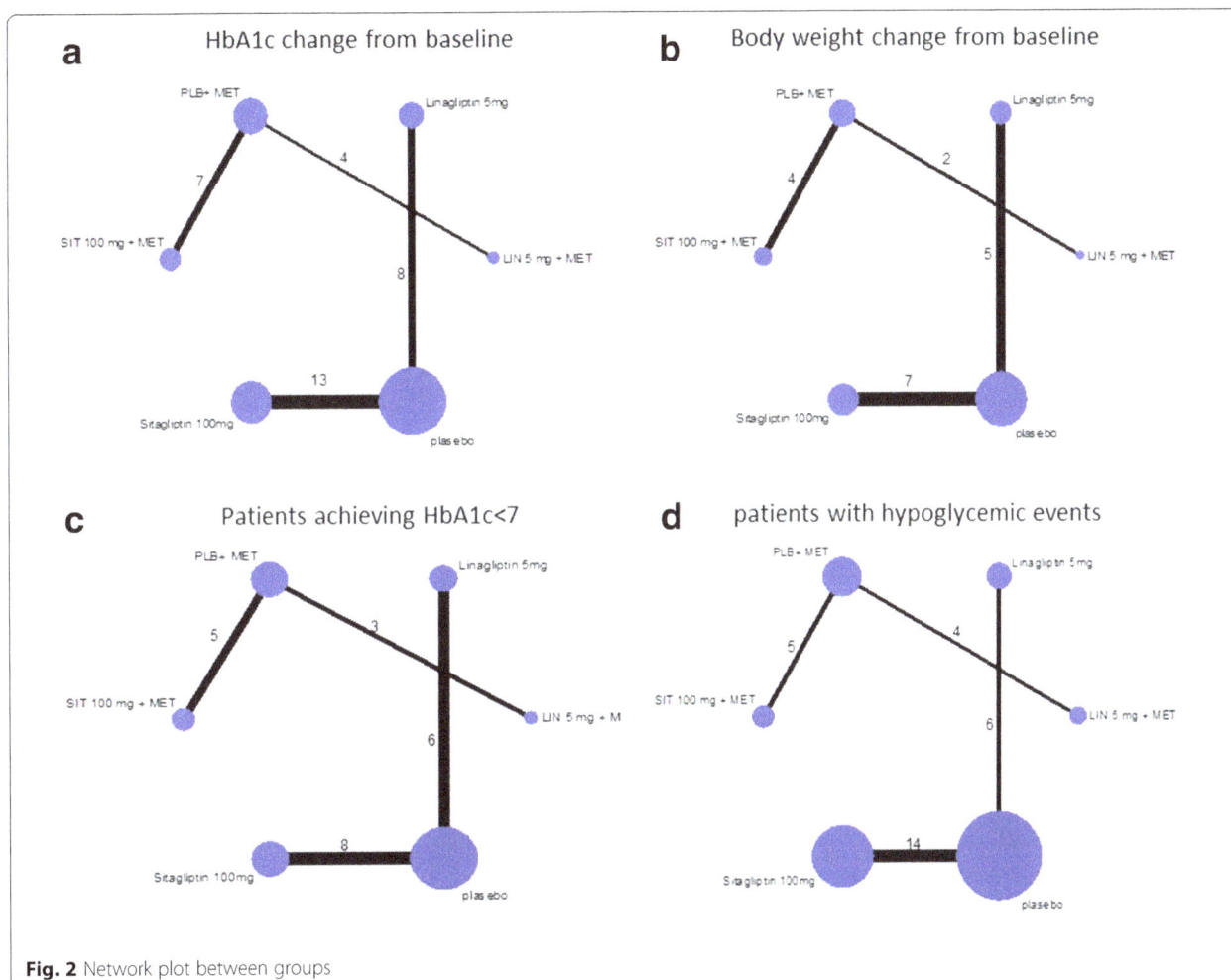

Fig. 2 Network plot between groups

the linagliptin and sitagliptin groups, as compared with the placebo group; the odds ratio of hypoglycemic events in the two groups was 0.53 and 0.44, respectively, as compared with the placebo group (comparisons 1 and 2). Moreover, the percentage of hypoglycemic events significantly decreased in the LIN 5 mg + MET group, as compared with the PLB + MET group; the odds ratio of hypoglycemic events in the LIN 5 mg + MET group was OR = exp.(−1.853) = 0.15 times more than that in the PLB + MET group (comparison 3). However, there was no significant difference between the SIT 100 mg + MET group and PLB + MET group (comparison 4). Then, the results of reported meta-analyses were combined and an indirect comparison of hypoglycemic events showed no significant difference between the linagliptin group and sitagliptin group (comparison 5). However, it significantly decreased in the LIN 5 mg + MET group, as compared with the SIT 100 mg + MET group; the odds ratio of hypoglycemic events in the LIN 5 mg + MET group was OR = exp.(−1.426) = 0.24 times more than that in the SIT 100 mg + MET group (comparison 6).

As shown in Table 3, considering the similarities between comparisons 1 and 3 and between comparisons 2 and 4, there was a significant difference in HbA1c changes from baseline in the linagliptin and sitagliptin groups (with and without MET), as compared with the placebo group; the mentioned drugs, respectively, reduced HbA1c by 0.495 and 0.375 units, as compared with the placebo group (comparisons 7 and 8). However, finally, there was no significant difference between the linagliptin group (with and without MET), as compared with the sitagliptin group (with and without MET) (comparison 9).

Comparing the groups in terms of body weight changes from baseline showed that there was no significant difference between the linagliptin and sitagliptin groups (with and without MET), as compared with the placebo group (with and without MET) (comparisons 7 and 8). In addition, finally, there was no significant difference between the linagliptin group (with and without MET), as compared with the sitagliptin group (with and without MET) in terms of body weight changes from baseline (comparison 9).

Table 2 Network meta-analysis for comparison of HbA1c changes from baseline, Body weight change from baseline, Percentage of patients achieving HbA1c <7 and Percentage of patients experiencing hypoglycemic events between the 2 groups

Comparison	Drug1	Drug2	HbA1c change from baseline			Body weight change from baseline			Percentage of patients achieving HbA1c <7%			Percentage of patients experiencing hypoglycemic events		
			Freq[1]	Mean difference (SE)	p-value	Freq	Mean difference (SE)	p-value	Freq	Odds Ratio (SE)	p-value	Freq	Odds Ratio (SE)	p-value
Direct (1)	Linagliptin 5 mg	placebo	8	−0.644(.045)	0	5	0.348(.283)	0.217	6	0.712 (.153)	0	6	−0.625 (.244)	0.01
Direct (2)	Sitagliptin 100 mg	placebo	13	−0.284(.125)	0.022	7	−0.925 (.795)	0.244	8	0.440(.261)	0.091	14	−0.820(.287)	0.004
Direct (3)	LIN 5 mg + MET	PLB+ MET	4	−.247(.283)	0.383	2	−2.489 (.191)	0	3	0.924(.701)	0.188	4	−1.853 (.119)	0
Direct (4)	SIT 100 mg + MET	PLB+ MET	7	−.555(.157)	0	4	−0.201 (.839)	0.811	5	0.667 (.446)	0.135	5	−0.427(.525)	0.417
Indirect (5)	Linagliptin 5 mg	Sitagliptin 100 mg	–	−0.359(.133)	<.05	–	1.273(.843)	>0.05	–	0.272 (.302)	>.05	–	0.195 (.377)	>.05
Indirect (6)	LIN 5 mg + MET	SIT 100 mg + MET	–	0.308(.324)	>.05	–	−2.288(.860)	<0.05	–	0.257(.830)	>.05	–	−1.426(.538)	<.05

1- Freq: frequency

Table 3 Network meta-analysis for comparison HbA1c changes from baseline, Body weight change from baseline, Percentage of patients achieving HbA1c <7 and Percentage of patients experiencing hypoglycemic events between 2 groups (If in Table 2 pairs (1 similar 3) & (2 similar 4))

Comparison	Drug1	Drug2	HbA1c change from baseline			Body weight change from baseline			Percentage of patients achieving HbA1c <7%			Percentage of patients experiencing hypoglycemic events		
			Freq	Mean difference (SE)	p-value	Freq	Mean difference (SE)	p-value	Freq	Ln(OR) (SE)	p-value	Freq	Ln(OR) (SE)	p-value
Direct (7)	Linagliptin 5 mg	placebo	12	−.495(.119)	0	7	−0.211(.701)	0.764	9	0.711 (.257)	0.006	10	−1.250 (.271)	0
Direct (8)	Sitagliptin 100 mg	placebo	20	−.375(.072)	0	11	−0.664 (.553)	0.229	13	0.514 (.209)	0.014	19	−0.753 (.228)	0.001
Indirect (9)	Linagliptin 5 mg	Sitagliptin 100 mg	–	−0.12(.139)	>.05	–	0.454 (.893)	>0.05	–	0.197 (.332)	>.05	4	−0.497(.354)	>0.05

Comparing the groups in terms of the percentage of HbA1c <7 revealed that there was a significant difference between the linagliptin and sitagliptin groups (with and without MET), as compared with the placebo group (with and without MET) as the odds ratio of HbA1c in the linagliptin and sitagliptin groups, respectively, was 2.03 and 1.67, as compared with the placebo group (comparisons 7 and 8). However, finally, there was no significant difference between the linagliptin group (with and without MET), as compared with the sitagliptin group (with and without MET) (comparison 9).

Comparing the groups in terms of hypoglycemic events showed that there was a significant difference between the linagliptin and sitagliptin groups (with and without MET), as compared with the placebo group (with and without MET) as the odds ratio of hypoglycemic events in the linagliptin and sitagliptin groups, respectively, was 0.28 and 0.47, as compared with the placebo group (comparisons 7 and 8). However, there was no significant difference between the linagliptin group (with and without MET), as compared with the sitagliptin group (with and without MET) (comparison 9).

Discussion

Using meta-analyses approach, we performed a direct-comparison between the drugs and placebo that the results were different. The results of the meta-analysis showed a significant difference in HbA1c changes from baseline in the linagliptin group and sitagliptin group (with and without MET), as compared with the placebo group, because HbA1c was reduced by these drugs, as compared with the placebo. It is in the same line with the results of the study of Gross JL et al. [20] However, there was no significant difference in the LIN 5 mg + MET group, as compared with the PLB + MET group.

Considering body weight changes from baseline revealed that there was no significant difference between the linagliptin and placebo groups and between the sitagliptin groups (with and without MET) and placebo group. However, it showed a significant difference in the LIN 5 mg + MET group,

as compared with the PLB + MET group, so that the drug reduced body weight, compared with the PLB + MET group.

As to the percentage of patients achieving HbA1c <7, it significantly increased in the linagliptin group, as compared with the placebo group; the odds ratio of HbA1c <7 in this group was two times more than that of the placebo group. However, there was no significant difference in the LIN 5 mg + MET and sitagliptin groups (with and without MET), as compared with the placebo group. Moreover, as to the percentage of hypoglycemic events, there was a significant difference in the linagliptin (with and without MET) and sitagliptin groups, as compared with the placebo group. The odds ratio of hypoglycemic events in the two groups was less than that in the placebo group. Nevertheless, there was no significant difference in the SIT 100 mg + MET group, as compared with PLB + MET group.

The results of network meta-analysis showed no significant difference in HbA1c changes from baseline, body weight changes from baseline, percentage of HbA1c <7, and percentage of hypoglycemic events in the linagliptin group (with and without MET), as compared with the sitagliptin group (with and without MET); thus, the efficiency of the two drugs are identical. Therefore, the results of this study are consistent with those of the studies conducted in other countries [20–22].

As noted in the results, in certain cases linagliptin has a relative advantage in pharmacokinetic superiority over sitagliptin; thus, it can be considered as a suitable alternative. Non-renal clearance is one of the pharmacokinetic features of linagliptin which makes it different from other gliptins available on the market. Therefore, its use in patients with renal insufficiency is safe and does not have any restriction [16]. Therefore, this drug is more advantageous, as compared with other drugs in this category, and is considered to be the treatment of choice in patients with renal insufficiency because kidney dysfunction is quite common in diabetic patients [23–26].

Although the efficacy of linagliptin and sitagliptin is the same, because the use of linagliptin has no restrictions in patients with renal dysfunction, and this drug is a better alternative for patients with renal dysfunction, it is necessary to make it accessible in Iran pharmaceutical market along with sitagliptin so that the physicians have an opportunity to prescribe thesedrugs for patients with different background diseases.

The results of meta-analysis can be different from those of indirect comparisons; however, we should be more cautious when interpreting the results of indirect comparisons. Systematic reviews and evaluation of the quality of clinical trials can help reduce the errors in the results of network meta-analysis but when there is a difference between the results of direct-comparison meta-analysis and indirect meta-analysis, it is necessary to re-examine the validity and generalizability of clinical trials to find the reason for the error. On the other hand, recent experimental results indicate the match between these two types of comparisons [27]. When using studies with a low quality, the results of indirect-comparison meta-analysis may be incomplete [28, 29]; on the other hand, it might be considered incomplete due to inherent differences caused via choosing the right plan, or due to limitations in comparing all the items one by one [30]. However, in this study, all the studies were examined in detail by expert people and they underwent quality assessment. At the end, this study compared linagliptin and sitagliptin drugs in terms of main efficacy and safety outcomes mentioned above. The results of this study showed no significant difference between linagliptin and sitagliptin in terms of clinical efficiency. Therefore, given their similar level of efficacy, the use of these two drugs depends on their availability and cost. According to this fact that efficacy of Linagliptin and sitagliptin is not statistically different in terms of main outcomes, any recommendation for use of each of them could be only based on cost and renal functionality of patients. For patients with renal impairments who cannot use sitagliptin and are preferred to use DPP4 inhibitors, linagliptin is a good choice. But for other patients, an economic study should be performed on the results of this study to consider economic perspective in decision making.

Conclusion

The results showed no significant difference between linagliptin and sitagliptin in terms of clinical efficacy and they had the same effect. However, as there is no restriction on the use of linagliptin in patients with renal dysfunction, it might be considered as a treatment of choice. Hence, it is recommended to include this drug, along with sitagliptin, in the list of pharmaceuticals in Iran.

Abbreviations

DALYs: Disability adjusted life years; DPP- 4: Dipeptidyl peptidase-4 inhibitors; IDF: International diabetes Federation; LIN: Linagliptin; MET: Metformin; OR: Odds Ratio; PICO: Population; Intervention; Comparators; Outcomes; PLB: Placebo; SIT: Sitagliptin

Acknowledgements

The authors would like to thank Shafayab Gostar Company for cooperation and providing data; Shiraz University of Medical Sciences, Shiraz, Iran and also Center for Development of Clinical Research of Nemazee Hospital and Dr. Nasrin Shokrpour for editorial assistance.

Funding

This paper was supported by Shafayab Gostar Company, Tehran, Iran.

Authors' contributions

KHK: Study concept and design, participated in literature bibliography, Acquisition of data, Analysis and interpretation of data, Drafting of the manuscript, Critical revision of the manuscript for important intellectual content. ES: Drafting of the manuscript, Acquisition of data. MS: Drafting of the manuscript and Statistical analysis. FL: Drafting of the manuscript, revised the paper critically for important intellectual content. AHM and BN: participate in design of study and final revision of the manuscript. MJ and MM: participated in literature bibliography and collecting clinical data. SHN: participate in design of study and supervised whole study and revised the paper critically for important intellectual content. All authors read and approved the final manuscript.

Competing interests

The authors declare that they have no competing interests.

Author details

[1]Health Human Resources Research Center, Department of Health Economics, School of Management and Information Sciences, Shiraz University of Medical Sciences, Shiraz, IR, Iran. [2]Department of Pharmacoeconomics and Pharmaceutical Administration, Faculty of Pharmacy, Tehran University of Medical Sciences, Tehran, IR, Iran. [3]Atherosclerosis Research center, Baqiyatallah University of Medical Sciences, Tehran, IR, Iran. [4]Iranian center of Excellence in health management, Department of health services management, School of management and medical informatics, Tabriz University of medical sciences, Tabriz, Iran. [5]Department of Pharmacoeconomics and Pharmaceutical Administration, Faculty of Pharmacy and Evidence-Based Medicine Group, Pharmaceutical Sciences Research Center, Tehran University of Medical Sciences, Tehran, Iran.

References

1. American Diabetes A. Economic costs of diabetes in the U.S. in 2012. Diabetes Care. 2013;36(4):1033–46.

2. Wong J, Constantino M, Yue DK. Morbidity and mortality in young-onset type 2 diabetes in comparison to type 1 diabetes: where are we now? Curr Diab Rep. 2015;15(1):566.

3. International Diabetes Federation: IDF Diabetes. 7th ed. 2015. Available at: http://www.diabetesatlas.org/component/attachments/?task=download&id=116.

4. Najafi B, Farzadfar F, Ghaderi H, Hadian M. Cost effectiveness of type 2 diabetes screening: a systematic review. Med J Islamic Repub Iran. 2016;30:326.

5. Boyle JP, Honeycutt AA, Narayan KM, Hoerger TJ, Geiss LS, Chen H, et al. Projection of diabetes burden through 2050. Diabetes Care. 2001;24(11):1936.

6. Bener A, Al-Hamaq AO. Predictions burden of diabetes and economics cost: contributing risk factors of changing disease prevalence and its pandemic impact to Qatar. Exp Clin Endocrinol Diabetes. 2016;124(8):504–11.

7. Marshall JA, Hamman RF, Baxter J, Mayer EJ, Fulton DL, Orleans M, et al. Ethnic differences in risk factors associated with the prevalence of non-insulin-dependent diabetes mellitus. The San Luis Valley diabetes study. Am J Epidemiol. 1993;137(7):706–18.

8. Korner J, Aronne LJ. The emerging science of body weight regulation and its impact on obesity treatment. J Clin Invest. 2003;111(5):565–70.

9. Zhong Y, Lin PJ, Cohen JT, Winn AN, Neumann PJ. Cost-utility analyses in diabetes: a systematic review and implications from real-world evidence. Value Health. 2015;18(2):308–14.

10. Ulrich S, Holle R, Wacker M, Stark R, Icks A, Thorand B, et al. Cost burden of type 2 diabetes in Germany: results from the population-based KORA studies. BMJ Open. 2016;6(11):e012527.

11. Scheen AJ. Pharmacokinetics of dipeptidylpeptidase-4 inhibitors. Diabetes Obes Metab. 2010;12:648–58.

12. Romero M, Marrugo R, Sanchez O, Lopez S, Alvis N. Cost-effectiveness analysis of using hypoglycemic agents (Linagliptin, Saxagliptin, Sitagliptin, Vildagliptin, Glimepiride and Glibenclamide) with Metformin in diabetes in Colombia. Value Health, 16. (3):A163.

13. Scheen AJ, Charpentier G, Ostgren CJ, et al. Efficacy and safety of saxagliptin in combination with metformin compared with sitagliptin in combination with metformin in adult patients with type 2 diabetes mellitus. Diabetes Metab Res Rev. 2010;26:540–9.

14. Park H, Park C, Kim Y, Rascati KL. Efficacy and safety of dipeptidyl peptidase-4 inhibitors in type 2 diabetes: meta-analysis. Ann Pharmacother. 2012;46(11):1453–69.

15. Wu D, Li L, Liu C. Efficacy and safety of dipeptidyl peptidase-4 inhibitors and metformin as initial combination therapy and as monotherapy in patients with type 2 diabetes mellitus: a meta-analysis. Diabetes Obes Metab. 2014;16(1):30–7.

16. McKeage K. Linagliptin: an update of its use in patients with type 2 diabetes mellitus. Drugs. 2014;74(16):1927–46.

17. Kavosi Z, Khorrami MS, Keshavarz K, Jafari A, Meshkini AH, Safaei HR, Nikfar S. Is Taurolidine-citrate an effective and cost-effective hemodialysis catheter lock solution? A systematic review and cost-effectiveness analysis. Med J Islamic Repub Iran. 2016;30:347.

18. Keshavarz K, Hashemi-Meshkini A, Gharibnaseri Z, Nikfar S, Kebriaeezadeh A, Abdollahi M. A systematic cost-effectiveness analysis of pregabalin in the management of fibromyalgia: an Iranian experience. Archives Med Sci. 2013;9(6):961.

19. Bucher HC, Guyatt GH, Griffith LE, Walter SD. The results of direct and indirect treatment comparisons in meta-analysis of randomized controlled trials. J Clin Epidemiol. 1997;50:683–91.

20. Gross JL, Rogers J, Polhamus D, Gillespie W, Friedrich C, Gong Y, et al. A novel model-based meta-analysis to indirectly estimate the comparative efficacy of two medications: an example using DPP-4 inhibitors, sitagliptin and linagliptin, in treatment of type 2 diabetes mellitus. BMJ Open. 2013;3(3):e001844.

21. Craddy P, Palin HJ, Johnson KI. Comparative effectiveness of Dipeptidylpeptidase-4 inhibitors in type 2 diabetes: a systematic review and mixed treatment comparison. Diabetes Ther 2014;5(1):1–41. PubMed PMID: 24664619.

22. Kamatani N, Katoh T, Sawai Y, Kanayama H, Katada N, Itoh M. Comparison between the clinical efficacy of linagliptin and sitagliptin. J Diabetes. 2013;4(4):51–4.

23. McGill JB. Linagliptin for type 2 diabetes mellitus: a review of the pivotal clinical trials. Ther Adv Endocrinol Metab. 2012;3(4):113–24.

24. Gupta V, Kalra S. Choosing a Gliptin. Indian J Endocrinol Metab. 2011;15(4):298–308. PubMed PMID: 22029001

25. Deacon C. Dipeptidyl peptidase-4 inhibitors in the treatment of type 2 diabetes: a comparative review. Diabetes Obes Metab. 2011;13(1):7–18.

26. Fuchs H, Tillement JP, Urien S, Greischel A, Roth W. Concentration-dependent plasma protein binding of the novel dipeptidyl peptidase 4 inhibitor BI 1356 due to saturable binding to its target in plasma of mice, rats and humans. J Pharm Pharmacol. 2009;61(1):55–62.

27. Bucher HC, Guyatt GH, Griffith LE, Walter SD. The results of direct and indirect treatment comparisons in meta-analysis of randomized controlled trials. J Clin Epidemiol. 1997;50(6):683–91.

28. Song F, Glenny AM, Altman DG. Indirect comparison in evaluating relative efficacy illustrated by antimicrobial prophylaxis in colorectal surgery. Control Clin Trials. 2000;21(5):488–97.

29. Song F, Xiong T, Parekh-Bhurke S, Loke YK, Sutton AJ, Eastwood AJ, et al. Inconsistency between direct and indirect comparisons of competing interventions: meta-epidemiological study. BMJ. 2011;343:d4909.

30. Glenny AM, Altman DG, Song F, Sakarovitch C, Deeks JJ, D'Amico R, et al. Indirect comparisons of competing interventions. Health Technol Assess. 2005;9(26):1–134. iii-iv

31. Del Prato S, Barnett AH, Huisman H, Neubacher D, Woerle HJ, Dugi KA. Effect of linagliptin monotherapy on glycaemic control and markers of b-cell function in patients with inadequately controlled type 2 diabetes: a randomized controlled trial. Diabetes Obes Metab. 2011;13(3):258–67.

32. Haak T, Meinicke T, Jones R, Weber S, Von Eynatten M, Woerle HJ. Initial combination of linagliptin and metformin improves glycaemic control in type 2 diabetes: a randomized, double-blind, placebocontrolled study. Diabetes Obes Metab. 2012;14(6):565–74.

33. Kawamori R, Inagaki N, Araki E, et al. Linagliptin monotherapy provides superior glycaemic control versus placebo or voglibose with comparable safety in Japanese patients with type 2 diabetes: a randomized, placebo and active comparatorcontrolled, double-blind study. Diabetes Obes Metab. 2012;14(4):348–57.

34. Barnett AH, Patel S, Harper R, et al. Linagliptin monotherapy in type 2 diabetes patients for whom metformin is inappropriate: an 18-week randomized, double-blind, placebo-controlled phase III trial with a 34-week active-controlled extension. Diabetes Obes Metab. 2012;14:1145–54.

35. Lajara R, Aguilar R, Hehnke U, Woerle HJ, Eynatten M. Efficacy and safety of Linagliptin in subjects with long standing type 2 diabetes mellitus (>10 Years): evidence from pooled data of randomized, doubleblind, placebo-controlled, phase III trials. Clinical Therapeutics. 2014;36(11):1595–605.

36. Chen Y, Ning G, Wang C, Gong Y, Patel S, Zhang C, Izumoto T, Woerle HJ, Wang W. Efficacy and safety of linagliptin monotherapy in Asian patients with inadequately controlled type 2 diabetes mellitus: a multinational, 24-week, randomized, clinical trial. J Diabetes Investig. 2015;6:692–8.

37. Taskinen MR, Rosenstock J, Tamminen I, et al. Safety and efficacy of linagliptin as add-on therapy to metformin in patients with type 2 diabetes: a randomized, double-blind, placebo-controlled study. Diabetes Obes Metab. 2011;13(1):65–74.

38. Inzucchi SE, Nauck MA, Hehnke U, Woerle HJ, Eynatten M, Henry RR. Improved glucose control with reduced hypoglycaemic risk when linagliptin is added to basal insulin in elderly patients with type 2 diabetes. Diab. Obes Metab. 2015;17:868–77.

39. Barzilai N, Guo H, Mahoney EM, et al. Efficacy and tolerability of sitagliptin monotherapy in elderly patients with type 2 diabetes: a randomized, double-blind, placebo-controlled trial. Curr Med Res Opin. 2011;27(5):1049–58.

40. Nonaka K, Kakikawa T, Sato A, et al. Efficacy and safety of sitagliptin monotherapy in Japanese patients with type 2 diabetes. Diabetes Res Clin Pract. 2008;79(2):291–8.

41. Aschner P, Kipnes MS, Lunceford JK, Sanchez M, Mickel C, Williams-Herman DE. Effect of the dipeptidyl peptidase-4 inhibitor sitagliptin as monotherapy on glycemic control in patients with type 2 diabetes. Diabetes Care. 2006;29(12):2632–7.

42. Goldstein BJ, Feinglos MN, Lunceford JK, Johnson J, Williams-Herman DE. Effect of initial combination therapy with sitagliptin, a dipeptidyl peptidase-4 inhibitor, and metformin on glycemic control in patients with type 2 diabetes. Diabetes Care. 2007;30(8):1979–87.

43. Hanefeld M, Herman GA, Wu M, Mickel C, Sanchez M, Stein PP. Once-daily sitagliptin, a dipeptidyl peptidase-4 inhibitor, for the treatment of patients with type 2 diabetes. Curr Med Res Opin. 2007;23(6):1329–39.

44. Scott R, Loeys T, Davies MJ, Engel SS. Efficacy and safety of sitagliptin when added to ongoing metformin therapy in patients with type 2 diabetes. Diabetes Obes Metab. 2008;10(10):959–69.

45. Raz I, Chen Y, Wu M, et al. Efficacy and safety of sitagliptin added to ongoing metformin therapy in patients with type 2 diabetes. Curr Med Res Opin. 2008;24(2):537–50.

46. Charbonnel B, Karasik A, Liu J, Wu M, Meininger G. Efficacy and safety of the dipeptidyl peptidase-4 inhibitor sitagliptin added to ongoing metformin therapy in patients with type 2 diabetes inadequately controlled with metformin alone. Diabetes Care. 2006;29(12):2638–43.

47. Pérez-Monteverde A, Seck T, Xu L, et al. Efficacy and safety of sitagliptin and the fixed-dose combination of sitagliptin and metformin vs. pioglitazone in drug-naïve patients with type 2 diabetes. Int J Clin Pract. 2011;65(9):930–8.

48. Russell-Jones D, Cuddihy RM, Hanefeld M, et al. Efficacy and safety of exenatide once weekly versus metformin, pioglitazone, and sitagliptin used as monotherapy in drug-naive patients with type 2 diabetes (DURATION-4): a 26-week double-blind study. Diabetes Care. 2012;35(2):252–8.

49. Nauck MA, Meininger G, Sheng D, Terranella L, Stein PP. Efficacy and safety of the dipeptidyl peptidase-4 inhibitor, sitagliptin, compared with the sulfonylurea, glipizide, in patients with type 2 diabetes inadequately controlled on metformin alone: a randomized, double-blind, non-inferiority trial. Diabetes Obes Metab. 2007;9(2):194–205.

50. Arechavaleta R, Seck T, Chen Y, et al. Efficacy and safety of treatment with sitagliptin or glimepiride in patients with type 2 diabetes inadequately controlled on metformin monotherapy: a randomized, doubleblind, non-inferiority trial. Diabetes Obes Metab. 2011;13(2):160–8.

51. Bergenstal RM, Wysham C, Macconell L, et al. Efficacy and safety of exenatide once weekly versus sitagliptin or pioglitazone as an adjunct to metformin for treatment of type 2 diabetes (DURATION-2): a randomised trial. Lancet. 2010;376(9739):431–9.

52. Forst T, Uhlig-Laske B, Ring A, et al. Linagliptin (BI 1356), a potent and selective DPP-4 inhibitor, is safe and efficacious in combination with metformin in patients with inadequately controlled Type 2 diabetes. Diabet Med. 2010;27(12):1409–19.

53. Gallwitz B, Rosenstock J, Rauch T, et al. 2-year efficacy and safety of linagliptin compared with glimepiride in patients with type 2 diabetes inadequately controlled on metformin: a randomised, double-blind, noninferiority trial. Lancet (North American Edition). 2012;380(9840):475–83.

54. Ross SA, Rafeiro E, Meinicke T. Efficacy and safety of linagliptin 2.5 mg twice daily versus 5 mg once daily in patients with type 2 diabetes inadequately controlled on metformin: a randomised, double-blind, placebocontrolled trial. Curr Med Res Opin. 2012;28(9):1465–74.

55. Aaboe K, Knop FK, Visbøll T, et al. Twelve weeks treatment with the DPP-4 inhibitor, sitagliptin, prevents degradation of peptide YY and improves glucose and non-glucose induced insulin secretion in patients with type 2 diabetes mellitus. Diabetes Obes Metab. 2010;12(4):323–33.

56. Derosa G, Carbone A, Franzetti I, et al. Effects of a combination of sitagliptin plus metformin vs metformin monotherapy on glycemic control, b-cell function and insulin resistance in type 2 diabetic patients. Diabetes Res Clin Pract. 2012;98(1):51–60.

57. Hermansen K, Kipnes M, Luo E, Fanurik D, Khatami H, Stein P. Efficacy and safety of the dipeptidyl peptidase-4 inhibitor, sitagliptin, in patients with type 2 diabetes mellitus inadequately controlled on glimepiride alone or on glimepiride and metformin. Diabetes Obes Metab. 2007;9(5):733–45.

^{99m}Tc-radiolabeled GE11-modified peptide for ovarian tumor targeting

Najmeh Rahmanian[1,2], Seyed Jalal Hosseinimehr[2], Ali Khalaj[3*], Zohreh Noaparast[2], Seyed Mohammad Abedi[4] and Omid Sabzevari[5]

Abstract

Background: Ovarian cancer is a serious threat for women health and the early diagnosis of this cancer might improves the survival rate of patients. The use of the targeted radiopharmaceuticals could be a non-invasive and logical method for tumor imaging. The aim of this study was to radiolabel GE11 peptide as a new specific probe for imaging of ovarian tumor.

Methods: HYNIC-SSS-GE11 peptide was labeled with ^{99m}Tc using tricine as a coligand. The ^{99m}Tc-tricine-HYNIC-SSS-GE11 peptide was evaluated for specific cellular binding in three cell lines with different levels of EGFR expression. Tumor targeting was assessed in SKOV3 tumor bearing mice.

Results: By using tricine as a coligand, labeling yield was more than 98% and the stability of the radiolabelled peptide in human serum up to 4 h was 96%. The in vitro cell uptake test showed that this radiolabeled peptide had a good affinity to SKOV3 cells with dissociation constant of 73 nM. The in vivo results showed a tumor/muscle ratio of 3.2 at 4 h following injection of ^{99m}Tc-tricine-HYNIC-SSS-GE11 peptide.

Conclusions: Results of this study showed that ^{99m}Tc-tricine-HYNIC-SSS-GE11 peptide could be a promising tool for diagnosis and staging of ovarian cancer.

Keywords: GE11 peptide, ^{99m}Tc, Molecular imaging, HYNIC, Radiopharmaceuticals

Background

Ovarian cancer has been reported as the fifth major cause of cancer related death and the eight most common cancer among women. Since the symptoms of the ovarian cancer in early stages are not clear, nearly 50% of patients are diagnosed in advanced stages (stage III/IV) whereas patient are over 65 years old [1, 2]. While early diagnosis may increase survival times of 90% of patients to 5 years, late diagnosis at stage 3 increases survival times of only 33% of patients to 5 years. Considering that ovarian cancer is frequently diagnosed at stage III or IV, a convenient screening method for early detection is highly desirable [3]. Recent approaches have focused attention to tumor targeting agents for identification of tumor cells. It has been shown that in approximately 70% of ovarian cancers there is an overexpression of Epidermal Growth Factor Receptors (EGFRs) which belongs to receptor kinase family and consist of 4 members, namely: HER1 (Human Epidermal Growth Factor Receptor 1; EGFR), HER2/neu, HER3 and HER4 [4]. Binding of EGF to EGFR is followed by homo or heterodimerization of the receptors which activate intracellular cascades and as a consequence result in cellular responses such as proliferation, differentiation and survival [5]. Overexpression of EGFR family which has been found in many human malignancies such as gastric, Non-Small Cell Lung Cancer (NSCLC), Squamous Cell Carcinoma of the Head and Neck (SCCHN), breast, ovarian, prostate, colorectal, esophageal, bladder and renal cancers result in tumor recurrence which decreases patient survival [6, 7]. Currently monoclonal Antibodies (mAbs) such as trastuzumab, pertuzumab and cetuximab are being used for treatment of tumors associated with overexpression of EGFR [8]. Measurement of EGFR levels have been described as a reliable method to follow up patient responses and to evaluate treatment efficacy

* Correspondence: khalaj@ams.ac.ir
[3]Department of Medicinal Chemistry, Faculty of Pharmacy, Tehran University of Medical Sciences Tehran, Iran
Full list of author information is available at the end of the article

following therapy with EGFR inhibitors. The radionuclide molecular imaging as a non-invasive method has been used to detect EGFR expression [9]. Radiolabeled peptides, proteins and antibodies such as [111In] Bz-DTPA-hEGF, 99mTc-EGF, 64Cu-DOTA-cetuximab, 111In-DTPA-CHX-A''-cetuximab, 111In-MAb 225, 99mTc-8B6 nanobody, and 111In-DOTA-Affibody molecule are some examples of EGFR specific radionuclide imaging agents. While 99mTc-radiolabeled antibodies have advantages of using readily available radionuclide through a generator at low cost which emits only gamma radiation of low energy of 140 Kev, they have some limitations such as slow tumor accumulation, slow blood clearance rate and high abdominal accumulation and as a result diminished target-non target contrast. Small molecular size peptides which have low side effects and good clearance pattern from blood are good targeting and imaging agents [10]. In 2005 Li et al. reported a novel dodecapeptide YHWYGYTPQNVI (GE11) as an EGFR targeting ligand which binds effectively to epithermal growth factor receptor without activating EGFR-mediated signaling pathway [11]. Selectivity and sensitivity of GE11 for EGFR makes it as a promising vector for systematic delivery of therapeutic pharmaceuticals [12–15] and also for specific delivery of imaging agents such as radioactive tracers including 18F, 64Cu and 131I [16–18]. Since high resolution for tumor visualization depends on high radioactivity uptake in the tumor and low uptakes in non-target tissues such as liver which might also blind metastatic lesions [19] several studies have indicated that pharmacokinetic modification of the imaging contrast through the use of an appropriate linker result in increased tumor uptake, reduced non-target tissues uptake and better tumor visualization [20, 21]. Among different linkers the use of Seryl-Seryl-Serine (SSS) sequence as spacer has shown remarkable effects on biodistribution by reducing liver accumulation and rapid clearance of the radiolabelled peptides [20, 21]. In this study SSS-GE11 was conjugated with hydrazinenicotinamide (HYNIC) and labeled with 99mTc using tricine as a coligand. The in vitro specificity of the radiolabelled peptide for binding to EGFR was determined in SKOV3, A549, and MCF-7 cell lines, of which SKOV3 ovarian carcinoma cells accumulated higher amount of the radiolabeled peptide and was used for in vivo tumor targeting in nude mice. In addition, biodistribution of the radiolabeled peptide was investigated in both normal and nude mice in order to determine the effects of Seryl-Seryl-Serine (SSS) sequence as spacer on liver accumulation and renal clearance of the radiolabeled peptide.

Methods

Instrumentation and materials

The HYNIC-SSS-GE11 was purchased from ProteoGenix (Schiltigheim, France). 99mTc was obtained from a 99Mo/ 99mTc radionuclide generator (Pars Isotope, Iran). Ammonium acetate, sodium citrate, acetonitrile (HPLC grade), and Methyl Ethyl Ketone (MEK) were obtained from Merck company (Darmstadt, Germany). Trifluoroacetic acid (TFA), anhydrous tin (II)-chloride and tricine were from Sigma-Aldrich company (St. Louis, MO, USA). Double distilled deionized water were used for the preparation of aqueous solutions. Lablogic mini scan TLC scanner (Sheffield, UK) was used for quantification of the distribution of radioactivity which was determined by Instant Thin Layer Chromatography on Silica Gel (ITLC-SG) strips and the resulting data were analyzed by Laura image analysis software. Radioactivity in the sample was measured using a gamma counter with a NaI(Tl) gamma detector (Delshid, Tehran, Iran). Knauer HPLC system (Berlin, Germany) was used for analytical reversed-phase high-performance liquid chromatography (RP-HPLC) and the HPLC analyses of the radiolabeled peptides were performed on a Lablogic radioactivity gamma detector with a Eurospher 100–5 C18, 4.6×250 mm (Knauer, Berlin, Germany) column. Elution of RP-HPLC was performed with a solvent system consisting of: 0.1% TFA in acetonitrile (solvent A) and 0.1% TFA in water (solvent B).

Human ovarian cancer (SKOV3), Non–Small Cell Lung Cancer (NSCLC) (A549) and human breast cancer cell lines (MCF-7) were obtained from the Pasture Institute of Iran and Iranian Genetic and Biological Resource Center and cultured at 37 °C in the presence of 5% CO_2 in Dulbecco's Modified Eagle's Medium (DMEM) (Gibco, Paisley, UK) supplemented with 10% Fetal Bovine Serum (FBS) and 100 μg/mL penicillin–streptomycin (Gibco, UK). HER2-specific antibody (trastuzumab), EGFR-specific antibody (cetuximab), and a CD20-specific antibody (rituximab) were from Roche (Switzerland).

All animal studies were carried out in accordance with the national animal protection regulation and approved by the Research Committee of Tehran University of Medical Sciences with approval code of 9112080151–131701.

Radiolabeling of HYNIC-SSS-GE11 conjugate with 99mTc

Radiolabeling of the peptide was performed according to the reported procedure with some modifications [22]. Briefly, 10 μg of HYNIC-SSS-GE11 was dissolved in 100 μL of 0.5 M ammonium acetate buffer of pH 6. Solution of tricine (10 mg in 0.5 M ammonium acetate buffer of pH 6) as a coligand for HYNIC was added to the HYNIC-SSS-GE11 and mixed with 100–1480 MBq of fresh 99mTc-pertecnetate solution and 40 μg of SnCl₂. 2H₂O (1 mg/mL in 0.1 N HCl). The mixture was incubated at room temperature for 30 min.

Quality control assessment

The labeling yield and radiochemical purity were assessed by analytical HPLC and Instant Thin Layer

Chromatography on Silica Gel (ITLC-SG). For analytical HPLC a gradient elution of 0.1% TFA in acetonitrile (A) and 0.1% TFA in water (B) was employed as follows: 0–10 min: (10–25% A and 90–75% B); 10–15 min: (25–50% A and 75–50% B); 15–20 min: (50–90% A and 50–10% B) for a total time of 20 min and flow rate of 1.0 mL min^{-1}. All solvents were filtered and degassed prior to passage through the column. ITLC-SG was run alongside by the use of different mobile phases such as methyl ethyl keton for free pertechnetate ($R_f = 1$), acetonitrile 50% for reduced hydrolyzed technetium ($R_f = 0$) and 0.1 M sodium citrate buffer of pH 5.5 for free ^{99m}Tc-coligand ($R_f = 1$) [23].

Stability assessment

The stability of ^{99m}Tc-tricine-HYNIC-SSS-GE11 peptide in solution at different time intervals (shelf life) was evaluated by dilution of the reaction mixture up to 1 ml with ammonium acetate buffer of pH 6 and incubation at ambient temperatures up to 24 h. The radiochemical purity of the diluted reaction mixture was analyzed by ITLC. All experiments were carried out in triplicates.

Serum stability of the peptide was also determined following addition of 100 μl of fresh human serum to 20 μl of the reaction mixture and incubation for 1 and 4 h at 37 °C. Plasma samples were then treated with 500 μl of a mixture of acetonitrile and ethanol (1:1), centrifuged (14,000 rpm, 6 min), filtered (0.22 μm) and degradation of the radiolabeled peptide was assessed in supernatant by RP-HPLC [24].

Cellular specific binding

The in vitro specificity of ^{99m}Tc-tricine-HYNIC-SSS-GE11 for binding to EGFR was determined by using three cell lines in SKOV3, A549, and MCF-7 according the reported method with some modifications [25]. Briefly, the cell lines were cultivated in Dulbecco's DMEM-high glucose supplemented with 10% (v/v) FBS at 37 °C in a humidified incubator in the presence of 5% CO_2. The cells were trypsinised using a trypsin-EDTA solution and seeded in 12 well plates with a cell density of 5×10^5 cells per dish and incubated for 24 h. On the day of experiment, cells were washed with cold serum-free medium or PBS and incubated with radiolabeled peptide at 37 °C for 2 h. Incubation was interrupted by the removal of the medium which was washed twice with 1 ml of incomplete cold medium. The cells were then trypsinized and diluted to 1 mL with complete medium. The supernatant was collected and the radioactivity was measured by a gamma counter. For determination of the specific binding of ^{99m}Tc-tricine-HYNIC-SSS-GE11, the SKOV3 cells were pre-incubated with 500-fold excess of the unlabeled peptide at 37 °C for 30 min prior to the addition of radiolabeled peptide. Blocking experiments were also performed in the

presences of trastuzumab, cetuximab and rituximab that are HER2, EGFR and CD20 specific antibodies respectively.

Cellular internalization

SKOV3 cells were seeded in the single well plates (1×10^6 per well) and incubated with 80 nM of the radioconjugated peptide at 37 °C for 5 min and 0.5, 1, 2 and 4 h. All experiment were performed in triplicates. Incubation was interrupted by the removal of the medium which was washed twice with ice-cold incomplete medium. The cells were then treated twice with 0.5 ml of urea buffer of pH 2.5 for 5 min on the ice to remove the surface receptor-bound fraction. Then, the cells were incubated with 0.5 mL of 1 M NaOH at 37 °C for 10 min. The cell debris were collected, and the dishes were washed with 0.5 mL of NaOH solution and the radioactivity of all collected supernatant were measured by the automated gamma counter. It should be noted that the radioactivity in the urea buffer and alkaline solution were considered as membrane bound and internalized, respectively [26, 27].

Dissociation constant

The affinity of ^{99m}Tc–tricine-HYNIC–SSS-GE11 was evaluated using saturation binding assay. For this purpose the SKOV3 cells were seeded in 24-well plates (25×10^4 cells/well), treated with increasing concentrations of ^{99m}Tc-tricine-HYNIC–SSS-GE11 (5, 10, 30, 65, 100, 150, 225 and 300 nM) and incubated at 37 °C in the presence (for non-specific binding) or absence (for total binding) of the unlabeled peptide. Three dishes were used for total binding and one dish containing 500-fold excess of highest concentration of radiolabeled peptide was used for non-specific binding. After 60 min of incubation, the cells were rinsed with cold serum-free medium and harvested by using a trypsin–EDTA solution. The bound radioactivity was determined with a gamma well counter and the binding data were analyzed by non-linear regression using GraphPad Software Prism version 5.04 for windows (GraphPad Software Inc., California, and USA). The equilibrium dissociation constant (Kd) and the maximum binding capacity (Bmax) of the receptor were obtained by saturation analysis. .

Biodistribution study in normal mice

Normal female NMRI mice (20–30 g, Mazandaran animal center institute, Sari, Iran) were used in this study and randomly divided into 3 groups of 4. 100 μL of the solution containing 1 μg of the radiolabeled peptide was intravenously injected to the tail vein of each mouse. Mice were euthanized through intraperitoneal injection of ketamine and xylazine at 1, 4 and 24 h after injection. Blood was collected from the heart after deep anesthesia by a syringe which had been washed with heparin. Thereafter, organ samples including; lungs, stomach, liver, kidneys, bone, muscle, salivary glands, heart, spleen and intestines were removed, weighted and the radioactivity of each sample was measured. The tissue uptake of all organs except intestine was calculated as percent of injected dose per gram tissue (% ID/g) and for the intestine was calculated as % ID of the whole sample.

Biodistribution study in nude mice bearing SKOV3 human ovarian cancer xenografts

The in vivo tumor-targeting of the radiolabeled peptide was studied in female nude mice bearing SKOV3 cancer xenografts. For tumor induction, 10×10^6 SKOV3 cells were subcutaneously injected into the right hind leg of nude mice and tumor was allowed to grow for about 4 weeks. In the day of experiment, the average tumor size was 0.63 ± 0.2 g and the mice were randomly divided into three groups of 4 mouse each. The mice were injected intravenously 1 µg of the radiolabelled peptide. At 1 h and 4 h after injection, the mice were sacrificed and the tumor and other tissues were dissected. Blocking experiment was also performed using three nude mice which were subjected to injection of the excess amount (500 µg/50 µl) of the unlabeled peptide 30 min before radioconjugate peptide injection.

Results

Radiolabeling of HYNIC-SSS-GE11 with ^{99m}Tc

HYNIC-SSS-GE11 was labeled with ^{99m}Tc using tricine as coligand and SnCl$_2$ as reducing agent (Fig. 1). Various factors such as pH and type of buffer, amount of SnCl$_2$, temperature and incubation time had influences on the radiochemical purity of ^{99m}Tc-HYNIC-SSS-GE11. Radiochemical yield was not greater than 80% in water, normal saline, phosphate-buffered saline of pH 7 and ammonium acetate of pH 5.2 but was higher than 98% in ammonium acetate buffer of pH 6 containing tricine

(10 mg), SnCl$_2$ (40 µg) and ^{99m}TcO$_4^-$Na (5–40 mCi). Radiochemical purity (RCP) determined after 1, 2 and 4 h by ITLC were found to be 97, 96 and 95% respectively. Also RCP assessed by radio HPLC was found to be 97 and 95% at 1 and 4 h respectively, considering 1–2% reduced hydrolyzed technetium (Fig. 2a). Experimental results showed acceptable radiochemical purity on the basis of the presence of a single radioactivity peak corresponding to ^{99m}Tc-HYNIC-SSS-GE11 with a retention time of 18–20 min.

Stability assessment in solution and serum

The radiolabeled conjugate solution showed a stability of approximately 93%, within 4 h, in solution (Fig. 3). Also, the stability of radiolabeled conjugate was evaluated in human serum for 1 and 4 h by radio HPLC (Fig. 2b). ^{99m}Tc-HYNIC-SSS-GE11 diluted in human serum showed stability of approximately 96% over 4 h. Based on the results, it can be concluded that the radiolabeled conjugate demonstrated acceptable stability in solution and human serum for 4 h.

Cellular specific binding

To confirm the specificity of the binding of radiolabeled peptide to EGFR receptor, three cell lines with different level of EGFR expression (A549: high EGFR, low HER2; SKOV3: high HER2; MCF-7: very low EGFR and HER2 expression) were used. Results showed that there was significant differences in in vitro tendency of different cells for binding to radiolabeled peptide. Based on the results, ^{99m}Tc-tricine-HYNIC-SSS-GE11 had higher tendency to bind to SKOV3 than A549 which in turn had higher tendency than MCF-7 cells. Accumulation of the radiolabeled peptide in SKOV3 cell line compared to MCF-7 cell line was 5 times higher and compared to A549 cells was 4.4 times higher (Fig. 4a). On the other

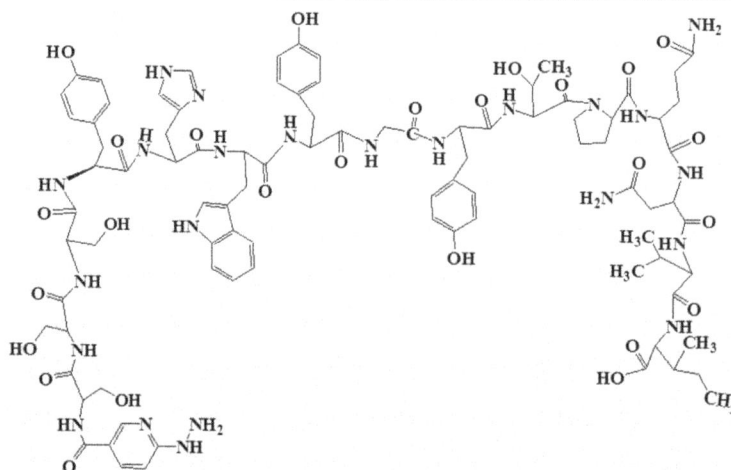

Fig. 1 Chemical structure of HYNIC-SSS-GE11

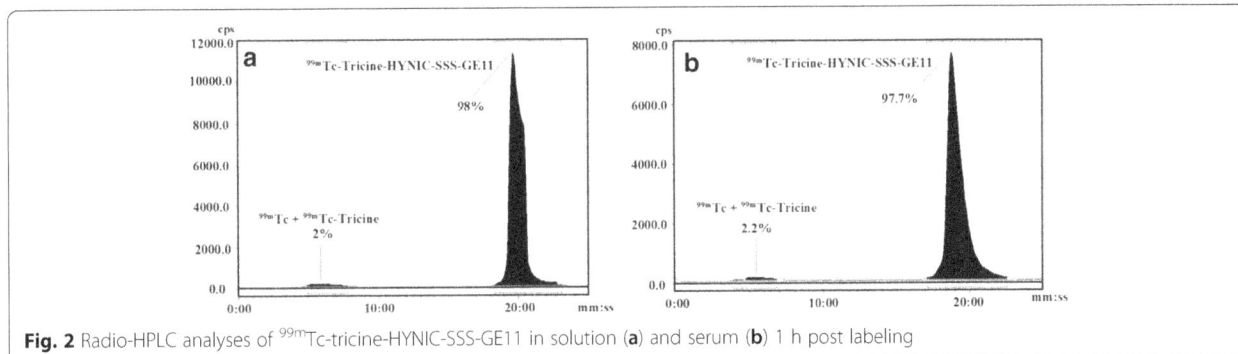

Fig. 2 Radio-HPLC analyses of ^{99m}Tc-tricine-HYNIC-SSS-GE11 in solution (**a**) and serum (**b**) 1 h post labeling

hand, the binding specificity tests demonstrated that the binding of ^{99m}Tc-HYNIC-SSS-GE11 was receptor mediated because pre-saturation of the SKOV3 cells with 500-fold excess molar of the cold peptide decreased the specific binding to 25% (Fig. 4a).

These results also revealed that the SKOV3 cells accumulated a higher amount of radioactivity resulting from receptor binding to the radiolabeled peptide. In addition, when SKOV3 cells pre-incubated with excess molar of antibodies such as cetuximab, trastuzumab and rituximab, specific binding decreased significantly by trastuzumab as a HER2 specific antibody (Fig. 4b).

Cellular internalization

The results of cellular internalization experiments are summarized in Fig. 5. The main source of the intracellular radioactivity was from the cell-bound radioactivity. Internalization of the radiolabeled peptide by SKOV3 cells was evaluated at 37 °C up to 4 h. Results showed that the fraction of internalized radioactivity increased with the time. Totally, about 52% of the radiolabeled peptide from membrane-bound conjugate internalized the cells up to 4 h.

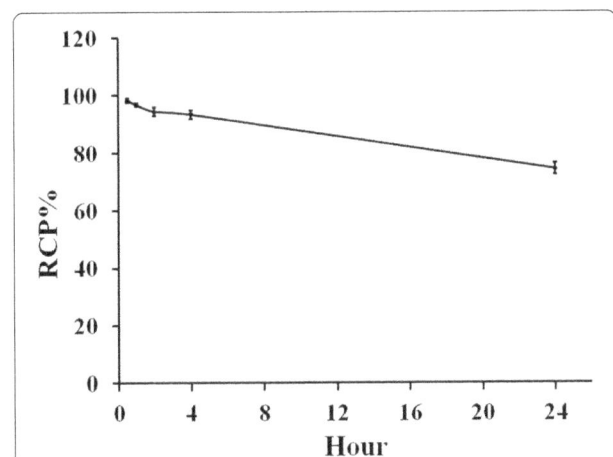

Fig. 3 Stability of ^{99m}Tc-tricine-HYNIC-SSS-GE11 in solution over time

Dissociation constant

The binding affinity of ^{99m}Tc-tricine-HYNIC-SSS-GE11 to SKOV3 cells was determined by treating cells with increasing concentration of radiolabeled peptide. The specific binding was calculated by subtracting the non-specific binding radioactivity from total binding activity. The saturation binding curve of ^{99m}Tc-tricine-HYNIC-SSS-GE11 to SKOV3 cells is shown in Fig. 6. The analysis of data revealed the radiolabeled peptide bound to receptors with a dissociation constant of 73 ± 17 nM and B_{max} of $(9 \pm 0.1) \times 10^5$.

Biodistribution in normal mice

The biodistribution of ^{99m}Tc-tricine-HYNIC-SSS-GE11 in normal female mice is represented in Table 1. Low accumulation of this radiolabeled peptide was observed in heart, lung, salivary gland, stomach, muscle and bone. Negligible amount of the radioactivity accumulation in stomach, thyroid and salivary gland indicated high in vivo stability of the radiolabeled peptide with low release of free ^{99m}Tc. Also the percent of the injected dose of the radiolabeled peptide that accumulated in the liver were 2.88, 2.05 and 0.33% at 1, 4 and 24 h, respectively. In addition, % ID/g values for radiolabeled peptide in the kidneys at 1, 4 and 24 h were 24.5, 17.5 and 3.5%, respectively. These findings showed that the radiolabeled peptide has low tendency for accumulation in liver and excretion by hepatobiliary system and as a result the kidney was the main excretion rout for the radiolabeled peptide. Also, the blood level of radioactivity was less than 1% ID/g at 1 and 4 h because the radiolabeled conjugate was cleared rapidly from the blood.

Biodistribution in nude mice bearing SKOV3 human ovarian cancer xenografts

To evaluate the uptake of radiolabeled peptide by ovarian tumor, additional biodistribution studies were performed in nude mice bearing SKOV3 xenografts (Table 2). Results compared to the normal mice showed similar patterns of low liver and high kidney uptakes and a fast clearance from the blood. Tumor uptake of

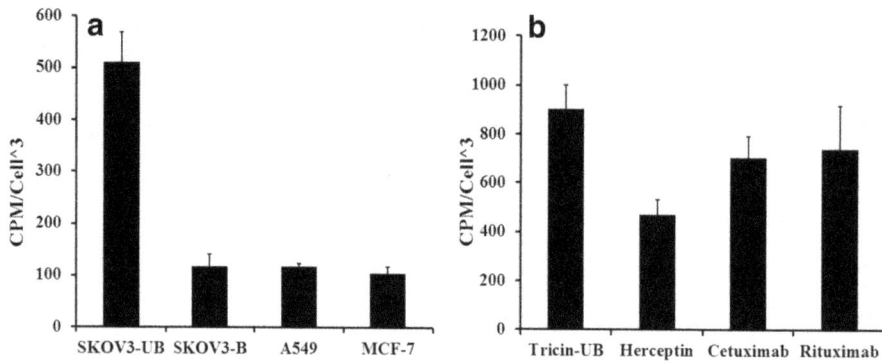

Fig. 4 a Specific binding of ^{99m}Tc-tricine-HYNIC-SSS-GE11 in three cell lines with different level of EGFR expression: SKOV3 (*high* HER2), A549 (*high* EGFR), MCF-7 (negative). Blocking experiment was performed in the presence of the excess (500-fold molar) of non-radiolabeled peptide. **b** Specific binding of ^{99m}Tc-tricine-HYNIC-SSS-GE11 in SKOV3 cells in the presence of (500-fold molar excess) and absence of the specific anti-body; trastuzumab (anti-HER2), cetuximab (anti-EGFR) and rituximab (anti-CD20)

radiolabeled conjugate were 2.33 and 1.66% at 1 and 4 h, respectively. The tumor/muscle ratios were 2.4 and 3.4 at 1 and 4 h, respectively. Also, tumor uptake was reduced significantly from 1.66% at 4 h to 0.93% in blocking study whereas 500-fold molar excess of cold peptide was injected 30 min prior injection of the related radioconjugated peptide.

Discussion

Radionuclide diagnostic strategy through utilization of molecular targeting probe is a simple and non-invasive method for diagnosis as well as treatment of cancers. EGFR has been reported to have a crucial role in initiation, progression and invasion of a variety of human malignancies with epithelial origin [28]. GE11 is a small peptide which was introduced by Li et al. during investigations on phage display techniques [11]. It has been shown that GE11 is able to bind EGFR efficiently with a K_D of 22nM without mitogencity. In this study GE11 was labeled with ^{99m}Tc to introduce a potential

radiolabelled peptide for in vivo targeting of tumors having overexpression of EGFR. Results of this study showed that radiolabeled GE11 peptide displays moderate tumor uptake, rapid blood clearance and high renal and low hepatobiliary excretion. Several chelators such as diaminedithiol (N_2S_2), triamidethiol (N_3S), PnAO (N_4) and HYNC have been used for labelling of a peptide with ^{99m}Tc. In this study HYNIC was used as chelator due to simple and high yield labeling and appropriate biological properties [29]. Tricine was selected as a coligand because it provides acceptable radiolabeling efficacy [22]. To improve pharmacokinetic properties and renal excretion of the labeled peptide, SSS linker was inserted between chelator and N-terminus of GE11 peptide [30]. This

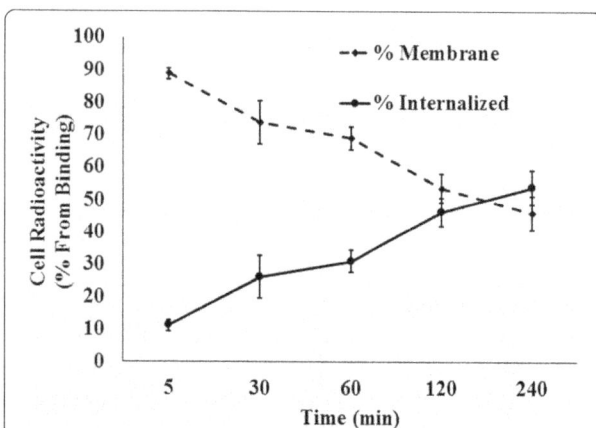

Fig. 5 Time dependency of internalization of ^{99m}Tc-tricine-HYNIC-SSS-GE11 in SKOV3 cells expressed as % of bound activity

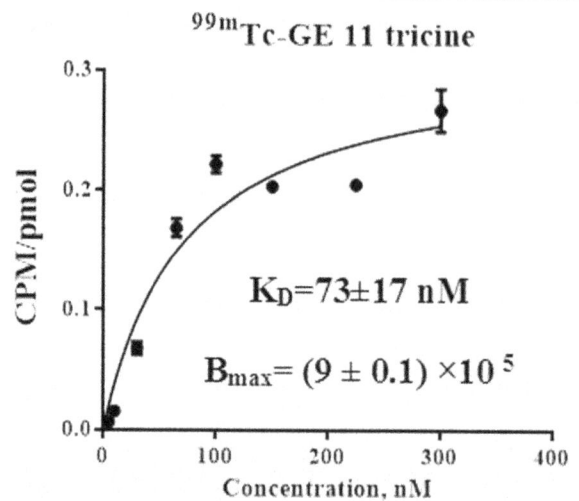

Fig. 6 Affinity assessment of ^{99m}Tc-tricine-HYNIC-SSS-GE11 in SKOV3 cell line by saturation binding analysis. Increasing concentration of ^{99m}Tc-tricine-HYNIC-SSS-GE11 were added to dishes with SKOV3 cells. The cells were then harvested and bound radioactivity (*y-axis*) was determined. The errors presented in the insert are standard errors of the curve fit

Table 1 Biodistribution of ^{99m}Tc-Tricine-HYNIC-SSS-GE11 peptide in normal female mice at 1, 4 and 24 h p.i.

Tissue	% ID/g ± SD		
	1 h	4 h	24 h
Blood	0.84 ± 0.04	0.39 ± 0.11	0.18 ± 0.05
Heart	0.76 ± 0.16	0.44 ± 0.18	0.40 ± 0.2
Lung	1.14 ± 0.63	0.68 ± 0.23	0.47 ± 0.09
s.g & Th.[a]	0.87 ± 0.15	0.46 ± 0.22	0.36 ± 0.12
Liver	2.88 ± 0.84	2.05 ± 0.39	0.33 ± 0.069
Spleen	0.61 ± 0.14	0.41 ± 0.13	0.20 ± 0.06
Kidney	24.5 ± 1.7	17.5 ± 1.25	3.55 ± 0.38
Stomach	0.91 ± 0.27	0.57 ± 0.15	0.32 ± 0.19
Muscle	0.52 ± 0.14	0.23 ± 0.11	0.19 ± 0.05
Bone	0.97 ± 0.14	0.57 ± 0.2	0.28 ± 0.05
Intestine	3.1 ± 0.91	1.89 ± 0.44	0.93 ± 0.28

Each mouse was administered 1 μg of radiolabeled peptide ($n = 4$) and sacrificed at 1, 4 and 24 h after injection. Data are mean ± SD
[a]Salivary gland and Thyroid are abbreviated as s.g and Th. respectively

approach resulted in generation of a radiolabeled peptide with high radiochemical yield (>98%) and acceptable stability in solution as it was verified by ITLC. Instability of ^{99m}Tc-tricine-complex due to multiple coordination isomerism have been described previously [31]. Assessment of the stability of the radiolabeled peptide of this investigation in human serum showed promising results. The

Table 2 Biodistribution of ^{99m}Tc-Tricine-HYNIC-SSS-GE11 peptide in mice bearing SKOV3 xenograft at 1 and 4 h after injection

Tissue	% ID/g ± SD		
	1 h	4 h	4 h-blocked[a]
Blood	2.53 ± 0.51	1.43 ± 0.18	0.99 ± 0.18
Heart	2.40 ± 0.96	1.56 ± 0.37	0.65 ± 0.1
Lung	3.39 ± 0.64	1.79 ± 0.34	1.24 ± 0.12
s.g & Th.[b]	2.52 ± 0.82	1.80 ± 0.21	0.89 ± 0.16
Liver	6.93 ± 0.95	4.64 ± 0.69	3.28 ± 0.93
Spleen	2.86 ± 0.17	1.49 ± 0.32	0.83 ± 0.1
Kidney	64.95 ± 7.81	57.90 ± 0.49	42.10 ± 4.39
Stomach	2.65 ± 0.66	1.53 ± 0.16	1.16 ± 0.11
Muscle	0.99 ± 0.21	0.51 ± 0.14	0.51 ± 0.07
Bone	1.91 ± 0.53	1.29 ± 0.29	1.01 ± 0.11
Intestine	8.38 ± 4.11	3.24 ± 0.9	3.83 ± 2.1
Tumor	2.33 ± 0.67	1.66 ± 0.41	0.93 ± 0.10
Tumor/Muscle Ratio	2.3	3.42	1.86
Tumor/Bone Ratio	1.2	1.3	0.92
Tumor/Blood Ratio	0.92	1.17	0.96

[a]To block receptors, mice were pretreated with excess of unlabeled peptides (500 μg) by intraperitoneal injection at 0.5 h before radiolabeled peptide injection ($n = 3$) Nude mice were administered 1 μg of radiolabeled peptide ($n = 4$) and sacrificed at 1 and 4 h after injection. Data are mean ± SD
[b]Salivary gland and Thyroid are abbreviated as s.g and Th. respectively

radiochemical purity was 95% within 4 h incubation time and no significant impurities including ^{99m}TcO$_4^-$, RHT and ^{99m}Tc-coligand were released.

It has been reported previously that GE11 is able to bind EGFR especially those of human hepatoma cell line SMMC-7721 [11], human non-small cell lung carcinoma cell line H1299 [12], human glioblastoma astrocytoma U87-MG [32], non-small cell lung cancer A549 [33], human ovarian adenocarcinoma SKOV3 [14, 16] and breast cancer HCC70 cells [34]. In this study the tendency of ^{99m}Tc-tricine-GE11 complex in binding to SKOV3, A549 and MCF-7 cell lines were compared. These cell lines have different levels of HER1 and HER2 expression. Several studies have shown that both epithermal growth factor 1 and 2 are associated and expressed at high levels in human ovarian cancer cell line SKOV3 and human non-small cell line cancer A549 but have lower expression of HER1 and HER2, respectively [17, 35, 36]. HER2 has important role in proliferation and progression of a variety of cancers such as breast, ovarian, non-small cell lung and hepatoma [37]. Therefore, several investigations have utilized different types of targeting biomolecules such as antibody, affibody, aptamer and peptide for diagnose and follow up of the treatments of cancers with high level of HER2 expression [38–45]. These targeting biomolecules have some disadvantages such as high molecular weight, high cost, long-half life in blood circulation, high immunogenicity and low stability. Recent studies have shown that the use of GE11 as an EGFR targeting biomolecule enhances the delivery of chemotherapeutic agents to ovarian cancer cells [14, 46].

In this work by competition and blocking experiments and using FDA approved antibodies it was shown that GE11 radioconjugate has high tendency to bind to HER2 in SKOV3 cell line. Saturation binding experiments showed that the ^{99m}Tc-tricine-HYNIC-SSS-GE11 complex was able to bind to SKOV3 with a K_D of 73 nM. The high in vivo stability was shown by biodistribution experiments in normal female mice where there was no significant release of the free ^{99m}Tc in salivary glands and stomach. The % ID/g values of the blood uptake of ^{99m}Tc-tricine-HYNIC-SSS-GE11 complex were 0.83, 0.39 and 0.18 at 1, 4 and 24 h respectively, indicating rapid clearance of the radioconjugate from the blood. In general, the high activity in gastrointestinal is very problematic and may mask metastatic lesions of other target organs. Several reports have shown the importance of linkers in modification of pharmacokinetic by reducing non-target uptake and improving tumor visualization [20, 21, 47]. In contrast to results of the first report on biodistribution of GE11 labeled with ^{125}I which showed high liver uptake [11], the kidney was the main route of excretion of radiolabeled GE11 peptide of this study due to the presence of seryl-seryl-serine as pharmacokinetic modifier linker. Results of in vivo biodistribution in nude mice bearing SKOV3 cancer xenografts, showed that the radioconjugated peptide had moderate tumor uptake with % ID/g values of 2.33 and 1.66 at 1 and 4 h after injection respectively. There was a significant statistical differences between concentration of the radiolabeled peptide in tumor and muscle in the way that the tumor-to-muscle ratio at 1 and 4 h of post-injection were 2.3 and 3.42, while tumor-to-blood ratio at these periods of time were 0.92 and 1.17 respectively. Results of this investigation shows that further optimization might be required to increase the clearance rate of the prepared radioconjugated peptide without reducing concentration of tumor radioactivity.

Conclusions

In this study the ^{99m}Tc-tricine-HYNIC-SSS-GE11 was prepared with highly radiochemical purity and good stability. The radioconjugated peptide showed specific binding mediated by HER2 on the cell surface. The biodistribution of the prepared radioconjugated peptide in normal and SKOV3 xenograft mice model showed that the renal system is the main route for excretion of the radioactivity due to presence of SSS linker which was used for modification of the pharmacokinetic. A tumor-to-muscle ratio of 3.4 was obtained with ^{99m}Tc-labeled peptide that showed HER2 targeting on SKOV3 tumor.

Abbreviations

^{99m}Tc: 99 m-Technetium; DMEM: Dulbecco's Modified Eagle's Medium; EGFR: Epidermal Growth Factor Receptor; FBS: Fetal Bovine Serum; HER: Human Epidermal growth factor Receptor; HYNIC: Hydrazinonicotinic acid; ITLC-SG: Instant Thin Layer Chromatography on Silica Gel; MAbs: Monoclonal Antibodies; MEK: Methyl Ethyl Ketone; NSCLC: Non-Small Cell Lung Cancer; RHT: Reduced Hydrolyzed Technetium; RP-HPLC: Reversed-Phase High-Performance Liquid Chromatography; SCCHN: Squamous Cell Carcinoma of the Head and Neck; SSS-GE11: Seryl-Seryl-Seryl-GE11 peptide; TFA: Trifluoroacetic acid

Acknowledgment

The authors are indebted to the Mazanderan University of Medical Sciences for providing laboratories and facilities to carry out this investigation.

Funding

This research was part of a Ph.D. thesis of the first author and was supported financially by the deputy of research of Tehran University of Medical Sciences and also by a grant (93025192) from Iran National Science Foundation (INSF).

Authors' contributions

NR participated in design of the study, carried out all experiments and drafted the manuscript. SJH participated in design of the study, interpretation and analysis of data and drafting the manuscript. AK participated in design and coordination of the study and was a major contributor in writing the manuscript. ZN supervised and participated in the biodistribution studies. SMA participated in preparation of ^{99m}Tc and supervised animal studies. OS supervised cellular studies. All authors read and approved the final manuscript.

Competing interests

The authors declare that they have no competing interests.

Author details

[1]Department of Radiopharmacy, Faculty of Pharmacy, Tehran University of Medical Sciences, Tehran, Iran. [2]Department of Radiopharmacy, Faculty of Pharmacy, Mazandaran University of Medical Sciences, Sari, Iran. [3]Department of Medicinal Chemistry, Faculty of Pharmacy, Tehran University of Medical Sciences Tehran, Iran . [4]Department of Radiology, Faculty of Medicine, Mazandaran University of Medical Sciences, Sari, Iran. [5]Department of Toxicology, Faculty of Pharmacy, Tehran University of Medical Sciences, Tehran, Iran.

References

1. Yancik R. Ovarian cancer: age contrasts in incidence, histology, disease stage at diagnosis, and mortality. Cancer. 1993;71(S2):517–23.
2. Goff BA, Mandel L, Muntz HG, Melancon CH. Ovarian carcinoma diagnosis. Cancer. 2000;89(10):2068–75.
3. Clarke-Pearson DL. Screening for ovarian cancer. New Engl J Med. 2009; 361(2):170–7.
4. Normanno N, De Luca A, Bianco C, Strizzi L, Mancino M, Maiello MR, et al. Epidermal growth factor receptor (EGFR) signaling in cancer. Gene. 2006; 366(1):2–16.
5. Boonstra J, Rijken P, Humbel B, Cremers F, Verkleij A,van Bergen en Henegouwen P. The epidermal growth factor. Cell Biol Int. 1995;19(5):413–30.
6. Alper Ö, Bergmann-Leitner ES, Bennett TA, Hacker NF, Stromberg K, Stetler-Stevenson WG. Epidermal growth factor receptor signaling and the invasive phenotype of ovarian carcinoma cells. J Natl Cancer Inst. 2001;93(18):1375–84.
7. Salomon DS, Brandt R, Ciardiello F, Normanno N. Epidermal growth factor-related peptides and their receptors in human malignancies. Crit Rev Oncol Hematol. 1995;19(3):183–232.
8. Herbst RS. Review of epidermal growth factor receptor biology. Int J Radiat Oncol Biol Phys. 2004;59(2):S21–6.
9. Abedi SM, Mardanshahi A, Shahhosseini R, Hosseinimehr SJ. Nuclear medicine for imaging of epithelial ovarian cancer. Future Oncol. 2016;12(9):1165–77.
10. Liu S, Edwards DS. 99mTc-labeled small peptides as diagnostic radiopharmaceuticals. Chem Rev. 1999;99(9):2235–68.
11. Li Z, Zhao R, Wu X, Sun Y, Yao M, Li J, et al. Identification and characterization of a novel peptide ligand of epidermal growth factor receptor for targeted delivery of therapeutics. FASEB J. 2005;19(14):1978–85.
12. Song S, Liu D, Peng J, Sun Y, Li Z, Gu J-R, et al. Peptide ligand-mediated liposome distribution and targeting to EGFR expressing tumor in vivo. Int J Pharm. 2008;363(1):155–61.
13. Master A, Malamas A, Solanki R, Clausen DM, Eiseman JL, Sen GA. A cell-targeted photodynamic nanomedicine strategy for head and neck cancers. Mol Pharm. 2013;10(5):1988–97.
14. Talekar M, Ganta S, Singh A, Amiji M, Kendall J, Denny WA, et al. Phosphatidylinositol 3-kinase inhibitor (PIK75) containing surface functionalized nanoemulsion for enhanced drug delivery, cytotoxicity and pro-apoptotic activity in ovarian cancer cells. Pharm Res. 2012;29(10):2874–86.
15. Ren H, Gao C, Zhou L, Liu M, Xie C, Lu W. EGFR-targeted poly (ethylene glycol)-distearoylphosphatidylethanolamine micelle loaded with paclitaxel for laryngeal cancer: preparation, characterization and in vitro evaluation. Drug Deliv. 2015;22(6):785–94.
16. Grünwald GK, Vetter A, Klutz K, Willhauck MJ, Schwenk N, Senekowitsch-Schmidtke R, et al. EGFR-targeted adenovirus dendrimer coating for improved systemic delivery of the theranostic NIS gene. Mol Ther Nucleic Acids. 2013;2(11):e131.
17. DeJesus OT. Synthesis of [64Cu] Cu-NOTA-Bn-GE11 for PET imaging of EGFR-rich tumors. Curr Radiopharm. 2012;5(1):15–8.
18. Dissoki S, Hagooly A, Elmachily S, Mishani E. Labeling approaches for the GE11 peptide, an epidermal growth factor receptor biomarker. J Label Compd Radiopharm. 2011;54(11):693–701.
19. Hosseinimehr SJ, Tolmachev V, Orlova A. Liver uptake of radiolabeled targeting proteins and peptides: considerations for targeting peptide conjugate design. Drug Discov Today. 2012;17(21):1224–32.
20. Alves S, Correia JD, Santos I, Veerendra B, Sieckman GL, Hoffman TJ, et al.

Pyrazolyl conjugates of bombesin: a new tridentate ligand framework for the stabilization of fac-[M (CO) 3] + moiety. Nucl Med Biol. 2006;33(5):625–34.

21. Parry JJ, Kelly TS, Andrews R, Rogers BE. In vitro and in vivo evaluation of 64Cu-labeled DOTA-linker-bombesin (7–14) analogues containing different amino acid linker moieties. Bioconjug Chem. 2007;18(4):1110–7.

22. Decristoforo C, Mather SJ. 99 m-Technetium-labelled peptide-HYNIC conjugates: effects of lipophilicity and stability on biodistribution. Nucl Med Biol. 1999;26(4):389–96.

23. von Guggenberg E, Sarg B, Lindner H, Melendez Alafort L, Mather SJ, Moncayo R, et al. Preparation via coligand exchange and characterization of [99mTc-EDDA-HYNIC-D-Phe1, Tyr3] Octreotide (99mTc–EDDA/HYNIC–TOC). J Label Compd Radiopharm. 2003;46(4):307–18.

24. Erfani M, Zarrabi Ahrabi N, Shafiei M, Shirmardi SP. A 99mTc-tricine-HYNIC-labeled peptide targeting the neurotensin receptor for single-photon imaging in malignant tumors. J Label Comp Radiopharm. 2014;57(3):125–31.

25. Wållberg H, Orlova A. Slow internalization of anti-HER2 synthetic affibody monomer 111In-DOTA-ZHER2: 342-pep2: implications for development of labeled tracers. Cancer Biother Radiopharm. 2008;23(4):435–42.

26. García-Garayoa E, Allemann-Tannahill L, Bläuenstein P, Willmann M, Carrel-Rémy N, Tourwé D, et al. In vitro and in vivo evaluation of new radiolabeled neurotensin (8–13) analogues with high affinity for NT1 receptors. Nucl Med Biol. 2001;28(1):75–84.

27. King R, Surfraz MB-U, Finucane C, Biagini SC, Blower PJ, Mather SJ. 99mTc-HYNIC-gastrin peptides: assisted coordination of 99mTc by amino acid side chains results in improved performance both in vitro and in vivo. J Nucl Med. 2009;50(4):591–8.

28. Grünwald V, Hidalgo M. The epidermal growth factor receptor: a new target for anticancer therapy. Curr Probl Cancer. 2002;26(3):114–64.

29. Liu Y, Liu G, Hnatowich DJ. A brief review of chelators for radiolabeling oligomers. Materials. 2010;3(5):3204–17.

30. Retzloff LB, Heinzke L, Figueroa SD, Sublett SV, Ma L, Sieckman GL, et al. Evaluation of [99mTc-(CO) 3-XY-bombesin (7–14) NH2] conjugates for targeting gastrin-releasing peptide receptors overexpressed on breast carcinoma. Anticancer Res. 2010;30(1):19–30.

31. Liu S, Edwards DS, Looby RJ, Harris AR, Poirier MJ, Barrett JA, et al. Labeling a hydrazino nicotinamide-modified cyclic IIb/IIIa receptor antagonist with 99mTc using aminocarboxylates as coligands. Bioconjug Chem. 1996;7(1):63–71.

32. Agnes RS, Broome A-M, Wang J, Verma A, Lavik K, Basilion JP. An optical probe for noninvasive molecular imaging of orthotopic brain tumors overexpressing epidermal growth factor receptor. Mol Cancer Ther. 2012;11(10):2202–11.

33. Colzani B, Speranza G, Dorati R, Conti B, Modena T, Bruni G, et al. Design of smart GE11-PLGA/PEG-PLGA blend nanoparticulate platforms for parenteral administration of hydrophilic macromolecular drugs: synthesis, preparation and in vitro/ex vivo characterization. Int J Pharm. 2016;511(2):1112–23.

34. S-i O, Takanashi M, Sudo K, Ueda S, Ishikawa A, Matsuyama N, et al. Systemically injected exosomes targeted to EGFR deliver antitumor microRNA to breast cancer cells. Mol Ther. 2013;21(1):185–91.

35. Bijman MN, van Berkel MP, Kok M, Janmaat ML, Boven E. Inhibition of functional HER family members increases the sensitivity to docetaxel in human ovarian cancer cell lines. Anticancer Drugs. 2009;20(6):450–60.

36. DeFazio-Eli L, Strommen K, Dao-Pick T, Parry G, Goodman L, Winslow J. Quantitative assays for the measurement of HER1-HER2 heterodimerization and phosphorylation in cell lines and breast tumors: applications for diagnostics and targeted drug mechanism of action. Breast Cancer Res. 2011;13(2):1.

37. Tai W, Mahato R, Cheng K. The role of HER2 in cancer therapy and targeted drug delivery. J Control Release. 2010;146(3):264–75.

38. Wållberg H, Orlova A, Altai M, Hosseinimehr SJ, Widström C, Malmberg J, et al. Molecular design and optimization of 99mTc-labeled recombinant affibody molecules improves their biodistribution and imaging properties. J Nucl Med. 2011;52(3):461–9.

39. Engfeldt T, Orlova A, Tran T, Bruskin A, Widström C, Karlström AE, et al. Imaging of HER2-expressing tumours using a synthetic Affibody molecule containing the 99mTc-chelating mercaptoacetyl-glycyl-glycyl-glycyl (MAG3) sequence. Eur J Nucl Med Mol Imaging. 2007;34(5):722–33.

40. Engfeldt T, Tran T, Orlova A, Widström C, Feldwisch J, Abrahmsen L, et al. 99mTc-chelator engineering to improve tumour targeting properties of a HER2-specific Affibody molecule. Eur J Nucl Med Mol Imaging. 2007;34(11):1843–53.

41. Varmira K, Hosseinimehr SJ, Noaparast Z, Abedi SM. An improved radiolabelled RNA aptamer molecule for HER2 imaging in cancers. J Drug Target. 2014;22(2):116–22.

42. Noaparast Z, Hosseinimehr SJ, Piramoon M, Abedi SM. Tumor targeting with a 99mTc-labeled AS1411 aptamer in prostate tumor cells. J Drug Target. 2015;23(6):497–505.

43. Varmira K, Hosseinimehr SJ, Noaparast Z, Abedi SM. A HER2-targeted RNA aptamer molecule labeled with 99 m Tc for single-photon imaging in malignant tumors. Nucl Med Biol. 2013;40(8):980–6.

44. Garmestani K, Milenic DE, Plascjak PS, Brechbiel MW. A new and convenient method for purification of 86 Y using a Sr (II) selective resin and comparison of biodistribution of 86 Y and 111 In labeled Herceptin™. Nucl Med Biol. 2002;29(5):599–606.

45. Tang Y, Wang J, Scollard DA, Mondal H, Holloway C, Kahn HJ, et al. Imaging of HER2/neu-positive BT-474 human breast cancer xenografts in athymic mice using 111 In-trastuzumab (Herceptin) Fab fragments. Nucl Med Biol. 2005;32(1):51–8.

46. Milane L, Duan Z, Amiji M. Development of EGFR-targeted polymer blend nanocarriers for combination paclitaxel/lonidamine delivery to treat multi-drug resistance in human breast and ovarian tumor cells. Mol Pharm. 2010;8(1):185–203.

47. Prasanphanich AF, Lane SR, Figueroa SD, Ma L, Rold TL, Sieckman GL, et al. The effects of linking substituents on the in vivo behavior of site-directed, peptide-based, diagnostic radiopharmaceuticals. In Vivo. 2007;21(1):1–16.

Fabrication and biological evaluation of chitosan coated hyaluronic acid-docetaxel conjugate nanoparticles in CD44$^+$ cancer cells

Nazanin Shabani Ravari[1], Navid Goodarzi[1*], Farhad Alvandifar[2], Mohsen Amini[3], Effat Souri[3], Mohammad Reza Khoshayand[4], Zahra Hadavand Mirzaie[2], Fatemeh Atyabi[1,2] and Rassoul Dinarvand[1,2]

Abstract

Background: Hyaluronic acid (HA) has been used for target-specific drug delivery because of strong affinity to CD44, a marker in which overexpressed in cancer cells and cancer stem cells. Conjugation of HA to the cytotoxic agents via active targeting can improve efficacy, biodistribution, and water solubility. To be able to benefit from passive targeting as well, a nanoparticulate system by counter ion using a polycation like chitosan may lead to a perfect delivery system.

Methods: Water soluble Hyaluronic acid-Docetaxel (HA-DTX) conjugate was prepared and used to formulate chitosan-coated HA-DTX nanoparticles by polyelectrolyte complex (PEC) method and optimized using Box-Behnken design. Biological evaluation of nanoparticles was done in CD44+ cancer cells.

Results and discussion: Biological evaluation of optimized formula showed IC50 of nanoparticles for 4 T1 and MCF-7 cell lines were 45.34 μM and 354.25 μM against 233.8 μM and 625.9 μM for DTX, respectively with increased cellular uptake showed by inverted confocal microscope.

Conclusion: Chitosan-coated HA-DTX nanoparticles were more effective against CD44+ cells than free DTX.

Keywords: Glyconanoparticles, Nanomedicine, Polyelectrolye Complex, Macromolecular Drug Delivery, Polysaccharides

Background

Most of the anticancer drug products have systemic toxicity because of the wide uncontrolled distribution in the body. Besides, their lack of tumor localization and short half-lives are considerable obstacle facing effective cancer chemotherapy. Development of nanoparticulate drug delivery systems and polymer-drug conjugates of low molecular weight cytotoxic drug molecules to macromolecular carriers are effective ways to address these problems by enhanced permeation and retention (EPR) effect [1, 2]. In addition, conjugation of cytotoxic drugs to hydrophilic macromolecules can increase the water solubility of insoluble drugs

such as docetaxel (DTX) and will enhance their biodistribution and therapeutic efficacy [3, 4].

DTX is an anticancer agent belongs to the Taxanes family and is a semi-synthetic derivative from the *Taxus brevifolia* [5] DTX shows its cytotoxic effect by inhibiting the depolymerization of microtubules and M-phase cell arrest [6]. The conventional formulations of DTX in drug market suffering from low solubility of the active pharmaceutical ingredient which has been resolved using tween 80 as surfactant. This issue led to some complications in the clinic to control formulation-related adverse drug reactions [7]. Due to the importance of this drug molecule in chemotherapy protocols, a lot of efforts dedicated to address novel formulations of DTX. In one of these approaches water-soluble macromolecular drug conjugates has been proposed to prepare tween-free

* Correspondence: goodarzi_n@razi.tums.ac.ir
[1]Nanotechnology Research Centre, Faculty of Pharmacy, Tehran University of Medical Sciences, Tehran 1417614411, Iran
Full list of author information is available at the end of the article

formulations along with targeted drug delivery such as hyaluronic acid-docetaxel (HA-DTX) conjugates. In our previous report [4], although prepared conjugate had better solubility profile but the efficacy did not benefit from its polysaccharide CD44-targeting properties and heparine like effects of hyaluronic acid in blood circulation. Therefore this report is an attempt to add passive targeting enhanced permeation and retention of nanoparticulate system while keeping hyaluronate moiety. For this purpose, the water soluble conjugate became coated with chitosan by polyelectrolyte complex (PEC) method to prepare a nanoparticulate drug delivery system to improve pharmacokinetic features and efficacy.

For this purpose, hyaluronic acid (HA) as one of the common polysaccharides carriers has been used for conjugation of low molecular weight cytotoxic drugs such as DTX. HA is biocompatible, biodegradable and non-immunogenic [8]. The most considerable advantage of HA is its strong affinity for CD44, a cell surface protein which is overexpressed in many cancer cells and cancer stem cells [9, 10]. CD44 is a specific biological receptor for HA [11, 12]. HA could have an enhanced attachment and uptake into malignant cells with metastatic activities [13] and has been used for target-specific drug delivery [14, 15]. We hypothesized using HA as carrier and targeting moiety simultaneously may reverse the multiple drug resistance of cancer stem cells via affecting CD44 and regarding physical correlation of P-gp and these markers [16]. In this regard, HA-DTX conjugates has been prepared and evaluated which showed suitable efficacy and safety profile. This research reports optimized polyelectrolyte complex nanoparticles using HA-DTX as cationic part.

Polyelectrolyte complexes which were prepared by electrostatic interaction between unlike charged polyions have received substantial attention in drug delivery systems. The synthesis of PEC nanoparticles is simple and can be easily carried out under mild conditions without using toxic organic solvents or chemical cross-linkers [17]. In the present study, chitosan as a N-deacetylated derivative of chitin has been used extensively as a biocompatible polysaccharide [18] with a cationic nature that can be protonated in weak acidic environment [19], and therefore it can improve the bioavailability of DTX [20].

Achieving optimization of the nanoparticle preparation could be performed by classical method of changing one variable at a time while others have been remained constant. However this method needs lots of series of experiments and time. Moreover in this approach the possible interaction between independent factors will not be observed. Therefore, the fine optimized formulation will not be achieved.

Design-of-experiment (DoE) method has been used in pharmaceutical studies to solve this problem. Optimization by response surface methodology including Box-Behnken method is considered as the major application of DoE [21, 22].

In the present study, the water soluble conjugated HA-DTX was synthesized. Then, chitosan coated HA-DTX nanoparticles were prepared by PEC method considering the anionic structure of HA-DTX and cationic chitosan. Box-Behnken statistical design using a response surface methodology has been employed to obtain the optimized condition in terms of particle size, size distribution, drug loading and zeta potential. For determination of efficacy of optimized chitosan coated HA-DTX conjugate nanoparticles, 3-(4,5-dimethylthiazol-2-yl)-2,5-diphenyltetrazolium bromide (MTT) assay was performed on MCF-7, human cancer cell line, and 4 T1 mouse breast cancer cell line. MCF-7 and 4 T1 cell lines were also used for cell uptake study.

Materials and methods
Materials
Sodium hyaluronate (MW 25 kDa) was purchased from GuangLong (Shandong, China). Anhydrous DTX was purchased from Jiangsu Yew (Jiangsu, China). Chitosan (MW 50 kDa, (Primex, Karmoy, Norway), 1-Ethyl–3-[3-(dimethylamino)-propyl] carbodiimide (EDC), N-hydroxy succinimide (NHS), 4′,6-diamidino-2-phenylindole (DAPI) and triethylamine were purchased from Sigma Aldrich (Seelze, Germany). MTT dye was from Merck (Darmstadt, Germany). Dulbecco's Modified Eagle Medium (DMEM) with high glucose, RPMI 1640, FBS (Fetal Bovine Serum), trypsin, penicillin and streptomycin were purchased from Biosera (Vienna, Austria). Ultra-purified water was used throughout the analysis and all other chemicals were of analytical grade. 4 T1 and MCF-7 cell lines were obtained from National Cell Bank of Iran (Pasteur Institute of Iran, Tehran, Iran).

Methods
Synthesis of hyaluronic acid-docetaxel (HA-DTX) conjugates
At first for preparing desalted HA, HA (MW 25 kDa) (1 g) was dissolved in 100 mL of deionized water, then the solution was dialyzed (MWCO 12 kDa) in deionized water for 24 h and lyophilized [23].

Desalted-HA (400 mg) was dissolved in 80 mL of deionized water. Then EDC and NHS were added to the solution in 11 and 10 molar ratios of carboxyl groups of HA, respectively. The mixture was stirred at 40 °C for 3 h. Then 80 mL dimethylformamide (DMF) containing 400 mg of DTX and 20 mL of triethylamine were added. After 24 h the mixture was refluxed at 70 °C and after cooling to room temperature was transferred to pretreat dialysis tubing (MWCO 3500 kDa). The mixture was purified by dialysis against water-acetone solution (50:50, v/v) for 1 h, water-acetone (75:25, v/v) for 1 h and water for 1 h, respectively. The obtained HA-DTX conjugate is water soluble. To eliminate the remained DTX, the mixture was transferred to a separating funnel and extracted three times with dichloromethane. The aqueous phase was lyophilized. Chemical integrity of the resulted product was checked by ^{1}H-NMR (Bruker AC 500 Spectrophotometer, Germany) and fourier transform infra-red (FTIR) spectroscopy (Nicolet Magna-FTIR 550 Spectrometer, WI, USA). The concentration of DTX was measured by UV Spectrophotometry (UV-visible Spectrophotometer, 160A, SHIMADZU, Japan) at 229 nm versus a suitable blank solution containing the appropriate concentration of HA.

Preparation of chitosan coated HA-DTX conjugate nanoparticle

Chitosan coated HA-DTX conjugate nanoparticles were prepared by PEC method, considering the anionic structure of HA-DTX conjugates and cationic chitosan [24]. As a representative example, 1 mL of aqueous solution of HA-DTX (4.25 mg/mL) was added slowly to 1 mL of dilute chitosan solution (0.250 mg/mL of 1 % acetic acid) in 1 min while stirring at 370 rpm at room temperature. It should be mentioned that during the screening and optimization procedure, various factors including ratios of HA-DTX conjugate to chitosan, stirring rate and temperature were evaluated.

DTX determination in the conjugates and nanoparticles

The concentration of DTX in conjugate was measured by UV spectrophotometry. Determination of DTX in prepared nanoparticles was performed by UV absorbance at 229 nm to determine drug loading and entrapment efficiency. The final solution of chitosan coated HA-DTX nanoparticles were transferred to microtubes and centrifuged by an ultracentrifuge (Optima MAX-XP Ultracentrifuge, Beckman Coulter, USA) at 22000 rpm (150700 g) for 20 min at 10 °C. After collecting the supernatant, the free remaining non-conjugated DTX in the reaction medium was measured by UV spectrophotometry. The encapsulated efficiency and DTX loading in nanoparticles were calculated, applying the following equations:

Fourier transform infra-red spectroscopy of conjugates

Freeze-dried conjugated HA-DTX, HA, DTX were analyzed by FTIR Spectrometer. The data was achieved in the range of 400–4000 cm^{-1} for each sample. The FTIR spectra of conjugated HA-DTX were compared with pure substances.

Experimental design studies

Box-Behnken statistical design which is a response surface methodology has been employed in the present study. In this study the effect of three quantitative independent variables consisting of stirring rate (rpm), ratio of HA-DTX conjugate to chitosan and temperature (°C) were investigated on dependent variables and responses, including particle size (nm), zeta potential (mv), polydispersity index (PdI) and DTX loading in nanoparticles with Design Expert software (V. 7.0.0, Stat-Ease Inc., Minneapolis, USA). Dependent and independent variables were elucidated based on the preliminary studies which are shown in Table 1.

The aim of the design was to achieve to the optimum formulation, with both minimum size and maximum loading. The PdI factor should be at possible lowest level and zeta potential should be appropriate to have stable nanoparticles. Obtained responses from three optimized formulations were compared with the suggested experimental responses to evaluate the precision of model.

Characterization of the nanoparticles

The size and zeta potential of the nanoparticles were determined using a Zetasizer Nano ZS Analyzer (Malvern Instruments, UK) with a He-Ne laser beam at wavelength of 633 nm at 25 °C.

Surface morphology of the nanoparticles observed using Scanning Electron Microscopy (SEM) (Philips Xl30, The Netherlands) and Atomic Force Microscopy (AFM) (dualscope™ DS 95-200/50, Denmark) microscopy. For AFM evaluation, one drop of nanoparticle suspension was dried on the surface of clean silicon wafer at room temperature. AFM study was performed with 20 μm scanner in tapping mode. For SEM imaging, dried nanoparticles were gently coated by gold layer with a sputter coater and evaluated at 30 kV using a 6300 field emission scanning electron microscope.

Differential scanning calorimetry (DSC) was performed using Mettler-Toledo DSC822^e (Greifensec, Switzerland) and data acquisition and analysis was carried out by a software package of STAR^e 9.01. The

$$Entrapment\ efficiency\ (\%) = \frac{Total\ amount\ of\ DTX - Amount\ of\ DTX\ in\ supernatant}{Total\ amount\ of DTX} \times 100$$

$$Drug\ loading\ (\%) = \frac{Weight\ of\ drug\ found\ loaded}{Weight\ of\ nanoparticle} \times 100$$

Table 1 Variables used in Box-Behnken experimental design

Independent factors	Factor level			Dependent factors
Numeric Factors	−1	0	1	Particle size (nm)
Stirring rate (rpm)	300	800	1300	Zeta potential (mv)
Ratio of HA-DTX conjugate to chitosan	13	17	21	Polydispersity index (Pdl)
Temperature (°C)	0	25	50	Drug content or DTX loading (%)

system was conducted by using 8 mg of sample, deposited in 40 μL aluminum pans and hermetically sealed, under a nitrogen gas dynamic flow at a scanning heating rate of 10 °C/min over a range of 20 °C to 300 °C. Empty hermetically sealed aluminum pan was used as a control.

Cytotoxicity evaluation of nanoparticles

For cytotoxicity study of nanoparticles, MTT assay was performed on MCF-7, human breast cancer cell line, and 4 T1 mouse breast cancer cell line [25]. Cell culture medium was DMEM with 10 % FBS and 5 % penicillin-streptomycin. Cells maintained at 37 °C and humidified environment with 5 % CO_2. Cells were seeded into 96-well plate separately at a seeding density of 5000 cell/well. After 24 h incubation, various concentrations of free DTX and nanoparticles (0.1, 10, 100, 500, 1000, and 1500 μM) (based on DTX equivalent concentration) were used as treatments and incubated for 48 h. Then 50 μL MTT (1 mg/mL) solution in PBS was added to each well and incubated for 4 h. Formazan precipitates dissolved by 150 μM dimethyl sulfoxide (DMSO). The absorption was measured at 570 nm and reference well at 620 nm by ELISA reader [26]. Cell viability was calculated by the following equation where OD is optical density:

$$\text{Cell viability\%} = (OD_{\text{test well}} / OD_{\text{reference well}}) \times 100$$

Preparation of fluorescent-labeled HA

To prepare fluorescent-labeled HA conjugate, HA was labeled with fluorescamine. One hundred mg of HA was dissolved in 10 mL water and 61.5 mg of EDC and 45.5 mg of NHS were added. The mixture was stirred for 3 h and then 45.84 mg fluorescamine was added and stirred for 24 h. The reaction flask was protected from light by covering with an aluminum foil. After 24 h the mixture was purified by dialysis (MWCO 3500) against deionized water and finally the product was freeze-dried. Fluorescent-labeled nanoparticles were also prepared by fluorescent-labeled HA conjugate instead of HA-DTX conjugate and the nanoparticle preparation method was the same as the optimized method used for normal nanoparticles.

Cell uptake studies

In order to study the cellular uptake of the nanoparticles, 4 T1 and MCF-7 cell lines were seeded at 1×10^5 cell/well in a cover glass and incubated at 37 °C with 5 % CO_2 atmosphere for 24 h. After complete adhesion, the medium was carefully removed and replaced with fresh medium containing fluorescent-labeled nanoparticles and incubated for 2 h. In this stage, the medium containing drug was removed and cells were washed 4 times with PBS and fixed with formaldehyde 4 % for 4 min. Nuclear coloring was performed with DAPI (0.5 mg/mL) in 5 min and then cells were washed 4 times with PBS using inverted confocal microscope (Nikon ECLIPSE Ti, Tokyo, Japan) cell images were taken [27].

Statistical analysis

SPSS 20.0 statistical software and one-way analysis of variance (ANOVA) were used to assess the data groups. All the results were evaluated as mean ± standard deviation (SD). Significance difference of $p < 0.05$ was accepted.

Results and discussion
Synthesis and characterization of water-soluble HA-DTX direct conjugate

Indirect HA-DTX conjugate was synthetized previously in our group. Conjugation of DTX in these studies needs preparation of succinyl DTX [4, 28]. The direct formation of conjugated HA-DTX has been reported for the first time with fewer procedure steps (Fig. 1). An esteric bound formed between 2′-OH of DTX and COOH of HA [29]. Formation of conjugated HA-DTX was confirmed by the presence of aromatic protons in ^{1}H-NMR spectra (Fig. 2). FTIR of freeze-dried HA-DTX conjugate, pure HA, pure DTX were also obtained (Fig. 3). DTX had a specific peak in 1242 cm^{-1} which had no interaction with HA specific peak. This peak has been repeated in HA-DTX conjugate spectrum with a little shift to 1249 cm^{-1}. Presence of this peak and HA related peaks in conjugate spectrum confirms the formation of HA-DTX conjugate.

The absorption of DTX in conjugate was measured by UV spectroscopy. According to UV absorption, it was shown that 1 mg of HA-DTX conjugate contains 69 μg of DTX.

Preparation of chitosan coated HA-DTX conjugate nanoparticle

Publications reported several nanoparticular based methods to improve DTX drug delivery to cancer cells (DTX loaded chitosan nanoparticle [30], targeted DTX nanoparticles with different targeting agents like folic acid [2] and albumin nanoparticles of DTX [28]). HA

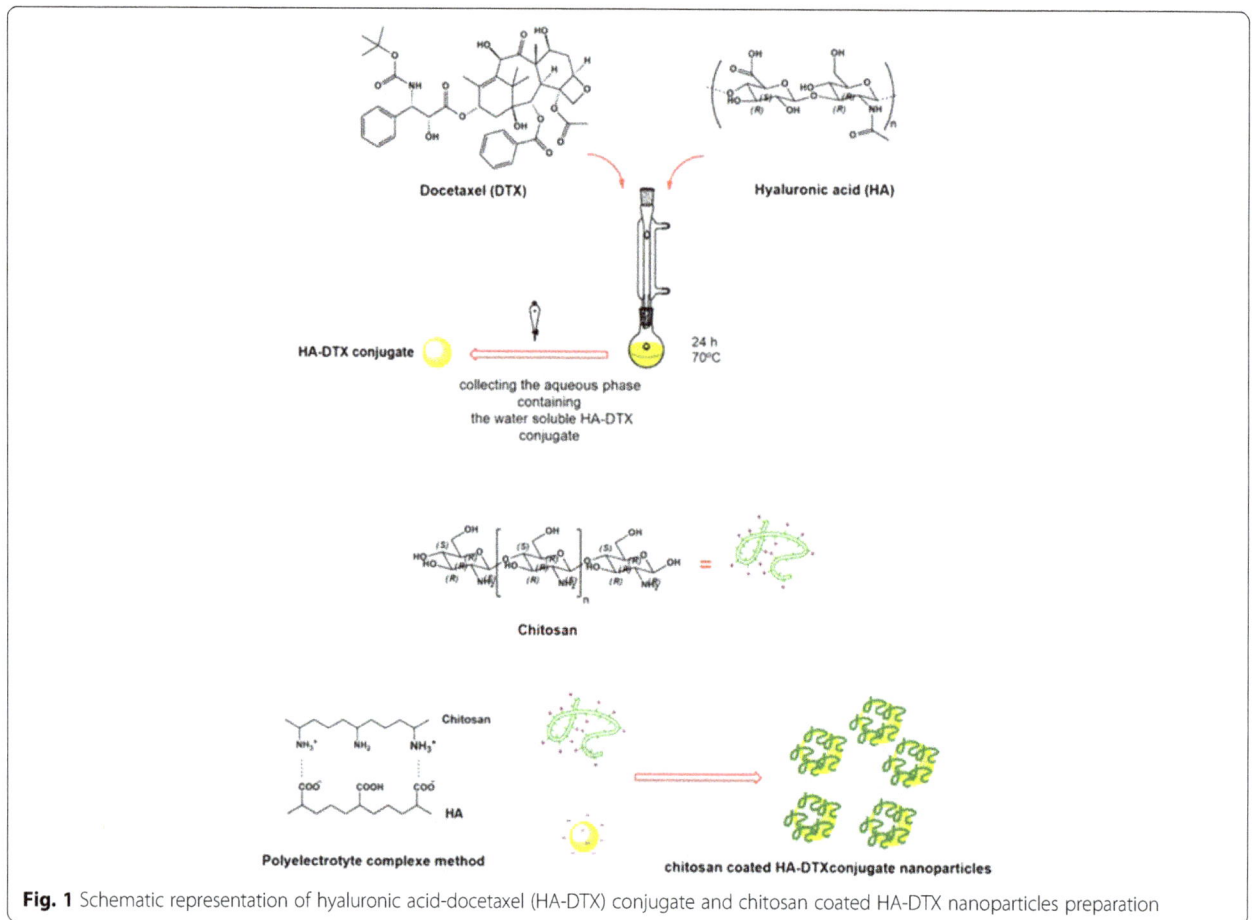

Fig. 1 Schematic representation of hyaluronic acid-docetaxel (HA-DTX) conjugate and chitosan coated HA-DTX nanoparticles preparation

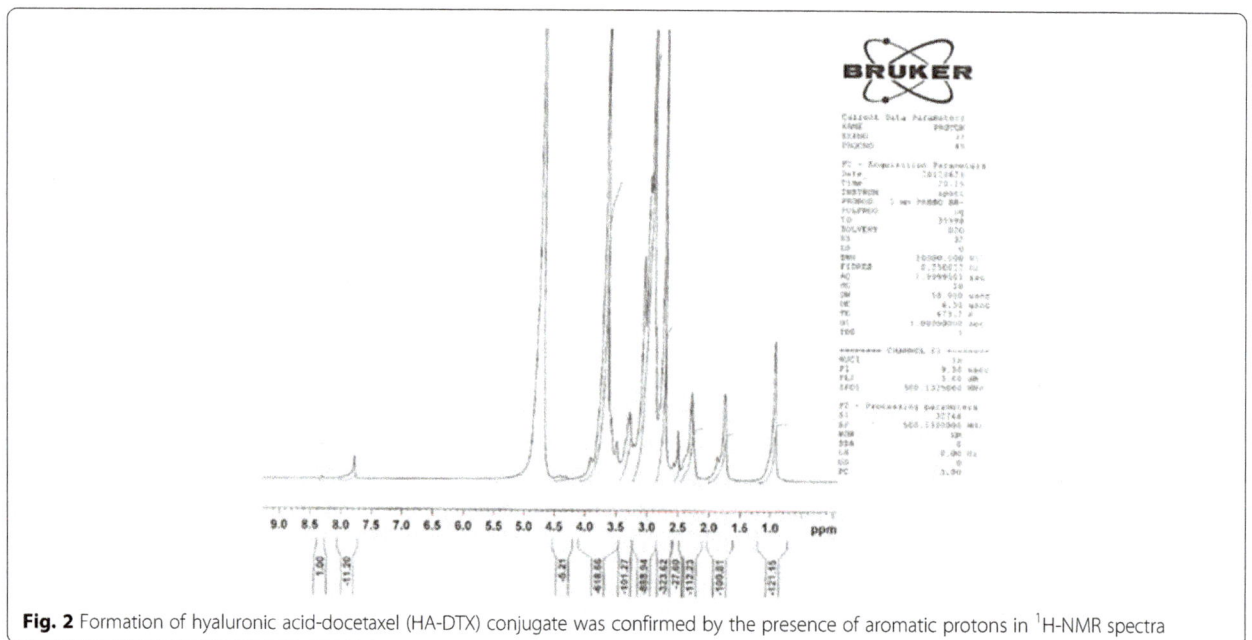

Fig. 2 Formation of hyaluronic acid-docetaxel (HA-DTX) conjugate was confirmed by the presence of aromatic protons in ^{1}H-NMR spectra

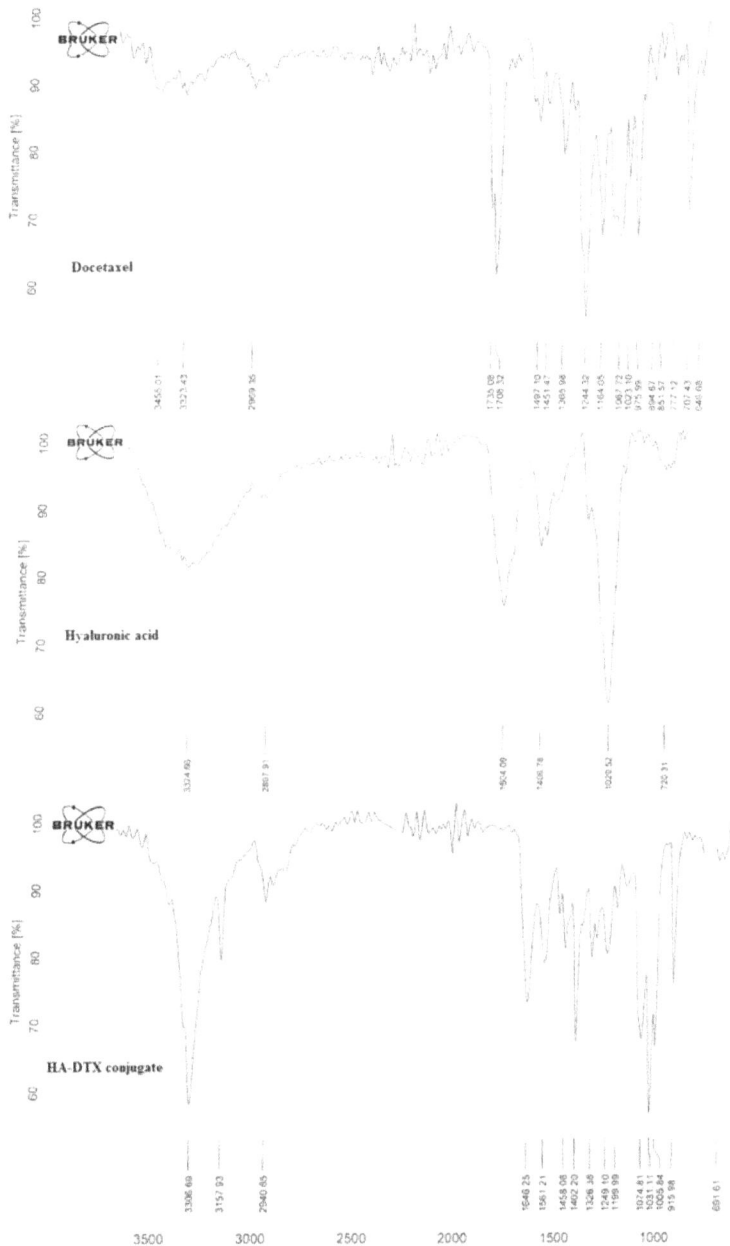

Fig. 3 FTIR spectrum of (**a**) docetaxel (DTX); **b** hyaluronic acid (HA); **c** hyaluronic acid-docetaxel (HA-DTX) conjugate

could cause heparin-induced thrombocytopenia because of its nature as a polysaccharide [31]. This event should be considered if the HA-DTX used alone. Coating the HA-DTX conjugate with chitosan may limit the exposure of HA with platelet in blood circulation and reduce thrombocytopenia. Chitosan-coated HA-DTX conjugate nanoparticles were prepared based on these findings.

Optimization studies

To obtain an optimized formulation of HA-DTX nanoparticles, Box-Behnken statistical design was used. Table 2 shows 17 runs based on Box-Behnken design to analyze

the effects of independent variables on dependent variables and the data achieved to find out optimized formulation.

As a result, 17 runs were needed to achieve the optimized formulation and the second-order polynomial functions explained the relationship between the dependent and the independent variable as following equation:

$$Y_{1,2,3} = b_0 + b_1 A + b_2 B + b_3 C + b_{11} A^2 + b_{22} B^2 + B_{33} C^2 + b_{12} AB + b_{13} AC + b_{23} BC$$

Table 2 The effect of independent variables on dependent variables

Run	Independent variables			Dependent variables			
	Stirring rate (rpm)	Ratio of HA-DTX conjugate to chitosan	Temperature (°C)	Particle size (nm)	Zeta potential (mv)	Polydispersity index (PdI)	DTX loading (%)
1	300.00	13.00	25.00	195	21.7	0.128	3.043
2	300.00	21.00	25.00	444	18.6	0.065	3.257
3	1300.00	13.00	25.00	176	22.3	0.129	3.034
4	1300.00	21.00	25.00	269	17.4	0.030	3.235
5	800.00	13.00	0.00	174	22.3	0.120	3.042
6	800.00	21.00	0.00	280	18.0	0.019	3.235
7	800.00	13.00	50.00	182	21.9	0.086	3.048
8	800.00	21.00	50.00	246	19.2	0.019	3.233
9	300.00	17.00	0.00	210	21.3	0.083	3.159
10	1300.00	17.00	0.00	199	19.6	0.033	3.161
11	300.00	17.00	50.00	210	21.3	0.031	3.157
12	1300.00	17.00	50.00	194	24.1	0.070	3.160
13	800.00	17.00	25.00	195	21.3	0.061	3.160
14	800.00	17.00	25.00	191	21.6	0.039	3.160
15	800.00	17.00	25.00	179	22.7	0.064	3.159
16	800.00	17.00	25.00	193	21.1	0.045	3.159
17	800.00	17.00	25.00	197	21.3	0.067	3.159

which A, B and C are independent variables, and Y is the predicted dependent factor, b_0 is the intercept, b_1, b_2, and b_3 are linear coefficients, b_{11}, b_{22}, and b_{33} are squared coefficients, and b_{12}, b_{13}, and b_{23} are the interaction coefficients of equation.

Size of nanoparticles

Size is the most important parameter in determining the nanoparticles cellular uptake. Nanoparticles were optimized to achieve minimum size while the PdI kept at minimum and loading maximum. As seen in Fig. 4a in the middle range of stirring rate, size of nanoparticles would be reduced. Higher stirring rate could generate bubble and solution splashing so it could not prepare suitable particles. It seems stirring rate at lower limit do not supply enough energy to product small particles, so enlargement has seen in this rate. Figure 4b represents that by increasing the ratio of HA-DTX to chitosan, the size of nanoparticles would be increased. Temperature had minor effect on the size of nanoparticles.

$$\text{Particle size} = 191 + 64A\text{-}27.63B\text{-}3.87C + 48.62A^2 + 31.38B^2\text{-}19.13C^2$$

Polydispersity index

Polydispersity index represents the homogeneity of nanoparticles and changs between of 0 to 1 with a desire to be

near 0. The less PdI value indicates the more size uniformity in nanoparticle. As shown in Fig. 4c by increasing the temperature, PdI reduced and it would be at minimum of 50 °C. On the other hand, lower PdI is observed in the middle range of stirrer rate. Figure 4d represents that by increasing the ratio of HA-DTX to chitosan, PdI would be decreased.

$$\text{PdI} = 0.055\text{-}0.041A\text{-}0.00563B\text{-}0.00613C + 0.022BC + 0.02A^2 + 0.013B^2\text{-}0.014C^2$$

Drug content

Higher amount of drug content is desired and represented an acceptable formulation strategy. HA-DTX to chitosan ratio was the most important factor in drug content. By increasing the ratio of HA-DTX to chitosan, higher drug content would be obtained.

$$\text{Drug content} = 3.16 + 0.099A + 0.000125C\text{-}0.018A^2\text{-}0.00138C^2$$

Confirmation of designed optimized experiments

After analyzing data and 3D diagrams by utilizing Box-Behnken method, an optimized formulation achieved which the independent variables were 18.5 for ratio of HA-DTX to chitosan, 723 rpm for stir rate and 50 °C for temperature. It also predicted the amount of

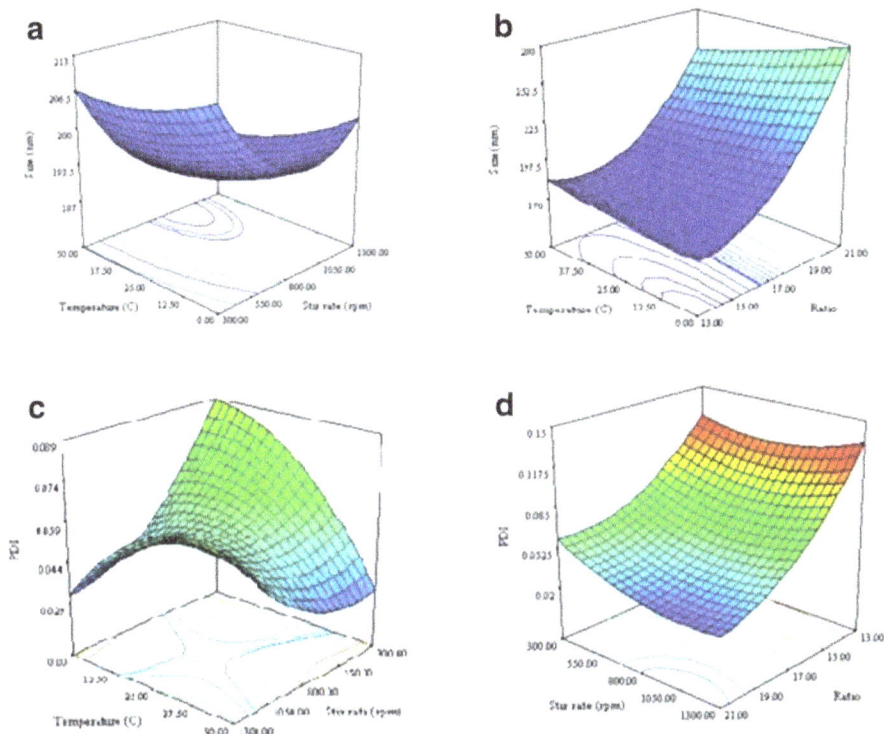

Fig. 4 Response surface plots showing the effect of different independent factors on (**a**) (**b**) size of nanoparticles; **c, d** polydispersity index

dependent factors would be 205 nm for size of nano-particles, 0.02 for PdI and 3.19 % for DTX content and +21.5 mV for zeta potential. Analysis of variance (ANOVA) and lack of fit parameters for the responses according to quadratic model is provided in Table 3.

Three experiments were performed in the lab ac-cording to the optimized formulation and there was no significant difference between the obtained and predicted results. The mean amount obtained in these experiments was 234 nm for size of nanoparticles, 0.088 for PdI and 3.18 % for DTX content and +20.03 mV for zeta potential. The mean entrapment efficiency for these experiments was 62.78 %. The

entrapment efficiency showed that nanoparticles could be an effective carrier for DTX.

Characterization of nanoparticles
Particle size,distribution and zeta potential
Particle size and size distribution of nanoparticles were measured by dynamic light scattering (DLS). The mean obtained size and PdI of the optimized chitosan coated HA-DTX conjugate nanoparticles were 234 nm and 0.088 respectively (Fig. 5a). Zeta potential of optimized nanoparticles was +20.03 mV which showed complete chitosan coating (Fig. 5b). This amount of zeta potential could provide the appropriate repulsive force to prevent

Table 3 Analysis of variance (ANOVA) and lack of fit parameters for the responses according to quadratic model

Parameters	Source	Sum of squares	Degrees of freedom (df)	Mean squares	F value	P-value
Particle Size	Quadratic vs 2FI	15730.13	3	5243.38	4.93	0.0378
Zeta Potential	Quadratic vs 2FI	8.71	3	2.9	5.3	0.0321
PdI	Quadratic vs 2FI	3.11E-03	3	1.04E-03	9.9	0.0065
Drug Loading	Quadratic vs 2FI	1.46E-03	3	4.86E-04	9.99	0.0063
Lack of Fit						
Particle Size	Quadratic	7239.25	3	2413.08	48.26	0.0013
Zeta Potential	Quadratic	2.2	3	0.73	1.79	0.2889
PdI	Quadratic	1.16E-04	3	3.86E-05	0.25	0.8579
Drug Loading	Quadratic	3.39E-04	3	1.13E-04	376.94	0.0001

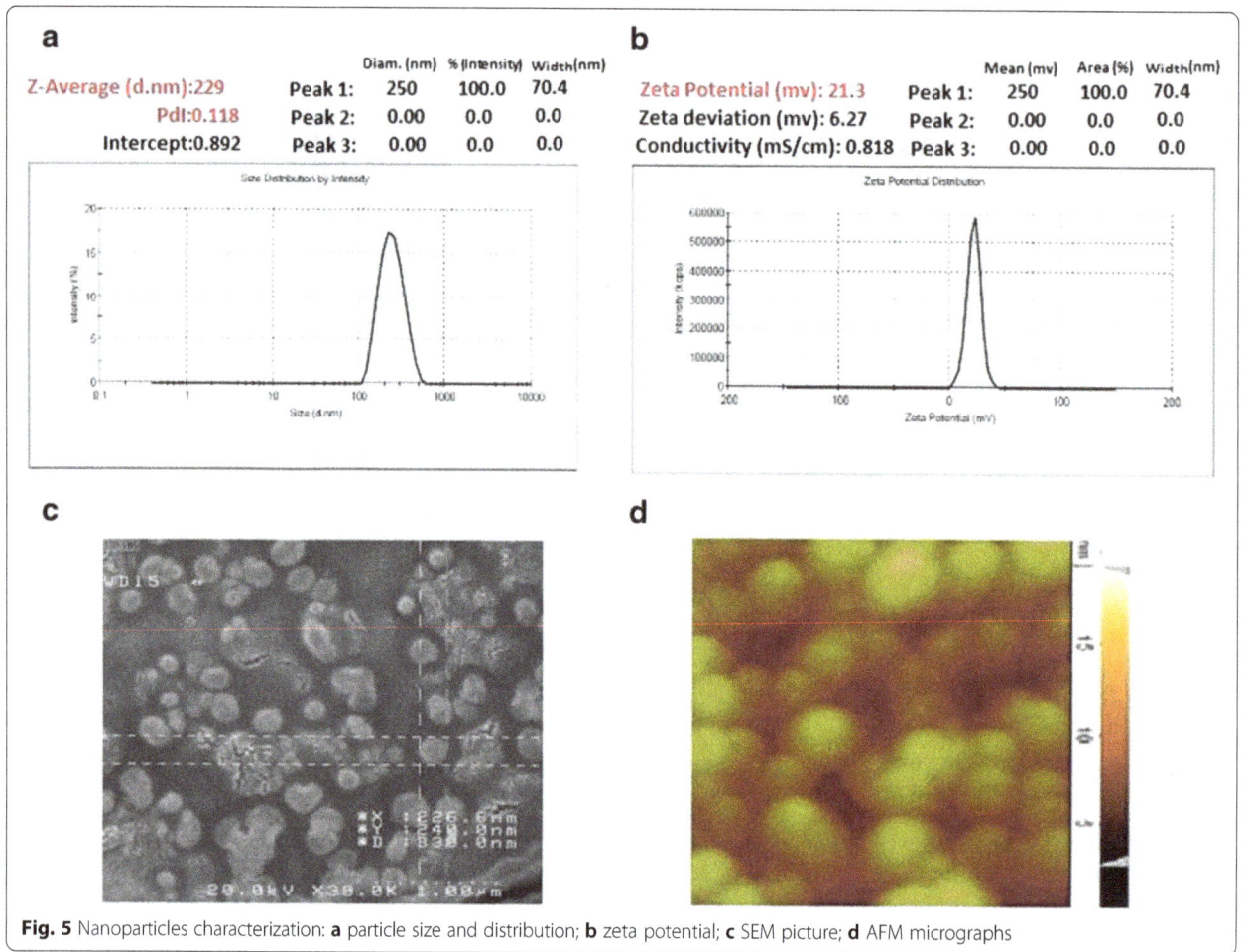

Fig. 5 Nanoparticles characterization: **a** particle size and distribution; **b** zeta potential; **c** SEM picture; **d** AFM micrographs

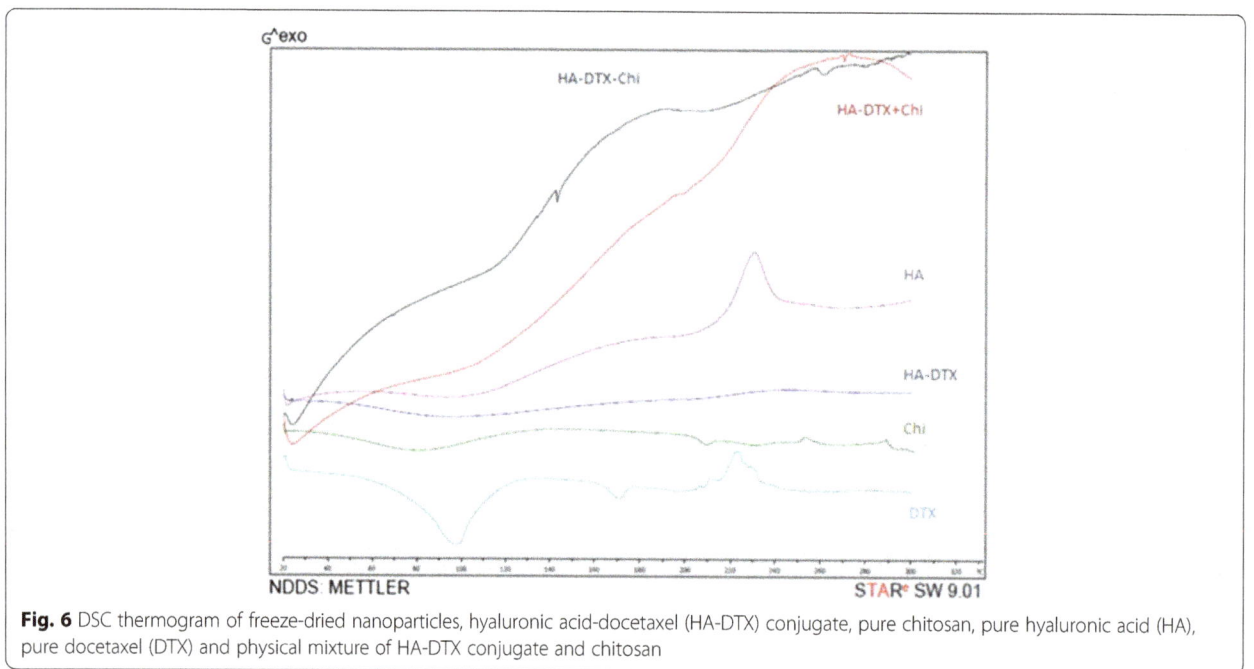

Fig. 6 DSC thermogram of freeze-dried nanoparticles, hyaluronic acid-docetaxel (HA-DTX) conjugate, pure chitosan, pure hyaluronic acid (HA), pure docetaxel (DTX) and physical mixture of HA-DTX conjugate and chitosan

nanoparticle aggregation and improv the stability of formulation.

Differential scanning calorimetry

Freeze-dried nanoparticles, conjugated HA-DTX, chitosan, HA, DTX and physical mixture of HA-DTX conjugate and chitosan was analyzed during predetermined increasing temperature rate to obtain DSC thermogram.

The DSC thermograms of DTX exhibit an endothermic peak showed melting around 170 °C. HA exhibited one exothermic peak presenting crystallization around 230 °C. Characteristic peaks of DTX and HA were not exist in the thermograms of conjugated HA-DTX. These findings confirm the development of HA-DTX conjugate (Fig. 6) [32].

DSC thermogram specificities of HA has an influence on DSC thermogram of physical mixture of HA-DTX

conjugate and chitosan. Because of the ionic charge of the chitosan (cationic) and HA (anionic), these two compounds can form a charge-transfer bond (the same as PEC formation) which may attenuate the difference in comparing these physical mixture and polyelectrolyte complex. So, DSC thermogram of nanoparticles may not express this influence. These results revealed that chitosan coated nanoparticles protected conjugated HA-DTX and weakened the effect of temperature, which showed the formation of chitosan coated HA-DTX nanoparticles.

Nanoparticle morphology

Chitosan coated HA-DTX nanoparticles were morphologically studied by SEM and AFM. SEM showed (Fig. 5c) that nanoparticles are uniform spheres and

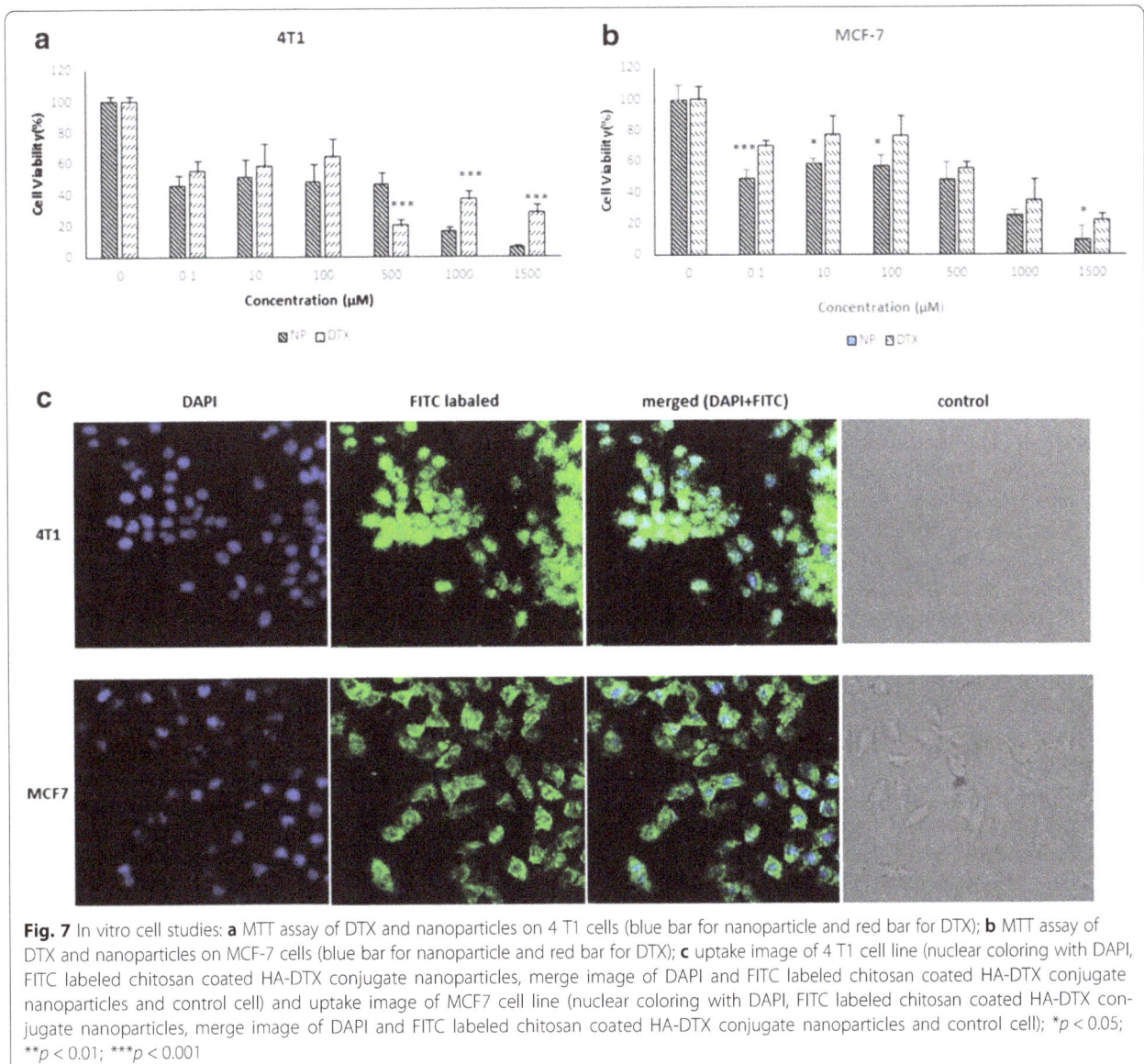

Fig. 7 In vitro cell studies: **a** MTT assay of DTX and nanoparticles on 4 T1 cells (blue bar for nanoparticle and red bar for DTX); **b** MTT assay of DTX and nanoparticles on MCF-7 cells (blue bar for nanoparticle and red bar for DTX); **c** uptake image of 4 T1 cell line (nuclear coloring with DAPI, FITC labeled chitosan coated HA-DTX conjugate nanoparticles, merge image of DAPI and FITC labeled chitosan coated HA-DTX conjugate nanoparticles and control cell) and uptake image of MCF7 cell line (nuclear coloring with DAPI, FITC labeled chitosan coated HA-DTX conjugate nanoparticles, merge image of DAPI and FITC labeled chitosan coated HA-DTX conjugate nanoparticles and control cell); $^*p < 0.05$; $^{**}p < 0.01$; $^{***}p < 0.001$

non-aggregated. AFM micrographs (Fig. 5d) confirmed the spherical shape of nanoparticles too.

In vitro cytotoxicity

The cytotoxicity of chitosan coated HA-DTX nanoparticles and DTX were assessed by MTT assay on 4 T1 and MCF-7 cell lines. By increasing the amount of nanoparticles or free DTX the cytotoxicity increased. The calculated IC50 of chitosan coated HA-DTX conjugate nanoparticles for 4 T1 and MCF-7 cell lines were 45.34 μM and 354.25 μM respectively while 233.8 μM and 625.9 μM for DTX on 4 T1 and MCF-7 cell lines after 48 h incubation. DTX loaded chitosan nanoparticles were more effective against cancer cells than free DTX drug [30]. Being agree to this result in our study cell viability (%) and IC50 of optimized nanoparticles were less than free drug. It may be because of higher DTX concentration which was available in intracellular space. Small size of nanoparticle as a passive targeting, effect of HA and the adhesive effect of chitosan coat may cause this availability. Therefore, nanoparticles were more potent than free DTX in cytotoxic effect on 4 T1 and MCF-7 cells (Figures 7a, b).

Cell uptake studies

Entrance of nanoparticles in cancer cells had a direct relation with their observed cytotoxic effect. Free DTX molecules could be transported out by P-glycoprotein (P-gp) pumps, but drug loaded nanoparticles were taken up by cells through an endocytosis pathway. The result represented higher cellular uptake of nanoparticles because of their ability to escape from the effect of P-gp pumps [33]. The uptake of optimized FITC-labeled chitosan-coated HA-DTX conjugate nanoparticles by 4 T1 and MCF-7 after 24 h incubation is shown in Fig. 7c. No treatment cells of each cell line are presented in Fig. 7c as a control. Based on fluorescence intensity, FITC-labeled chitosan-coated HA-DTX nanoparticles showed appropriate entrance into 4 T1 and MCF-7 cells. As a result it can be proposed that developed nanoparticles could bring loaded drug molecules effectively to cell cytoplasm as a novel drug delivery system.

Conclusion

Water soluble HA-DTX conjugate was prepared according to HA strong affinity for CD44, a cell surface protein which is overexpressed in many cancer cells and cancer stem cells. Chitosan-coated HA-DTX nanoparticles by polyelectrolyte complex method improved DTX availability. The fine optimized formulation was achieved with proper particle size, PdI, zeta potential and drug loading. The biological evaluation of nanoparticles showed they were more potent than free DTX in cytotoxic effect on MCF-7 and 4 T1 cells beside of their appropriate entrance

in to cells. These findings need further evaluation to take into account potential improved pharmacokinetic of nanoparticulate drug delivery system.

Authors' contributions
NSR carried out all experiments and drafted the manuscript. NG supervised and finalized the paper. FA participated in nanoparticles fabrication. MA conducted structure elucidation. EF revised the manuscript and helped in analysis. MRK lead statistical analysis and DOE. ZHM helped in cellular studies. FA supervised all pharmaceutical and cellular studies. RD supervised all experiments and approved the manuscript. All authors read and approved the final manuscript.

Competing interests
The authors declare that they have no competing interests.

Author details
[1]Nanotechnology Research Centre, Faculty of Pharmacy, Tehran University of Medical Sciences, Tehran 1417614411, Iran. [2]Nanomedicine and Biomaterial Lab, Department of Pharmaceutics, Faculty of Pharmacy, Tehran University of Medical Sciences, Tehran, Iran. [3]Department of Medicinal Chemistry, Faculty of Pharmacy, Tehran University of Medical Sciences, Tehran, Iran. [4]Department of Drug and Food Control, Faculty of Pharmacy and Pharmaceutical Quality Assurance Research Center, Tehran University of Medical Sciences, Tehran, Iran.

References

1. Goodarzi N, Varshochian R, Kamalinia G, Atyabi F, Dinarvand R. A review of polysaccharide cytotoxic drug conjugates for cancer therapy. Carbohydr Polym. 2013;92:1280–93.
2. Tavassolian F, Kamalinia G, Rouhani H, Amini M, Ostad SN, Khoshayand MR, Atyabi F, Tehrani MR, Dinarvand R. Targeted poly (l-γ-glutamyl glutamine) nanoparticles of docetaxel against folate over-expressed breast cancer cells. Int J Pharm. 2014;467:123–38.
3. Dosio F, Stella B, Arpicco S, Cattel L. Macromolecules as taxane delivery systems. Expert Opin Drug Deliv. 2011;8:33–55.
4. Goodarzi N, Ghahremani MH, Amini M, Atyabi F, Ostad SN, Shabani Ravari N, Nateghian N, Dinarvand R. CD44-targeted docetaxel conjugate for cancer cells and cancer stem-like cells: A novel hyaluronic acid-based drug delivery system. Chem Biol Drug Des. 2014;83:741–52.
5. Mugabe C, Liggins RT, Guan D, Manisali I, Chafeeva I, Brooks DE, Heller M, Jackson JK, Burt HM. Development and in vitro characterization of paclitaxel and docetaxel loaded into hydrophobically derivatized hyperbranched polyglycerols. Int J Pharm. 2011;404:238–49.
6. Akhlaghi SP, Saremi S, Ostad SN, Dinarvand R, Atyabi F. Discriminated effects of thiolated chitosan-coated pMMA paclitaxel-loaded nanoparticles on different normal and cancer cell lines. Nanomedicine. 2010;6:689–97.
7. Cho HJ, Yoon HY, Koo H, Ko SH, Shim JS, Lee JH, Kim K, Chan Kwon I, Kim DD. Self-assembled nanoparticles based on hyaluronic acid-ceramide (HA-CE) and Pluronic ® for tumor-targeted delivery of docetaxel. Biomaterials. 2011;32:7181–90.
8. Menzel EJ, Farr C. Hyaluronidase and its substrate hyaluronan: Biochemistry, biological activities and therapeutic uses. Cancer Lett. 1998;131:3–11.
9. Dalerba P, Cho RW, Clarke MF. Cancer stem cells: models and concepts. Annu Rev Med. 2007;58:267–84.
10. Aruffo A, Stamenkovic I, Melnick M, Underhill CB, Seed B. CD44 is the principal cell surface receptor for hyaluronate. Cell. 1990;61:1303–13.
11. Auzenne E, Ghosh SC, Khodadadian M, Rivera B, Farquhar D, Price RE, Ravoori M, Kundra V, Freedman RS, Klostergaard J. Hyaluronic acid-paclitaxel: antitumor efficacy against CD44 (+) human ovarian carcinoma xenografts. Neoplasia. 2007;9:479–86.
12. Stamenkovic I, Aruffo A, Amiot M, Seed B. The hematopoietic and epithelial forms of CD44 are distinct polypeptides with different adhesion potentials for hyaluronate-bearing cells. EMBO J. 1991;10:343.
13. Herrlich P, Sleeman J, Wainwright D, König H, Sherman L, Hilberg F, Ponta H. How tumor cells make use of CD44. Cell Commun Adhes. 1998;6:141–7.

14. Kurisawa M, Chung JE, Yang YY, Gao SJ, Uyama H. Injectable biodegradable hydrogels composed of hyaluronic acid–tyramine conjugates for drug delivery and tissue engineering. Chem Commun (Camb). 2005;14:4312–4.

15. Lee H, Mok H, Lee S, Oh Y-K, Park TG. Target-specific intracellular delivery of siRNA using degradable hyaluronic acid nanogels. J Control Release. 2007; 119:245–52.

16. Misra S, Ghatak S, Toole BP. Regulation of MDR1 expression and drug resistance by a positive feedback loop involving hyaluronan, phosphoinositide 3-kinase, and ErbB2. J Biol Chem. 2005;280:20310–5.

17. Polexe RC, Delair T. Elaboration of stable and antibody functionalized positively charged colloids by polyelectrolyte complexation between chitosan and hyaluronic acid. Molecules. 2013;18:8563–78.

18. Park JH, Kwon S, Lee M, Chung H, Kim J-H, Kim Y-S, Park R-W, Kim I-S, Seo SB, Kwon IC. Self-assembled nanoparticles based on glycol chitosan bearing hydrophobic moieties as carriers for doxorubicin: in vivo biodistribution and anti-tumor activity. Biomaterials. 2006;27:119–26.

19. Kim SJ, Yoon SG, Lee KB, Park YD, Kim SI. Electrical sensitive behavior of a polyelectrolyte complex composed of chitosan/hyaluronic acid. Solid State Ion. 2003;164:199–204.

20. Saremi S, Dinarvand R, Kebriaeezadeh A, Ostad SN, Atyabi F. Enhanced oral delivery of docetaxel using thiolated chitosan nanoparticles: preparation, in vitro and in vivo studies. Biomed Res Int. 2013;2013:150478.

21. Jafari Malek S, Khoshchehreh R, Goodarzi N, Khoshayand MR, Amini M, Atyabi F, Esfandyari-manesh M, Tehrani S, Mohammad Jafari R, Maghazei MS, et al. Cis-Dichlorodiamminoplatinum (II) glyconanoparticles by drug-induced ionic gelation technique targeted to prostate cancer: Preparation, optimization and in vitro characterization. Colloids Surf B Biointerfaces. 2014; 122:350–8.

22. Azadi A, Hamidi M, Khoshayand M-R, Amini M, Rouini M-R. Preparation and optimization of surface-treated methotrexate-loaded nanogels intended for brain delivery. Carbohydr Polym. 2012;90:462–71.

23. Lee H, Lee K, Park TG. Hyaluronic acid – paclitaxel conjugate micelles: Synthesis, characterization, and antitumor activity. Bioconjug Chem. 2008;19: 1319–25.

24. Denuziere A, Ferrier D, Damour O, Domard A. Chitosan–chondroitin sulfate and chitosan–hyaluronate polyelectrolyte complexes: biological properties. Biomaterials. 1998;19:1275–85.

25. Luo Y, Prestwich GD. Synthesis and selective cytotoxicity of a hyaluronic acid-antitumor bioconjugate. Bioconjug Chem. 1999;10:755–63.

26. Manoochehri S, Darvishi B, Kamalinia G, Amini M, Fallah M, Ostad SN, Atyabi F, Dinarvand R. Surface modification of PLGA nanoparticles via human serum albumin conjugation for controlled delivery of docetaxel. Daru. 2013; 21:58.

27. Lee JY, Choi YS, Suh JS, Kwon YM, Yang VC, Lee SJ, Chung CP, Park YJ. Cell-penetrating chitosan/doxorubicin/TAT conjugates for efficient cancer therapy. Int J Cancer. 2011;128:2470–80.

28. Nateghian N, Goodarzi N, Amini M, Atyabi F, Khorramizadeh MR, Dinarvand R. Biotin/folate-decorated human serum albumin nanoparticles of docetaxel: comparison of chemically conjugated nanostructures and physically loaded nanoparticles for targeting of breast cancer. Chem Biol Drug Des. 2015; 87(1):69–82.

29. Li C, Yu D-F, Newman RA, Cabral F, Stephens LC, Hunter N, Milas L, Wallace S. Complete regression of well-established tumors using a novel water-soluble poly (L-glutamic acid)-paclitaxel conjugate. Cancer Res. 1998;58: 2404–9.

30. Jain A, Thakur K, Kush P, Jain UK. Docetaxel loaded chitosan nanoparticles: Formulation, characterization and cytotoxicity studies. Int J Biol Macromol. 2014;69:546–53.

31. Gandhi NS, Mancera RL. The structure of glycosaminoglycans and their interactions with proteins. Chem Biol Drug Des. 2008;72:455–82.

32. Saremi S, Atyabi F, Akhlaghi SP, Ostad SN, Dinarvand R. Thiolated chitosan nanoparticles for enhancing oral absorption of docetaxel: Preparation, in vitro and ex vivo evaluation. Int J Nanomedicine. 2011;6:119–28.

33. Panyam J, Labhasetwar V. Dynamics of endocytosis and exocytosis of poly (D, L-lactide-co-glycolide) nanoparticles in vascular smooth muscle cells. Pharm Res. 2003;20:212–20.

Permissions

All chapters in this book were first published in DARUJPS, by BioMed Central; hereby published with permission under the Creative Commons Attribution License or equivalent. Every chapter published in this book has been scrutinized by our experts. Their significance has been extensively debated. The topics covered herein carry significant findings which will fuel the growth of the discipline. They may even be implemented as practical applications or may be referred to as a beginning point for another development.

The contributors of this book come from diverse backgrounds, making this book a truly international effort. This book will bring forth new frontiers with its revolutionizing research information and detailed analysis of the nascent developments around the world.

We would like to thank all the contributing authors for lending their expertise to make the book truly unique. They have played a crucial role in the development of this book. Without their invaluable contributions this book wouldn't have been possible. They have made vital efforts to compile up to date information on the varied aspects of this subject to make this book a valuable addition to the collection of many professionals and students.

This book was conceptualized with the vision of imparting up-to-date information and advanced data in this field. To ensure the same, a matchless editorial board was set up. Every individual on the board went through rigorous rounds of assessment to prove their worth. After which they invested a large part of their time researching and compiling the most relevant data for our readers.

The editorial board has been involved in producing this book since its inception. They have spent rigorous hours researching and exploring the diverse topics which have resulted in the successful publishing of this book. They have passed on their knowledge of decades through this book. To expedite this challenging task, the publisher supported the team at every step. A small team of assistant editors was also appointed to further simplify the editing procedure and attain best results for the readers.

Apart from the editorial board, the designing team has also invested a significant amount of their time in understanding the subject and creating the most relevant covers. They scrutinized every image to scout for the most suitable representation of the subject and create an appropriate cover for the book.

The publishing team has been an ardent support to the editorial, designing and production team. Their endless efforts to recruit the best for this project, has resulted in the accomplishment of this book. They are a veteran in the field of academics and their pool of knowledge is as vast as their experience in printing. Their expertise and guidance has proved useful at every step. Their uncompromising quality standards have made this book an exceptional effort. Their encouragement from time to time has been an inspiration for everyone.

The publisher and the editorial board hope that this book will prove to be a valuable piece of knowledge for researchers, students, practitioners and scholars across the globe.

List of Contributors

Hassan Hashemi, Mohammad Amin Seyedian, Mohammad Miraftab, Hooman Bahrmandy and Soheila Asgari
Noor Ophthalmology Research Center, Noor Eye Hospital, No. 96 Esfandiar Blvd., Vali'asr Ave., Tehran, Iran

Araz Sabzevari
Faculty of Pharmacy, Tehran University of Medical Sciences, Tehran, Iran

Shadi Mahdizadeh
Department of Cell and Molecular Biology, Kish International Campus, University of Tehran, Kish, Iran

Gholamreza Karimi
Medical Toxicology Research Center, School of Pharmacy, Mashhad University of Medical Sciences, Mashhad, Iran

Sepideh Arabzadeh
Biotechnology Research Center, School of Pharmacy, Mashhad University of Medical Sciences, Mashhad, Iran

Javad Behravan
Biotechnology Research Center, School of Pharmacy, Mashhad University of Medical Sciences, Mashhad, Iran
Department of Pharmaceutical Biotechnology, School of Pharmacy, Mashhad University of Medical Sciences, Mashhad, Iran

Fatemeh Kalalinia
Biotechnology Research Center, School of Pharmacy, Mashhad University of Medical Sciences, Mashhad, Iran
Medical Genetic Research Center, Mashhad University of Medical Sciences, Mashhad, Iran

Hermann Lage
Institute of Pathology, Charite University, Campus Mitte, Humboldt, Berlin, Germany

Massoud Amanlou
Department of Medicinal Chemistry, Faculty of Pharmacy and Pharmaceutical Sciences Research Center, Tehran University of Medical Sciences, Tehran, Iran

Anahita Johari
Department of Medicinal Chemistry, Faculty of Pharmacy and Pharmaceutical Sciences Research Center, Tehran University of Medical Sciences, Tehran, Iran
Institute of Biochemistry and Biophysics, University of Tehran, Tehran, Iran

Ali Akbar Moosavi-Movahedi
Institute of Biochemistry and Biophysics, University of Tehran, Tehran, Iran

Mehdi Esfandyari-Manesh, Nazanin Shabani Ravari, Fatemeh Atyabi and Rassoul Dinarvand
Nanotechnology Research Centre, Faculty of Pharmacy, Tehran University of Medical Sciences, Tehran, Iran
Novel Drug Delivery Lab, Department of Pharmaceutics, Faculty of Pharmacy, Tehran University of Medical Sciences, Tehran, Iran

Behrad Darvishi
Nanotechnology Research Centre, Faculty of Pharmacy, Tehran University of Medical Sciences, Tehran, Iran
Medical Nanotechnology Department, School of Advanced Technologies in Medicine, Tehran University of Medical Sciences, Tehran, Iran

Mona Noori Koopaei
Novel Drug Delivery Lab, Department of Pharmaceutics, Faculty of Pharmacy, Tehran University of Medical Sciences, Tehran, Iran

Seyed Hossein Mostafavi
Novel Drug Delivery Lab, Department of Pharmaceutics, Faculty of Pharmacy, Tehran University of Medical Sciences, Tehran, Iran
Department of Bioengineering, University of California, Riverside, CA, USA

Medical Nanotechnology Department, School of Advanced Technologies in Medicine, Tehran University of Medical Sciences, Tehran, Iran

Reza Faridi Majidi
Medical Nanotechnology Department, School of Advanced Technologies in Medicine, Tehran University of Medical Sciences, Tehran, Iran

Mohsen Amini
Department of Medicinal Chemistry, Faculty of Pharmacy, Tehran University of Medical Sciences, Tehran, Iran

Seyed Nasser Ostad
Department of Toxicology and Pharmacology, Faculty of Pharmacy, Tehran University of Medical Science, Tehran, Iran

Zahra Alam-mehrjerdi and Kate Dolan
Program of International Research and Training, National Drug and Alcohol Research Centre, Faculty of Public Health and Community Medicine,, University of New South Wales, Sydney, Australia

Reza Daneshmand
Substance Abuse and Dependence Research Center, University of Social Welfare and RehabilitationSciences, Tehran, Iran

Mercedeh Samiei
Department of Psychiatry, School of Behavior Sciences, University of Social Welfare and Rehabilitation Sciences, Tehran, Iran

Roya Samadi
Psychiatry and Behavioral Sciences Research Center, Department of Psychiatry, Mashhad University of Medical Sciences, Mashhad, Iran

Mohammad Abdollahi
Department of Toxicology and Pharmacology, Faculty of Pharmacy and Pharmaceutical Sciences Research Center, Tehran University of Medical Sciences, Tehran, Iran

Monia Deghrigue and Abderrahman Bouraoui
Laboratoire de développement chimique, galénique et pharmacologique des médicaments (LR12ES09). Equipe de Pharmacologie marine, Faculté de pharmacie de Monastir, Université de Monastir, Monastir, Tunisie

Carmen Festa, Maria Valeria D'auria and Simona de Marino
Department of Pharmacy, University of Naples "Federico II", via D. Montesano 49, I- 80131 Napoli, Italy

Lotfi Ghribi and Hichem Ben Jannet
Laboratoire de chimie hétérocyclique, produits naturels et réactivité. Equipe de chimie médicinale et produits naturels (LR11ES39), Faculté des sciences de Monastir, Université de Monastir,= Monastir, Tunisie

Rafik Ben Said
Institut National des Sciences et Technologie de la Mer (INSTM), Salambo, Tunis, Tunisie

Arman Engheta and Ali Atri
Department of Plastic Surgery, Imam Khomeini Hospital, Tehran University of Medical Sciences, Tehran, Iran

Shahryar Hadadi Abianeh
Department of Plastic Surgery, Razi Hospital, Tehran University of Medical Sciences, Vahdat Eslami st, Tehran, Iran

Mehdi Sanatkarfar
Department of Anesthesiology, Razi Hospital, Tehran University of Medical Sciences, Tehran, Iran

Mohsen Zeeb and Behrooz Mirza
Department of Applied Chemistry, Faculty of science, Islamic Azad University, South Tehran Branch, Tehran, Iran

Seyedeh-Somayeh Zamani and Mahmoud Etebari
Department of Pharmacology and Toxicology, Isfahan Pharmaceutical Sciences Research Center, School of Pharmacy and Pharmaceutical Sciences, Isfahan University of Medical Sciences, Isfahan, Iran

Mohsen Hossieni
Department of Pharmaology, School of Medicine, Tehran University for Medical Sciences, Tehran, Iran

Pirooz Salehian
Sarem Fertility and Infertility Research Centre, Sarem Hospital, Shahrak-e-Ekbatan, Tehran, Iran

Soltan Ahmad Ebrahimi
Department of Pharmacology, Iran University for Medical Sciences, Tehran, Iran

Maryam Payan and Mohammad Reza Rouini
Biopharmaceutics and Pharmacokinetics Division, Department of Pharmaceutics, School of Pharmacy, Tehran University of Medical sciences, Tehran, Iran

Nader Tajik
Cellular and Molecular Research Center (CMRC), Iran University of Medical Sciences, Tehran, Iran

Mohammad Hossein Ghahremani
Department of Pharmacology and Toxicology, School of Pharmacy, Tehran University of Medical sciences,Tehran, Iran

Reza Tahvilian
Department of pharmaceutics, School of Pharmacy, Kermanshah University of Medical Sciences, Kermanshah, Iran

Gilda Kianimehr
Psychiatric Research Center, Roozbeh Hospital, Tehran University of Medical Sciences, Tehran 13337, Iran

Farzad Fatehi
Shariati Hospital, Neurology Department, Tehran University of medical Sciences, Tehran, Iran

Sara Hashempoor and Mohammad-Reza Khodaei-Ardakani
Razi Psychiatric Hospital, University of Social Welfare and Rehabilitation, Tehran, Iran

Farzin Rezaei and Ali Nazari
Qods Hospital, Kurdistan University of Medical Sciences, Sanandaj, Iran

Ladan Kashani
Infertility Ward, Arash Hospital, Tehran University of Medical Sciences, Tehran, Iran

Shahin Akhondzadeh
Psychiatric Research Center, Roozbeh Psychiatric Hospital, Tehran University of Medical Sciences, South Kargar Street 13337, Tehran, Iran

Nasser Nassiri Koopaei
Department of Pharmaceutics, School of Pharmacy, University of Florida, Orlando, USA.

Mohammad Abdollahi
Department of Toxicology & Pharmacology, Faculty of Pharmacy and Pharmaceutical Sciences Research Center, Tehran University of Medical Sciences, Tehran, Iran
Endocrinology and Metabolism Research Center, Endocrinology and Metabolism Clinical Sciences Institute, Tehran University of Medical Sciences, Tehran, Iran
Toxicology Interest Group, Universal Scientific Education and Research Network, Tehran University of Medical Sciences, Tehran, Iran

Pilar Pérez Lozano, Encarna García Montoya, Montserrat Miñarro, Josep R Ticó, and Josep M Suñe Negre
Pharmacy and Pharmaceutical Technology Department, Faculty of Pharmacy, University of Barcelona, Avda Joan XXIII s/n 08028, Barcelona, Spain

Paloma Flórez Borges
Pharmacy and Pharmaceutical Technology Department, Faculty of Pharmacy, University of Barcelona, Avda Joan XXIII s/n 08028, Barcelona, Spain
Reig Jofre Group, c. Gran Capitá 6 08970, Sant Joan Despi, Barcelona, Spain

Enric Jo
Reig Jofre Group, c. Gran Capitá 6 08970, Sant Joan Despi, Barcelona, Spain

Masoomeh Yosefifard and Majid Hassanpour-Ezatti
Department of Biology, Sciences School, Shahed University, Tehran, IRAN

Atousa Ziaei and Shamim Sahranavard
Traditional Medicine and Material Medical Research Center; Department of Traditional Pharmacy, School of Traditional Medicine, Shahid Beheshti University of Medical Sciences, Tehran, Iran

Mohammad Javad Gharagozlou
Department of Pathology, Faculty of Veterinary Medicine, University of Tehran, Tehran, Iran

Mehrdad Faizi
Department of Pharmacology and Toxicology, School of Pharmacy, Shahid Beheshti University of Medical Sciences, Tehran, Iran

Renata Cavalcanti Carnevale, Caroline de Godoi Rezende Costa Molino, Marília Berlofa Visacri and Priscila Gava Mazzola
Department of Clinical Pathology, Faculty of Medical Sciences (FCM), University of Campinas (UNICAMP), Alexander Fleming, 105, 13083-881 Campinas, SP, Brazil

Patricia Moriel
Department of Clinical Pathology, Faculty of Medical Sciences (FCM), University of Campinas (UNICAMP), Alexander Fleming, 105, 13083-881 Campinas, SP, Brazil
Faculty of Pharmaceutical Sciences (FCF), University of Campinas (UNICAMP), Sérgio Buarque de Holanda, 25, 13083-859 Campinas, SP, Brazil

Durdana Waseem, Ihsan-ul Haq and Gul Majid Khan
Department of Pharmacy, Quaid-i-Azam University, Islamabad 45320, Pakistan

Arshad Farooq Butt and Moazzam Hussain Bhatti
Department of Chemistry, Allama Iqbal Open University, H-8, Islamabad 44000, Pakistan

Parichehr Hassanzadeh, Morteza Azhdarzadeh and Meshkat Dinarvand
Nanotechnology Research Center, Faculty of Pharmacy, Tehran University of Medical Sciences, Tehran, Iran

Fatemeh Atyabi and Rassoul Dinarvand
Nanotechnology Research Center, Faculty of Pharmacy, Tehran University of Medical Sciences, Tehran, Iran
Department of Pharmaceutics, Faculty of Pharmacy, Tehran University of Medical Sciences, Tehran, Iran

Ahmad-Reza Dehpour
Department of Pharmacology, Faculty of Medicine, Tehran University of Medical Sciences, Tehran, Iran

Sanaz Jamshidfar, Yalda H. Ardakani, Hoda Lavasani and Mohammadreza Rouini
Biopharmaceutics and Pharmacokinetic Division, Department of Pharmaceutics, Faculty of Pharmacy, Tehran University of Medical Sciences, Tehran, Iran

Cuiwei Chen, Xiaowei Shi and Fanzhu Li
Department of Pharmaceutics, Zhejiang Chinese Medical University, Hangzhou 311042, China

Hongyue Zheng
Libraries of Zhejiang Chinese Medical University, Zhejiang Chinese Medical University, Hangzhou 310053, China

Junjun Xu
Department of Pharmacy, The Second Affiliated Hospital, School of Medicine, Zhejiang University, Hangzhou 310052, China

Xuanshen Wang
Department of Pharmacy, The Second Hospital of Dalian Medical University, Dalian 116027, China

Khosro Keshavarz, Farhad Lotfi and Mojtaba Jafari
Health Human Resources Research Center, Department of Health Economics, School of Management and Information Sciences, Shiraz University of Medical Sciences, Shiraz, IR, Iran

Ehsan Sanati, Amir Hashemi-Meshkini and Mohammad M. Mojahedian
Department of Pharmacoeconomics and Pharmaceutical Administration, Faculty of Pharmacy, Tehran University of Medical Sciences, Tehran, IR, Iran

Mahmood Salesi
Atherosclerosis Research center, Baqiyatallah University of Medical Sciences, Tehran, IR, Iran

Behzad Najafi
Iranian center of Excellence in health management, Department of health services management, School of management and medical informatics, Tabriz University of medical sciences, Tabriz, Iran

Shekoufeh Nikfar
Department of Pharmacoeconomics and Pharmaceutical Administration, Faculty of Pharmacy and Evidence-Based Medicine Group, Pharmaceutical Sciences Research Center, Tehran University of Medical Sciences, Tehran, Iran

Najmeh Rahmanian
Department of Radiopharmacy, Faculty of Pharmacy, Tehran University of Medical Sciences, Tehran, Iran
Department of Radiopharmacy, Faculty of Pharmacy, Mazandaran University of Medical Sciences, Sari, Iran

Seyed Jalal Hosseinimehr and Zohreh Noaparast
Department of Radiopharmacy, Faculty of Pharmacy, Mazandaran University of Medical Sciences, Sari, Iran.

Ali Khalaj
Department of Medicinal Chemistry, Faculty of Pharmacy, Tehran University of Medical Sciences Tehran, Iran

Seyed Mohammad Abedi
Department of Radiology, Faculty of Medicine, Mazandaran University of Medical Sciences, Sari, Iran

Omid Sabzevari
Department of Toxicology, Faculty of Pharmacy, Tehran University of Medical Sciences, Tehran, Iran

Nazanin Shabani Ravari and Navid Goodarzi
Nanotechnology Research Centre, Faculty of Pharmacy, Tehran University of Medical Sciences, Tehran 1417614411, Iran

Fatemeh Atyabi and Rassoul Dinarvand
Nanotechnology Research Centre, Faculty of Pharmacy, Tehran University of Medical Sciences, Tehran 1417614411, Iran
Nanomedicine and Biomaterial Lab, Department of Pharmaceutics, Faculty of Pharmacy, Tehran University of Medical Sciences, Tehran, Iran

Farhad Alvandifar and Zahra Hadavand Mirzaie
Nanomedicine and Biomaterial Lab, Department of Pharmaceutics, Faculty of Pharmacy, Tehran University of Medical Sciences, Tehran, Iran

Mohsen Amini and Effat Souri
Department of Medicinal Chemistry, Faculty of Pharmacy, Tehran University of Medical Sciences, Tehran, Iran

Mohammad Reza Khoshayand
Department of Drug and Food Control, Faculty of Pharmacy and Pharmaceutical Quality Assurance Research Center, Tehran University of Medical Sciences, Tehran, Iran

Index

www.ingramcontent.com/pod-product-compliance
Lightning Source LLC
Chambersburg PA
CBHW082044190326
41458CB00010B/3449